MENINGITIS

Edited by **George Wireko-Brobby**

Meningitis
Edited by George Wireko-Brobby

Published by InTech
Janeza Trdine 9, 51000 Rijeka, Croatia

Publishing Process Manager Tajana Jevtic

Technical Editor Teodora Smiljanic

Cover Designer InTech Design Team

Additional hard copies can be obtained from orders@intechopen.com

Meningitis, Edited by George Wireko-Brobby
p. cm.
ISBN 978-953-51-0383-7

For EU product safety concerns:
IN TECH d.o.o., Prolaz Marije Krucifikse Kozulić 3, 51000 Rijeka, Croatia,
info@intechopen.com or visit our website at intechopen.com.

Meet the editor

Professor Dr Sir George Wireko-Brobby was born in 1942 in Ghana. He studied at the University of Marbug, West Germany from 1964 to 1973. He graduated in Medicine and Dentistry by a double doctoral Dissertation with Magna cum Laude in both areas. George Wireko Brobby is a Professor of Otorhinolaryngology (ENT) and past Dean of the School of Medical Science KNUST Kumasi Ghana. He is the current President of the Ghana Postgraduate College of Physicians and Surgeons. He is a teacher at the undergraduate and postgraduate level and internal assessor at the West African College of Surgeons and the Ghana College of Physicians and Surgeons in his field of Ear, Nose and Throat Surgery. Prof Brobby was appointed as a WHO Consultant on Prevention of Deafness and Hearing Impairment in 1996. He has travelled far and wide and collaborated with Institutions, ENT Department of Kenya, Zambia, Ethiopia, Tanzania, Sheffield, UK, Liverpool, UK, Universities of Ulm and Dusseldorf, Germany, Cyprus, New Delhi, India and Malta. Sir George is Associate Editor in the Journal of Hearing International, Japan and a member of the Editorial Board of the Ghana Medical Association. He is also a co-Editor of the British Medical Journal - African Edition and a member of the AdvisoryBoard of KNUST Journal. His international experiences include his appointment as the President Initiative for Deaf Education in Commonwealth countries from 1990-1998, Secretary General of the Pan African Federation of Otolaryngological Societies (PAFOS), culminating in his election as President of PAFOS form 1999-2004.

Contents

Preface

This book focuses on two primary objectives. It aims to provide general practitioners, paediatricians, and specialist physicians with an essential text written in an accessible language, and also to highlight the differences in pathogenesis and causative agents of meningitis in the developed and the developing world.

Meningitis is a medical emergency requiring a rapid diagnosis and an immediate transfer to an institution supplied with appropriate antibiotic and supportive measures.

Especially in the developing world, where malaria is rampant, one must maintain a high level of caution when confronted with a febrile child or one who has an altered mental status, as the first ten hours of care may make a crucial difference in the outcome.

Bacterial or purulent meningitis is the most important form of infection in the United States in terms of incidence, sequela and ultimate loss of productive life.

Aseptic meningitis, usually caused by a virus, is also common, however significant sequela are rare and the disease is self-limiting.

In Sub-Saharan Africa, seasonal outbreaks and epidemics of meningitis and septicaemia numerically present the greatest public health impact on the continent.

The three polysacharide encapsulated bacteria for which licensed vaccines are curable are Pneumococcus, Haemophilius influenza type b (Hib) and the Neisseia Meningococcus. They are also the most common causative agents of bacterial meningitis in Sub Saharan Africa.

Especially in South Africa, granulomatous meningitis, caused either by *M. tuberculosis* or fungi is a major cause of neurologic injury and death.

The necessary factors to consider for the epidemiology of the disease include age, ethnicity, season, host factors and regional pattern of the antibiotic resistance among likely pathogens.

The first month after birth represents the period of highest attack rate for meningitis with likely pathogens including *S. agalactiae*(group B streptococcus), *E. coli*, other gram negative enteric organisms, and *L. monocytogenes*. Beyond the neonatal period the most important pathogens are *H. influenza* type B, 1 up to 6 years of age, *N. menigococcus* and *S. pneumoniae*.

In the US and Europe, the disease is reported with increased frequency among African Americans, Native Americans and individuals in rural areas.

Even in Africa, patients with poor socio-economic factors suffer more from the devastating effects of meningitis. In West Africa, the meningitis belt passes through the Northern part of the countries where people live in overcrowded huts. It has been documented that especially in the dry season, meningococcal, pneumococcal and Haemoiphilus infection spread by the respiratory route, which is aided by overcrowding. It has also been documented that host factors predisposing the infection include congenital or Acquired Immune Deficiency status, Sickling Haemoglobinopathies, chronic liver or renal disease. The classic triad of symptoms in meningitis is fever, headache, and stiff neck. However in children under 2 years of age, stiff neck or other signs of meningial irritation may be absent. Alterations level of consumers is a common finding present in up to 90% of patients.

In this book a detailed chapter on laboratory findings has also been provided.

Once meningitis is suspected, an immediate examination of the CSF is indicated, except if a strong suspicion of an intracranial mass lesion is present, where lumbar puncture may be delayed until a CT scan or an MRL has been done.

Effective treatment of meningitis depends on early aggressive supportive therapy and a selection of empiric antimicrobials appropriate for the likely pathogens.

In Europe and the USA, 1 third generation cephalosporine has become the first-line therapy, but while these drugs remain relatively expensive, it is probably reasonable for most African hospitals to continue with the combination of a peniciline and chloramphenicol as initial therapy as long as clinicans are aware of the risk of recondescences, particularly if steroids are used.

Common neurological complications in both adults and children are motor deficit, cognition deficit, hemiplegia epilepsy, developmental and learning disabilities, including blindness and deafness. A special chapter on the devastating effects of sensorineural hearing loss and the benefits of early rehabilitation is also included in this book.

Prof. Dr. Dr. Sir George Wireko-Brobby
President of the Ghana Postgraduate College of Physicians and Surgeons
Professor of Otorhinolaryngology, Department of Eye, Ear, Nose and Throat,
School of Medical Science, KNUST, Kumasi,
Ghana

1

Bacterial Meningitis and Deafness in Sub-Saharan Africa

George Wireko-Brobby
College of Health Science, School of Medical Sciences, KNUST, Kumasi Ghana

1. Introduction

Bacterial Meningitis is a leading cause of childhood Deafness in Ghana and the sub- Saharan Africa. Children are predominantly at risk of bacterial meningitis mainly because of their immature immune system, and malnutrition especially in our part of the world. Lack of immunization practices also makes them more susceptible to significantly high morbidity and mortality.

Even with the provision of highly effective antibiotic therapy, death and long-term disabilities are the common but still serious consequences of acute bacterial meningitis in developing countries.

Common neurological complications in both adult and children are motor deficit, cognition deficit, hemiplegia, epilepsy, developmental and learning disabilities, blindness and Deafness.

In this chapter, we shall focus more on the devastating effects of sensorineural Hearing loss or Deafness, after bacterial meningitis. Delay in the Diagnosis of Hearing loss occurs firstly because language development of Hearing impaired children, parallels that of normal infants till the age of nine months. Secondly, because children with profound hearing loss coo and bable until this age, the parents are likely to ignore any subtle evidence of hearing impairment such as lack of response to environmental sound. Damage to the Cochlea, occurs in the early stages of the illness and it is often permanent and irreversible. Woodrow & Brobby (1997); Daya et al. (1998).

Prevention of deafness relies on early treatment with appropriate antibiotics, but adjunctive treatment with dexametnasore though controversial may be useful in preventing the sequel of sensorineural Hearing loss. In the long term vaccinations may be the most practicable means to reducing the burden of meningitis in the developing countries of Africa.

Facilities for audiological assessment and management of children recovering from meningitis are crucial for the detection of significant hearing impairment and the implementation of rehabilitation programmes.

Our observation at our University Teaching Hospital (KATH) is that about 20% of patients who survive with neurological sequelae, permanent sensorineuraal Hearing loss, accounts for approximately 75% of these cases.

In a study on causes of Deafness in Ghana, Brobby (1998) Meningitis was rated the 3rd amongst other childhood infections. Recent observations predict that meningitis has taken the 2nd position after measles.

This is worrying because even a mild hearing loss of less than 40 Db may have long-term developmental consequences. Given the scale of this problem, there is the need to review critically our knowledge about the natural history of the hearing loss which may follow meningitis and to discuss the applicability of recent therapeutic interventions studied in industrial nations to the diseases in the African contest.

2. Microbiology

In Africa, acute bacterial meningitis has an overall annual endemic rate in the region of 10-50 per 10^5 populations, a figure at least 10 times that for Europe and the United States, and this disparity appears to be growing. Fortnum (1992). More than 70 per cent of cases are caused by either Streptococcus pneumonia (pneumococcal) or Neisseria meningitides (meningococcal). Haemophius influenza type b (Hib) is responsible for fewer cases in the population as a whole although it is a major problem in children less than 12 months of age, Airede (1993).

Epidemics of meningococcal meningitis sweep through the sub-Saharan 'meningitis belt' every 8 to 12 years. Annual incidence may reach 1 per cent of the population in certain areas.

Although this review concentrates on acute bacterial meningitis in Ghana, tuberculous meningitis is also relatively common in certain areas and is the leading cause of meningitis in the Western Cape Province of South Africa, where deafness. Deafness is a well-recognized complication. From our experience, viral meningitis has only rarely been associated with deafness.

In Africa seasonal outbreaks and epidemics of meningecal meningitis and septicaemia, numerically represent their greatest public health impact on the continent.

In Ghana, the three polysaccharide encapsulated bacteria for which licensed vaccines are curable are Pneumococcus, Haemophilus influenza type b (Hib) and the Neisseria Menigococcus. Our observation is that Haemophilus influenza type b is responsible for fewer cases of meningitis in our sub-region.

3. Epidemiology

A number of factors appear to influence the frequency of post-meningitis hearing loss but it is not possible to predict hearing loss accurately in individual cases. Factors affecting this figure including the causative organism, the pneumococcus causing the highest rate of deafness (31.8 per cent) in comparison with the meningococcus (7.5 per cent) and Hib (11.4 per cent) All ages may develop deafness – the fact that most cases occur in infants may reflect their greater susceptibility to severe infection rather than a particular vulnerability to hearing impairment. At a community level, meningitis is one of the most common causes of hearing loss. In Kumasi, Ghana, meningitis is responsible for 8.5 per cent of cases of sensorineural hearing impairment in children.Brobby (1998)

4. Natural history

Sensorineural heating loss is typically bilateral, and occurs within 48 hours of the development of meningitis, with the majority of children who go on to suffer permanent damage having abnormal hearing tests on admission to hospital. There appears to be an initial phase of mild, reversible damage. Significant sensorineural hearing loss persisting after the acute phase of the illness is characteristically permanent although cases of partial recovery have been documented on certain occasions. Mild, temporary, conductive deficits are common in the recovery phase. Pathological correlates for these clinical findings are still lacking but potential pathophysiological mechanisms are discussed below.DAYA et al (1997)

5. Pathology

The auditory lesion in post-meningitic hearing loss remains obscure. It is likely that more than one mechanism of auditory pathway damage occurs. A body of clinical and experimental evidence suggests that the cochlea is the most frequent site of sensorineural damage, bacteria gaining access to the labyrinth via the cochlear aqueduct. DAYA et al (1998) Cell wall components directly toxic to cochlear hair cells, setting up a serous labyrinthitis In addition, these components also stimulate the inflammatory response, leading to suppurative labyrinthitis and permanent damage; in severe cases the labyrinth may be completely obliterated and neo-ossification occurs. The vestibular apparatus is commonly damaged in conjunction with this process. Other potential mechanisms of deafness include septic thrombophlebitic or embolisation of blood vessels supplying the inner ear and damage to the VIIIth cranial never or central auditory pathways.

6. Diagnosis

Screening for deafness during hospitalization is an accurate predictor of hearing impairments at follow-up, and ideally should be performed on all cases. It is also important to examine the middle ear with tympanometry in order to assess conductive impairments, which can be expected to improve with time. A follow-up assessment at approximately 6 weeks, when acute inflammation has subsided, confirms the degree of sensorineural damage and allows appropriate rehabilitation to be instituted. Assessment of hearing loss following meningitis is currently based on audiometric methods. Unfortunately the inaccuracy of age-appropriate tests in healthy children, the infants' lack of consistent response to sound and the effect of associated motor disorders tend to impair the validity of audiometry. More objective methods such as Brainstem Audiometry Evoked Responses (BAERs) and Oto-Acoustic Emissions (OAEs) have yet to reach the clinic in most parts of the continent.

More objective methods such as Brainstean Auditory Evoked responses (BAERs) and Oto-Acustic Emulsions (OAEs) are the latest state of the art equipments for this purpose. (DAYA et, al 1998)

Fortunately, the Kumasi Hearing Assessments Centre established through the magnificent generosity of the Commonwealth Society for the Deaf is the only centre, recognized by the WHO, in Africa, South of the Sahara which has all these facilities.

7. Acute management

Prompt Empirical antibiotic treatment should include Agents active agent all main pathogens for the eradication of the infecting organism in order to ensure optimal outcome. The introduction of sulphonamides in the 1950s (primarily for meningococcal meningitis) and of penicillins in the 1960s had a striking effect on incidence of mortality and mobility. The spread of plasmid-borne betalactamases in Hib led to the addition of chloramphenicol to therapy. This combination is still standard in most African countries. The latest challenge to this regimen has been the relatively recent appearance of penicillin-resistant pneumococci and meningococci. Further, some pneumococci are also chloramphenicol-resistant. This will undoubtedly affect the choice of antibiotics although the number of studies documenting a worsening clinical outcome is still small. In Europe and the USA third-generation cephalosporins have become first-line therapy but while these drugs remain relatively expensive, it is probably reasonable for most African hospitals to continue with the combination of a penicillin and chloramphenicol as initial therapy as long as clinicians are aware of the risk of recrudescence, particularly if steroids are being used. Friedland 1998.

A large number of clinical trials have been performed addressing the issue of whether steroids reduce the frequency of adverse outcomes, particularly hearing loss. It is not possible to discuss these studies in detail here, but certain points should be borne in mind when considering the evidence for and against steroids. Most trials could be criticized on methodological grounds because data were analysed without pre-defined end-points, allowing multiple comparisons to be made. In the three trials where significant results have been obtained, there were unusually high incidences of adverse outcome in the placebo group. Furthermore, no study with a consistent antibiotic regimen throughout has shown statistically significant reduction in hearing loss. Despite these problems, the case for giving dexamethasone in Hib meningitis is felt by many authorities to be strong. The role for dexamethasone in pneumococcal and meningococcal disease is at present unresolved.

Many of the trials of both dexamethasone and antibiotic regimens have been performed in the United States, with Hib as the dominant aetiology and so considerable caution should be exercised when applying conclusion to the African setting A recent reported trial in Pakistan found no evidence that dexamethasone was beneficial and suggested that it may be deleterious in this setting. Quazy (1996) Airede (2008)

The finding of different outcomes in various settings is not uncommon. There are clearly huge differences in terms of population, genetics, and timing of presentation, microbiology and general supportive care which can explain this apparent discrepancy. Giving the added cost of dexamethasone to the family of a patient who has already begun receiving two antibiotics, we feel that there is insufficient evidence at this time to recommend routine use of dexamethasone for acute bacterial meningitis of unknown cause.

Currently, the recommended empirical treatment of meningitis is ampicillin plus an aminoglycoside and a third generation cephalosporin.

The use of dexamethasore remains controversial. But our experience at KATH suggests that initial Doses of 50mg Hydrocartison before the administration of the antibiotics help to reduce the occurance of Sensorineural hearing loss.

8. Discussion

The most common causes of bacterial Meningitis in the US, Europe and other developed countries since the 1980s have been the pneumococcus, Haemophilus influenza Type b, the meningococcus, Group B strepotococcus and Listeria monocytogenes.

Works on neonatal meningitis have also shown to involve Strept, agalaciac, Listeria monocytogene, and enteric gram neg. WAS E'coli and citrobacteria spp.Delourois (2009) Longe (1984) Laving (2003).

As already discussed under the epidemiology of meningitis in Africa, the three polysaccharide encapsulated bacteria most common in Ghana and Africa are Pheunococcus, Haemophilus influenza Type B and the Meningococcus.

The global epidemiology changed drastically during the 20th century as vaccines and antibiotics became available to prevent and treat the deadly disease.

Differential Diagonisis of Sensorineural Hearing loss in Ghanaian children revealed that, post-natal infections were the cause of about 60% of all Sensorineural Hearing loss in Ghanaian children, with measles leading with 30%, followed by malaria (Cerebral) with 14% and meningitis with 7.5%. See the Table Brobby (I986)[11] (1986)[1]

Recent observations have revealed that Bacterial meningitis is on the increase threatening to overtake cerebral malaria.

This may be due to better management, and increased awareness and prevention of malaria in the sub region.

It is interesting to note that deafness as a medical and social problem in the third world shows itself not very much differently from the image it portrays itself in the developed countries. However, in the developed countries deafness as a handicap has been made visible and effectively treated and prevented.

For example, all childhood infections like Measles, Meningitis, Mumps and Malaria (the four MS) have been eliminated in the developed countries, by immunization.

The main cause of Deafness in US and Europe is due to otoseclerosis and chromosomal anomalies. For example while as connexin 26 mutation causes only 18% of Deafness in Ghana; it is responsible for causing 50% and more of Sensorineural Hearing loss in US and Europe. Brobby (1986)[12] (1998)[13] Hammelman et al (2001)[14]

It is important to observe that deafness remains a hidden handicap. In Africa delay in diagnosis is common because the vocalization of hearing impaired children parallels that of normal infants until the age of nine months; all children co and bubble; parents are indeed likely to assume that speech is developing normally, ignoring any subtle evidence of hearing impatient such as lack of response to environmental sounds.

The effect of deafness on a child is devastating. Ability to participate in school activities or in a community life at a level commensurate with others has been the comparative benchmark for quality of life across the millennia. Participation in the world be it modern or ancient, centres on communication. In ancient Greece, deafness represented a curse, an absence of intelligence, an inability to participate in community life. Throughout mediaval times the inability to understand or express speech meant that an individual was not allowed to inherit the family fortune. Being unable to speak, i.e. to communicate was not allowed to receive the sacraments of the Church, which reflected one of the primary elements of full participation in community life. It is therefore our duty as crusaders for the prevention of deafness to summon all efforts to encourage all Third World Countries to extend their programme of Immunization of the 6 killer diseases which have been eliminated in developed countries, Tuberculosis, Tetanus, Diphtheria, Pertusis, Measles and Poliomyelitis.

The various National Governments should be made aware that Measles, Meningitis, Mumps, Tetanus and Rubellen, can be effectively prevented by cheap, readily available and non-toxic immunization.

9. Vaccination

In many industrialized nations Hib has been virtually eliminated by the use of a conjugated vaccine. Before these results can be applied in Africa the epidemiology of Hib disease (uncertain because of technical problems with culture, especially in the face of pre-treatment) must be characterized. A recent vaccine trial, in which Hib epidemiology in The Gambia was thoroughly assessed prior to the vaccination campaign, showed 95 per cent efficacy against invasive Hib disease and should serve as a model for future studies. Mulhdlland (1997)

At present, we are unaware of any African country which routinely vaccinates its children against Hib. Clearly, countries have many other health priorities, and the Hib vaccine is still relatively expensive although vaccination may actually be cost-effective in the long-term. Vaccination against group A and C meningococcal disease provides relatively short-lived immunity and has so far only been used to abort epidemics. Pneumococcal vaccine development has been hampered by the need to include a large number of serotypes.

10. Rehabilitation

Any sensorineural hearing loss is significant since even mild impairments may be of educational significance and subtle high-frequency deficits may interfere with the normal acquisition of language skills. Children with significant losses shuld be enrolled into a programme of rehabilitaition at a hearing assessment centre or a school for the deaf. Parental counselling is crucial for success. Most infants with even profound hearing loss retain some residual function, usually in the low frequencies. With early detection and management, this residual hearing can be harnessed by a comprehensive programme of amplification and auditory training (hearing aids and batteries should be commonplace commodities, affordable and available even in developing countries). This approach, in combination with simultaneous use of lip-reading and sign language, can transform the environment of a hearing-impaired child from a world of isolation, confusion and frustration to one of hope.

11. References

[1] Woodrow C.J, Brobby, G.W, deafnes, and meningitis in Africa, Postgraduate Doctor. Volume 19, M.4

[2] Daya, H, Woodrow, C.J, Brobby, G.W, et al 1997 pp 89-93, , Assessment of cochlear Damage after pneumococcal Meningitis using otoacustic Emissions. Trans Royal Soc of Tropical medicine and Hygiene 1997 Vol 91, pp 248-249,

[3] Brobby G.W, Causes of congenital and acquired Total Sensorineural Hearing loss in Ghana's children, Tropical Doctor Vol 18, pp30-32, 1988.

[4] Fortnum Hearing impairment after bacterial meningitis; a review Arch dis.cluld 1992 Vol 67, pp128-13, 3.

[5] Airede AI. Neoriatal bacterial meningitis in the middle belt of Nigeria, Developmental Medicine and child Neurology 1993, Vol 35, pp 424-430

[6] Daya, H, Amedofu, G.K. Woodrow, C.J Brobby.G.W. et al Deafness and Meningitis: what can otoacustic Emissions offer, Trans.Royal Soc of Trop.med and Hygiene Proceeding, Aspn Colorado 1997, 1998. pp.10-12,

[7] Fried land IR, klugman K.P. Failure of chloranplricol therapy in peniallure -resistant preumococcal meningitis. Lancet 1992, pp339, 405-408.

[8] Quazi .SA, Khan MA, Mughal etal; dexamethasone and bacterial meningitis in Pakistan Arch Dis chil 1916; Vol 75:pp 482-488

[9] Airede K, Adeyemi O, Ibrahim T, Neonatal bacterial meningitis and dexamethazore adjunctive usage in Nigeria. Nigeria journal of chemical Practice 2008, pp 235-245.

[10] Longe C, Omere J, Okoro A, Neonatal meningitis in Nigeria infants Acta padtatrical Scandinarica 1984, Vol 73:pp477-481

[11] Laving AMR, Musoke RN, Wasunna,AO Derathi G. Neonatal bacterial meningitis at the new born unit of Kenyatta national hospital, East Africa medical journal 2003,Vol 80. pp456-462

[12] Brobby G.W, Two cases of otosclciosis in Kumasi Ghana; Case Reports : Tropical and Geographical Medicine 1986 Vol 36 pp.292-295,

[13] Brobby G.W, Muller- Myshok, Horstman R, Connexin 26 R 143 Mutation Associated with Recessive Non-Syudromic Sensorinural Deafness in Africa. New England Journal of Medicine 1998 No 97 pp 3182-3183.

[14] Hammerlman, C, Amedofu, G.K. Brobby G.W. et al Distinct Pattern of Connexin 26 R mutation causing sensorineural Hearing impairment in Ghana. Journal of Human mutation 2000, Vol 9 pp 231-237

[15] Mulholland K, Hilton S, Adegbila R, et al randomised trial of Hemophilus influenza type-b tetanus/protean conjugate for prevention pneumonia and menigitis in Gambian infants lancet 1997:349(9060) pp 1191-1197.

2

Emerging Pathogens in Neonatal Bacterial Meningitis

Marisa Rosso, Pilar Rojas, Gemma Calderón and Antonio Pavón
UGC of Neonatology Hospital Virgen del Rocio, Spain

1. Introduction

Neonatal meningitis (NM) is a serious disease with substantial mortality and morbidity even among treated neonates (Overall, 1970; Harvey et al., 1999). Costs associated with treating false positive patients include prolonged hospital stay, exposure of the neonate to broad spectrum antibiotics, and insertion of central venous catheters for prolonged antibiotic administration.

The incidence of neonatal meningitis is difficult to accurately determine because of testing limitations. The incidence of bacterial meningitis is approximately 0.3 per 1000 live births in industrialized countries (Davies & Rudd, 1994). A recent study of neonatal infections in Asia (collecting data from China, Hong Kong, India, Iran, Kuwait, and Thailand), reported estimated incidence of neonatal meningitis from 0.48 per 1000 live births in Hong Kong to 2.4 per 1000 live births in Kuwait (Tiskumara et al., 2009). Another recent publication that looked at neonatal infections in Africa and South Asia found an incidence of neonatal meningitis ranging from 0.8 to 6.1 per 1000 live births (Thaver et al., 2009).

The rate of mortality from bacterial meningitis in developed countries among neonates has declined from almost 50% in the 1970s to less than 10% in the late 1990s due to advances in perinatal care over the last decades. However, a corresponding decrease in the morbidity rate has not occurred (Puopolo et al., 2005). Neonatal bacterial meningitis continues to be a serious disease with an unchanging rate of adverse outcome of 20-60%, despite a worldwide decline in mortality (Berardi et al., 2010). Morbidities related to neonatal bacterial meningitis continue to be a significant source of disability. In a prospective sample of more than 1500 neonates surviving until age 5 years, the prevalence of neuromotor disabilities including cerebral palsy was 8.1%, learning disability 7.5%, seizures 7.3%, and hearing problems 25.8%. No problems were reported in 65% of babies who survived group B streptococcal (GBS) meningitis and in 41.5% of those who survived *Escherichia coli (E.Coli)* meningitis (Bedford et al., 2001).

The three major pathogens in developed countries are: *Group B streptococcus*, gram negative rods and *Lysteria mococytogenes*. Group B streptococci are the most commonly identified organisms, implicated in roughly 50% of all cases of bacterial meningitis, and *E coli* accounts for another 20%; identification and treatment of maternal genitourinary infections is thus an important prevention strategy (Klinger et al., 2000). *Listeria monocytogenes* is the third most common pathogen, with 5-10% of cases; it is unique because it exhibits transplacental transmission (Heath et al., 2003). Historically regardless of the specific pathogen involved, neonatal meningitis is most often caused by vertical transmission during labor, but the increasing numbers of infants surviving premature delivery and advances in unit intensive care it is increasingly recognized as an emerging cause of hospital-acquired infection, particularly among severely debilitated or immunosuppressed patients. The accumulative incidence of meningitis is highest in the first month of life and is higher in preterm neonates than term neonates (Overall , 1970). For premature infants who develop meningitis, the neurodevelopmental consequences are often profound (Stoll et al., 2004). It occurs most frequently in the days following birth and is more common in premature infants than term infants (Davies & Rudd, 1994). Neonatal meningitis occurs in roughly 0.3 per 1000 live births; it is closely associated with sepsis, which is 5 times as common.

Risk factors for the development of meningitis include low birth weight (< 2500 g), preterm birth (< 37 weeks' gestation), premature rupture of membranes, traumatic delivery, fetal hypoxia, and maternal peripartum infection (including chorioamnionitis). Moreover neonates are at greater risk of sepsis and meningitis than other age groups because of deficiencies in humoral and cellular immunity and in phagocytic function. Infants younger than 32 weeks' gestation receive little of the maternal immunoglobulin received by full-term infants. (Volpe, 2008a,2008b). Inefficiency in the neonates alternative complement pathway compromises their defense against encapsulated bacteria (Krebs et al., 2007) T-cell defense and mediation of B-cell activity also are compromised. Finally, deficient migration and phagocytosis by neutrophils contribute to neonatal vulnerability to pathogens of even low virulence.

No one clinical sign is pathognomonic of meningitis. Because the signs of meningitis are subtle and nonspecific there may be delays in diagnosis and treatment (Feigin et al., 1992).

- Bacterial meningitis, early onset
  - Symptoms appearing within the first 72 hours of life are referable primarily to systemic illness rather than meningitis. These include temperature inestability, episodes of apnea or bradycardia, hypotension, feeding difficulty, hepatic dysfunction, and irritability alternating with lethargy. (Volpe, 2008 a,2008b)
  - Respiratory symptoms can become prominent within hours of birth in GBS infection; however, the symptom complex also is seen with infection by *Escherichia coli* or *Listeria* species.
- Bacterial meningitis, late onset
  - Late-onset bacterial meningitis (symptom onset beyond 72 hours of life) is more likely to be associated with neurologic symptoms. Most commonly seen are stupor and irritability, which Volpe describes in more than 75% of affected neonates.

Between 25% and 50% of neonates will exhibit the following neurological signs: seizures; bulging anterior fontanel; extensor posturing/ opisthotonus; focal cerebral signs including gaze deviation and hemiparesis; cranial nerve palsies. Nuchal rigidity per se is the least common neurologic sign in neonatal bacterial meningitis, occurring in fewer than 25% of affected neonates.

Interpretation of cerebrospinal fluid (CSF) findings is more difficult in neonates than in older children, especially in premature infants whose more permeable blood-brain barrier causes higher levels of glucose and protein (Smith et al., 2008). So when faced with the need to make therapeutic decisions on the interpretation of CSF parameters, pediatricians, family practice physicians, and neonatologists often use The Harriet Lane Handbook as their guide (Robertson & Shilkofski, 2005). The classic finding of decreased CSF glucose, elevated CSF protein, and pleocytosis is seen more with gram-negative meningitis and with late gram-positive meningitis; this combination also is suggestive of viral meningitis, especially HSV (Carges et al., 2006). The number of white blood cells found in the CSF in healthy neonates varies based on gestational age. Many authors use a cutoff of 20-30 WBC/µL. Only if all 3 parameters are normal does the lumbar puncture provide evidence against infection; no single CSF parameter exists that can reliably exclude the presence of meningitis in a neonate (Garges et al., 2006) .Bacterial meningitis commonly causes CSF pleocytosis greater than 100 WBC/µL, with predominantly polymorphonuclear leukocytes gradually evolving to lymphocytes (Garges et al., 2006).

Emerging pathogens are those that have appeared in a human population for the first time, or have occurred previously but are increasing in incidence or expanding into areas where they have not previously been reported, usually over the last 20 years (World Health Organization (WHO), 1997). In our patients, the reported risk factors associated with emerging pathogens infection are prematurity, neurosurgical procedures (especially shunts and drainages), intracranial haemorrhages. Our current patients have been undergone several neurosurgical procedures and also, importantly, have been treated with a previous broad-spectrum antibiotic, which is also a suggested risk factor for infection with these emerging pathogens (*Stenotrophomonas Maltophilia* (Rojas et al., 2009), *Kluyvera ascorbata* (Rosso et al., 2007), *Enterobacter sakazakii* (Hunter et al., 2008) and *Rhodococcus equi* (Strunk et al., 2007). Although these pathogens are considered an infrequent cause of meningitis, it has become a focus of interest not only due to increasing recognition of its pathogenic potential but also because of its marked antibiotic resistance.

2. Emerging pathogens and clinical case reports

In this chapter we report several cases of these emerging pathogens meningitis in newborns successfully treated. Two of them have been reported previously for us.

2.1 Rhodococcus equi (R. equi)

Rhodococcus equi is a Gram-positive, aerobic, pleomorphic, nonmotile, branching filamentous coccobacillus and was first isolated from the lungs of foals in Sweden in 1923 by Magnusson. Called *Rhodococcus* because of its ability to form a red (or salmon-colored) pigment, *R. equi* can be weakly acid-fast and bears a similarity to diphtheroids. *R. equi* primarily causes zoonotic infections that affect grazing animals. The first report of human infection occurred in the 1960s.The natural reservoir for this organism appears to be soil. The two main methods of acquiring this organism are inhalation and direct inoculation through trauma. Infections with *R. equi* have a significant potential for hematogenous dissemination, with bacteremia occurring in up to 80% of immunocompromised patients (Emmons et al., 1991).

2.1.1 Case report

Patient was born as the first of twin brothers at 27 +2 weeks. The pregnancy was complicated by twintwin-transfusion syndrome, with twin 1 being the recipient. Delivery was by cesarean section for fetal distress. The APGAR scores at 1 and 5 minutes were 8 and 9, respectively. Shortly after delivery, the baby developed respiratory distress syndrome requiring intubation and ventilation for 2 days. After that, respiratory support was by continuous positive airway pressure. On day 10, sepsis with coagulase-negative staphylococci was treated with intravenous vancomycin (10 days) and gentamicin (3 days). Head ultrasound examination on day 1 was normal, but a repeated scan on day 7 revealed a right-sided grade III intraventricular hemorrhage. Subsequent examinations demonstrated a slow increase of the size of the lateral ventricles and elevated resistive indices indicative of posthemorrhagic hydrocephalus. Therapeutic lumbar punctures performed 2–3 times per week yielded sterile cerebrospinal fluid (CSF). Cerebral magnetic resonance imaging on day 57 demonstrated post hemorrhagic aqueduct stenosis with dilated lateral and third ventricles. A ventriculoperitoneal-shunt was inserted on day 59 under perioperative antibiotic prophylaxis with intravenous vancomycin (1 dose) and cefotaxime (3 doses). On day 61, the baby developed apnea episodes and seizures requiring intubation and mechanical ventilation. A lumbar puncture was performed and CSF showed 24 106/L white cells (56% neutrophils) and 56 106/L erythrocytes. Gram-positive bacilli were seen in the CSF. Empiric antibiotic treatment with intravenous vancomycin (15 mg/kg/dose twice daily), meropenem (40 mg/kg/dose thrice daily), and ciprofloxacin (10 mg/kg/dose twice daily) was started. The VP-shunt was externalized on day 63 and removed on day 67. Cultures of the removed shunt and follow-up lumbar puncture CSF did not grow bacteria. The initial CSF culture had bacterial growth on day 68. CSF plated onto Blood Agar (Columbia agar base, Oxoid, Melbourne, Australia) and Chocolate Agar (GC agar base, Oxoid) and incubated at 35°C in a 5% CO2 atmosphere for 48 hours grew colonies 3–4 mm in diameter, irregularly round, smooth, and semitransparent. Production of salmon-colored pigmentation occurred after 4 days incubation. Gram stain revealed the presence of irregular shaped Gram-positive bacilli. Colonies were catalase- positive, oxidase negative, nitrate reduction positive, alkaline phosphatase positive, and urease negative. By the API Coryne system (Biomerieux, Marcyl'Etoile, France), the profile number was 1100004. The organism produced equi factors that interacted with the beta-toxin of *Staphylococcus aureus* to give an area of complete hemolysis on Sheep Blood Agar (Trypticase Soy agar base, Oxoid). Identification of *Rhodococcus equi* was confirmed by cellular fatty acid analysis and DNA sequencing. The antibiotic regimen was changed to intravenous vancomycin (15 mg/kg/dose twice daily) and rifampin (20 mg/kg once daily) and continued until day 90. This was followed by oral treatment with rifampin (10 mg/kg once daily) and azithromycin (10 mg/kg once daily) for a further 3 months. The baby's condition improved, and the CSF white cell count normalized. At the chronologic age of 6.5 months, a VP-shunt was reinserted without complications because of increasing hydrocephalus. When last seen at corrected age of 1 year, the boy had made good developmental progress with only slightly delayed motor skills.

2.2 Kluyvera ascorbata (K. ascorbata)

A new genus in the family *Enterobacteriaceae* in 1981 using molecular characterization and deoxyribonucleic acid (DNA)-DNA hybridation techniques. Strains of *Kluyvera* were divided into two named species, *Kluyvera ascorbata* and *Kluyvera cryocrescens,* and a third unnamed group, *Kluyvera* species group 3 (Farmer et al., 1981). The genus currently consists of 4 species, *K. ascorbata, K. cryocrescens, K. georgina* (formerly species group 3) and *K.cochleae* (Carter et al., 2005). It is a small, motile Gram-negative bacillus with peritrichous flagella that is oxidase- negative and catalase- positive, and it ferments glucose (Farmer et al., 1981; Brooks et al., 2003; Narchi et al., 2005; Paredes-Rodriguez et al., 2002). Confirmatory species identification of *Kluyvera* requires the demonstration of ascorbate utilization and glucose fermentation at 5°C. *Kluyvera* is present in the environment in water, soil, sewage, hospital sinks, and food products of animal origin (Brooks et al., 2003). It also has been isolated from a variety of human specimens (most commonly sputum, urine, stool, throat, and blood).It was initially considered to be a benign saprophyte predominantly colonizing the respiratory, gastrointestinal or urinary tract (Carter et al., 2005; Narchi et al., 2005;Sarria et al., 2001).

2.2.1 Case report

A male infant was born full term with a prenatally diagnosed lumbosacral myelomeningocele and dilated cerebral ventricles. The herniation was reduced and the defect repaired and a ventriculoperitoneal shunt was inserted. Five days following surgery he development fever, irritable crying and poor appetite. The physical examination was otherwise normal. Blood tests showed a peripheral white blood cell count of $4x10^9$ /L, normal hemoglobin and platelet count and a C-reactive protein of 148 mg/L. Urine analysis by the dipstick method was normal. Cerebrospinal fluid obtained by ventriculoperitoneal shunt puncture was yellow and turbid. Analysis of CSF revealed pleocytosis with a white blood cell count of 11664 cells/mm^3 (98% neutrophils), protein 3.4 g/l, glucose 0.01 g/l. The concomitant plasma glucose was normal. Blood, urine and CSF cultures were obtained. The Gram stain of CSF was negative. Empirical antibiotic therapy with meropenem was started. Blood and urine cultures were normal. *Kluyvera ascorbata* was isolated from CSF sample. It was susceptible in vitro to third generation cephalosporins, trimethoprim, aminoglycosides, aztreonam, fluorquinolones, imipenem and amoxicillin-clavulanate; it was resistant to first generation cephalosporins and with intermediate susceptibility to second generation cephalosporins. Despite treatment with antibiotics, the patient remained febrile and with poor appetite. A computed tomography brain scan showed a left dilated ventricle. The shunt was removed and a temporary external CSF drainage was inserted. Two days after external CSF drainage was inserted, he became afebrile and appeared better. CSF analyses performed after 21 days of treatment revealed clear CSF. There were no white blood cells and the protein and glucose values were 2.7 g/l and 0.34 g/l, respectively. Gram stain of that CSF specimen failed to reveal bacteria and the culture was sterile. He received antibiotic therapy for 28 days, a ventriculoperitoneal shunt was replaced after infection was eradicated.

2.3 Stenotrophomonas maltophilia (S. maltophilia)

Is a nonfermentative Gram-negative bacillus, previously known as *Pseudomonas maltophilia* and later *Xanthomonas maltophilia*. This bacterium is found in several environments such as water, soil, plants, food and hospital settings (Nicodemo & Garcia –Paez 2007; Yemisen et al., 2008). It is increasingly recognised as a significant cause of hospital acquired infection particularly among severely debilitated and immunosuppressed patients, those receiving longterm antimicrobial therapy and those with indwelling central venous catheters. The resultant infections are extensive, with the respiratory tract, soft tissues and the skin most frequently involved (Nicodemo & Garcia -Paez 2007; Denis et al., 1977).

2.3.1 Case report

A baby boy was delivered at 26 weeks of gestation after a spontaneous rupture of membranes. The patient was admitted to our neonatal intensive care unit with Apgar scores of two and eight at 1 and 5 minutes, respectively. On the 12th day of his life clinical and radiological signs of perforated necrotizing enterocolitis (NEC) occurred and required surgical intestinal resection. Cerebral ultrasound at day 15 of his life was performed and showed intraventricular haemorrhage and dilated cerebral ventricles. Because of NEC, temporary external CSF drainage was inserted. Two weeks after external CSF drainage was performed, he developed *Klebsiella Extended-spectrum beta-lactamase (ESBL)* meningitis. Antibiotic therapy with meropenem was started and the external CSF drainage was replaced. After 19 days of treatment with meropenem a new CSF sample from drainage revealed 1200 cells/mm3 (95% neutrophils), protein 3.4 g/L and glucose 0.03 g/L. Gramnegative bacillus were seen on gram strain in the CSF culture and it was positive for *S. maltophilia.* The strain was only susceptible in vitro to trimethoprimsulfamethoxazole (TMP-SMX), with a mean inhibitory concentration (MIC) of ≤2/38, minocycline and ciprofloxacin. TMP-SMX intravenous therapy (50 mg/kg per day in two divided doses) was commenced. The external ventricular drainage was not removed at this stage because the patient's state was critical. The next sample analysis of CSF from the drainage 14 days after starting TMP-SMX revealed the following profile: white blood cell count of 1300 cells/mm3 (90% neutrophils), protein 1.39 g/L and glucose 0.04 g/L. The CSF culture was still positive for *S. maltophilia* and consequently ciprofloxacin (15 mg/kg per day in two divided doses) was added to TMP-SMX. Furthermore, the external ventricular drainage was removed and after 7 days of therapy with ciprofloxacin in combination with TMP-SMX, the analysis of the CSF was normal and the culture was sterile. Finally, 21 more days of therapy were completed with both antibiotics. No adverse effects were found during ciprofloxacin treatment. There was no displacement of bilirubin with the use of sulfamethoxazole in our patient and the values were normal (maximum total bilirubin 127 mg/dL). A ventricular-peritoneal shunt was inserted after the infection was eradicated due to severe ventricular dilatation.

2.4 Enterobacter sakazakii (E. sakazakii)

Is a motile, non-sporeforming, Gramnegative facultative anaerobe. It was known as 'yellow pigmented Enterobacter cloacae' until 1980 when it was designated as a new species by Farmer, Asbury, Hickman and Brenner in honour of the Japanese bacteriologist Riichi Sakazaki. They reported that DNA–DNA hybridization studies found no clear generic assignment for *E. sakazakii* as it was 53–54% related to Enterobacter and *Citrobacter* species. A comparison of the type strains of these two genera showed that E. sakazakii was 41% related to *C. freundii* and 51% related to *E. cloacae.* Subsequently, since it was also phenotypically closer to E. cloacae, Farmer, Asbury, Hickman and Brenner (1980) assigned the organism to the *Enterobacter* genus.The natural habitat of *E. sakazakii* is unknown, but it has been isolated from a number of hospital sources (Farmer et al., 1980). Most of these reports describe single cases. Because pigment production, a distinguishing characteristic of *E. sakazakii*, is greatly diminished at the usual incubation temperature of 36°C, it seemed likely that a number of *E. sakazakii* isolates were not recognized as atypical *E. cloacae* in the past

2.4.1 Cases report

Infection of the newborn is probably through ingestion of contaminated infant milk formula and not through vertical transmission from the mother during birth (Muytjens & Kollee, 1990). The first reported association of *E. sakazakii* with contaminated Infant milk formula (IMF) powder was by (Muytjens et al., 1983) in the Netherlands studying eight cases of neonatal meningitis and sepsis. *E. sakazakii* was isolated from prepared milk formula, a dish brush and a stirring spoon. These isolateswere studied in more detail later by(Smeets et al., 1998). In Iceland three cases were reported linked to milk formula contaminated with *E. sakazakii* (Biering et al., 1989). US Centers for Disease Control and Prevention (Himelright et al., 2002) reported an investigation into the 2001 Tennessee outbreak of *E. sakazakii* in a neonatal intensive care unit in which 10 cases were identified. The index case was a male infant (born at 33.5 weeks) who had been admitted to the neonatal intensive care unit because of premature birth weight and respiratory distress. After 11 days the baby developed symptoms of meningitis (fever, tachycardia, decreased vascular perfusions and suspected seizure activity) and despite being given intravenous antibiotics the infant died after a further 9 days. *E. sakazakii* was cultured from the cerebrospinal fluid. Following increased surveillance a further 10 cases of *E. sakazakii* colonisation were found on the neonatal unit; 2 from 'non-sterile' site with clinical deterioration. The use of infant formula milk was the only factor associating the cases. More recently (Simon et al., 2010) described a case of meningitis in a neonatal intensive care unit occurred as a result of the use of a powered infant formula contaminated with *E. sakazakii* at manufacturing level, and an inadequate preparation and storing of the reconstituted product were identified as risk factors.

3. Discussion

The potential virulence of these pathogens above mentioned have been uncertain in the past, owing in part to its relatively recent characterization and the small number of reported clinical infections.

The reported risk factors associated with these pathogens infection are prematurity, neurosurgical procedures (especially shunts and drainages), intracranial haemorrhages and malignancies (Caylan et al., 2002). Our patients had undergone several neurosurgical procedures and also importantly, had been treated with a previous broad-spectrum antibiotic such as ampicillin, 3rd generation cephalosporins and carbapenem which is also a suggested risk factor for infection. Aggressive antimicrobial intervention is lifesaving in neonates with suspected meningitis.

These emergent pathogens are increasingly recognised as a cause of nosocomial infections of special interest because of its intrinsic resistance to multiple antimicrobial agents used to treat Gram-negative infections. So (Rojas et al., 2009) found *S. maltophilia* isolates were resistant to ampicillin, cefazolin and extended spectrum penicillins, but were susceptible to the aminoglycosides and trimethoprimsulfamethoxazole. It is resistant to a variety of antibiotics, for example aminoglycosides, ß-lactam agents and it is intrinsically resistant to carbapenems. Based on susceptibility studies, TMP-SMX is the drug of choice for treatment of *S. maltophilia* infections. However, recent data indicate that the percentage of strains resistant to TMPSMX may be increasing(Nicodemo & Garcia –Paez 2007; Wen-Tsung et al., 2002; Krcmery V et al., 1999; Van den Oever et al., 1998). In this patient the pathogen was susceptible to this antimicrobial therapy but CSF cultures only became sterile after removal of the external ventricular drainage and the addition of ciprofloxacin to TMP-SMX. We decided to add ciprofloxacin because TMP-SMX is bacteriostatic and the infant was seriously ill (Table1). The administration of sulfamethoxazole, which binds to albumin and competes with bilirubin, can increase the possibility of hyperbilirubinaemia and serious neurological complications such as kernicterus in neonates. This was not observed in our patient.

Little information is available regarding the in vitro antibiotic susceptibilities and clinical effectiveness of antibiotics in *Kluyvera* infections. The agents most consistently active in vitro against *Kluyvera* are third-generation cephalosporins, fluorquinolones, aminoglycosides, imipenem, chloramphenicol, and nitrofurantoin. Most strains are resistant to ampicillin, first and second-generation cephalosporins and ticarcillin. Agents with variable activity include ampicillin-sulbactam, aztreonam, piperacillin, tetracycline and trimethoprim-sulfamethoxazole. (Narchi et al., 2003; Sarria et al.,2001). In our case, above mentioned the *Kluyvera* species was also sensitive to third-generation cephalosporins, quinolones, aminoglycosides and carbapenems. We used meropenem with a good clinical response. We used this antibiotic because of predisposing factors for resistant hospital acquired microorganisms such as colonization with nosocomial pathogens, broad spectrum antibiotic usage, underlying disease and intensive care unit admission.

Case No	Reference/ Year	Age/sex	Neurosurgical procedure	Therapy	Outcome
1	1977	8 months/male	None	Ampicilin, colistin	Died
2	1977	13 months/ female	None	Chloramphenicol, sulphadoxine	Recovered
3	1984	7 days/ male	None	None	Died
4	2002	4 days/ female	None	Ciprofloxacin	Recovered
5	2009	69 days/ male	External (CSF) drainage	TMP-SMX, ciprofloxacin	Recovered

Table 1. Details of children with meningitis caused by *S. maltophilia*

(Lai, 2001) found all *E. sakazakii* isolates were resistant to ampicillin, cefazolin and extended spectrum penicillins, but were susceptible to the aminoglycosides and trimethoprimsulfamethoxazole. Whereas sensitivity to 3rd generation cephalosporins and the quinolones was variable. Subsequently (Lai, 2001) proposed the use of carbapenems or 3rd generation cephalosporins with an aminoglycoside or trimethoprim with sulfamethoxazole. This treatment regime has improved the outcome of E. sakazakii meningitis though the resistanceof *Enterobacter spp.* to these antibiotics is increasing (Lai, 2001; Dennison & Morris, 2002) have reported an *E. sakazakii* infection that was resistant to multiple antibiotics, including ampicillin, gentamicin and cefotaxamine.

Other hand selection of antibiotics should be determined based on likely pathogen, local patterns of antibacterial drug sensitivities, and hospital policies. When NM is suspected, treatment must be aggressive, as the goal is to achieve bactericidal concentration of antibiotics and to sterilize CSF as soon as possible with empiric antibiotic treatment should include agents active against all main pathogens; but we must be alert because these novel pathogens are resistant to a variety of antibiotics, for example aminoglycosides, ß-lactam agents and including to carbapenems. Here, we have reported our experience with these emerging pathogens in neonatal meningitis.

4. Conclusion

In summary we are witnessing new emerging pathogens causing potentially fatal bacterial neonatal meningitis. Here, we report our experience with these emerging pathogens. Given the expected increase in the future regarding the frequency of these emerging pathogens causing nosocomial infections including meningitis due to these organisms in neurosurgical patients and its marked resistance to antibiotics, they should be considered as a potential cause of meningitis in neonates with external ventricular drainage who are receiving long term broad spectrum antimicrobial therapy.

5. Acknowledgements

We would like to express our gratitude to Dr. Olaf Neth for technical support.

6. References

Bedford, H.; de Louvois, J; Halket, S.; Peckham, C.; Hurley, R. & Harvey, D.(2001). Meningitis in infancy in England and Wales: follow up at age 5 years. *BMJ*. Sep 8 323(7312), pp.533-6.

Berardi, A.; Lugli, L.; Rossi, C.; China, MC.; Vellani, G.; Contiero, R.; Calarca, F.; Carmelo, F.; Causula, F.; DiCarlo, C.; Rossi, Mr.; Chiarabini, R.; Ferrari, M.; Mininti, S.; Venturelli, C.; Silvestrini, D., Dodi, I., Zucchini, A. & Ferrari, F.(2010). Infezioni da Streptococco B Della Regione Emilia Romagna. Neonatal bacterial meningitis. *Minerva Pediatri*, Jun; Vol.62, (3 Suppl 1)pp.51-4

Biering, G.; Karlsson, S.; Clark, NC.; Jonsdottir, KE.; Ludvigson, P. & Streingrimsson, O.(1989). Three cases of neonatal meningitis caused by Enterobacter sakazakii in powdered milk. *J Clin Microbiol, Vol*, 27, pp. 2054–56

Brooks, T. & Feldman, S.(2003).Central venous catheter infection in a child: case report and review of *Kluyvera* infection in children. *South Med J*, Vol.96, pp.214-17.

Carter, JE. & Evans, TN.(2005). Clinically significant *Kluyvera* infections: a report of seven cases. *Am J Clin Pathol*, Vol.123, pp.34-338

Caylan, R.; Aydin, K. & Koksal, I.(2002). Meningitis cause by Stenotrophomonas maltophilia: case report and review of the literature. *Ann Saudi Med.*, Vol. 22, pp.216-8.

Davies, PA. & Rudd, PT.(1994). Incidence; The Developing Brain. In: *Neonatal Meningitis*. Cambridge, England: Cambridge University Press;

Dennison, S K. & Morris, J.(2002). Multiresistant Enterobacter sakazakii wound infection in an adult. *Infections in Medicine*, Vol.19, pp.533–35.

Denis, F.; Sow, A. & David M. (1977).Etude de deux cas de meningitis a Pseudomonas maltophilia observes au Senegal. *Bull Soc Med Afr Noire Lang Fr,* Vol. 22, pp.135-9.

Emmons, W.; Reichwein, B. & Winslow, DL (1991). *Rhodococcus equi* infection in the patient with AIDS: literature review and report of an unusual case. *Rev Infect Dis,* Vol.13, pp.91–6.

Farmer, JJ III.; Asbury, MA.; Hickmann, FW. & Brenner, DJ. (1980). *Enterobacter sakazakii*: a new species of "*Enterobacteriaceae*" isolated from clinical specimens. *Int. J. Syst. Bacteriol,* Vol.30, pp.569-84.

Farmer, JJ III.; Fanning, GR.; Huntley-Carter, GP.; Holmes, B., Hickman, FW.; Richard, C. & Brener, DJ. (1981) *Kluyvera,* a new (redefined) genus in the family Enterobacteriaceae: identification of *Kluyvera ascorbata* sp. nov. and *Kluyvera cryocrescens* sp. nov. in clinical specimens. *J Clin Microbiol,* Vol. 13, pp.919-933

Feigin, RD.; McCracken, GH Jr. & Klein, JO.(1992). Diagnosis and management of meningitis. *Pediatr Infect Dis J,* Vol.11, pp.785–814

Garges, HP.; Moody, MA.; Cotten, CM.; Smith, PB.; Tiffany, KF.; Lenfestey, R.; Li, JS.; Fowler, VG. & Benjamin, DK Jr.(2006). Neonatal meningitis: what is the correlation among cerebrospinal fluid cultures, blood cultures, and cerebrospinal fluid parameters?. *Pediatrics,* Apr; Vol. 117(4), pp. 1094-100

Heath, PT.; Nik Yusoff, NK. & Baker, CJ.(2003). Neonatal meningitis. *Arch Dis Child Fetal Neonatal **Ed***. May, Vol.88(3), pp.F173-8.

Himelright, I.; Harris, E.; Lorch, V.; Anderson, M.; Jones, T.; Craig; A.; Kuehnert, M.; Forster, T.; Arduino, M.; Jensen, B. & Jernigan, D.(2002). Enterobacter sakazakii infections associated with the use of powdered infant formula — Tennessee, 2001. *Morbidity Mortality Weekly Report,* Vol.51, pp. 298–300.

Iversen, C. S & Forsythe, J. (2003). Risk profile of *Enterobacter sakazakii,* an emergent pathogen associated with infant milk formula.*Trends Food Sci.Technol,* Vol.11, pp. 443-54

Klinger, G.; Chin, CN.; Beyene, J. & Perlman, N.(2000). Predicting the outcome of neonatal bacterial meningitis. *Pediatrics,* Sep Vol.106(3), pp.477-82

Krcmery, V Jr.; Filka, J.; Uher, J.; Kurak, H.; Sagat, T.; Tuharsky, J.; Novak, I.; Urbanova, T.; Kralinsky, K.; Mateicka, F.;, Krcméryová, T.; Jurga, L.; Sulcová, M.; Stencl, J. & Krúpová, I.(1999) Ciprofloxacin in treatment of nosocomial meningitis in neonates and in infants: report of 12 cases and review. *Diagn Microbiol Infect disease,* Vol.35, pp.75-80.

Krebs, VLJ. & Costa GAM. (2007). Clinical outcome of neonatal bacterial meningitis according to birth weight. *Arq,* December; Vol.65, pp.1149-1153.

Lai KK.(2001). Enterobacter sakazakii infections among neonates, infants, children, and adults: Case reports and a review of the literature. *Medicine,* Vol.80, pp.113–122

Magnusson, H(1923). Spezifische infektio¨se Pneumonie beim Fohlen: ein neuer Eitererreger beim Pferd. *Arch Wiss Prakt Tierheilkd,* Vol.50, pp.22–38

Muytjens, HL.; Zanen, HC.; Sonderkamp, HJ.; Kollee, LA.; Wachsmuth, IK. & Farmer, JJ.III.(1983) Analysis of eight cases of neonatal meningitis and sepsis due to Enterobacter sakazakii. *J Clin Microbiol,* Vol.18, pp.115–120

Muytjens, HL. & Kolee, LA. (1990). Enterobacter sakazakii meningitis in neonates: causative role of formula?. *Pediatric Infectious Disease,* Vol.9, pp. 372–73.

Narchi, H.(2005). *Kluyvera* urinary tract infection: case report and review of the literature. *Pediatr Infect Dis J,* Vol. 24, pp.570-572.

Nicodemo, AC. & García Paez JI.(2007). Antimicrobial therapy for Stenotrophomonas maltophilia infections. *Eur J Clin Microbiol Infect Dis,* Vol. 26, pp.229-37.

Overall, JC.Jr.(1970) Neonatal bacterial meningitis. Analysis of predisposing factors and outcome compared with matched control subjects. *J Pediatr, Vol.*76, pp.499–511.

Paredes-Rodriguez, D.; Villalobos-Vinda, J.; Avilés-Montoya, A. & Alvarado-Cerdas, E.(2002) Meningitis por *Kluyvera sp.* en una paciente con una derivación lumbo-peritoneal: reporte de un caso. *Acta Med Costarric,* pp.44.

Puopolo, KM.; Madoff, LC. & Eichenwald, EC. (2005) Early-onset group B streptococcal disease in the era of maternal screening. *Pediatrics.* May Vol.115(5), pp. 1240-6.

Robertson, J. & Shilkofski, N.(2005) *The Harriet Lane Handbook.* 17th (Ed). Mosby; Philadelphia, pp. 557.

Rojas, P.; Garcia, E.; Calderón, GM.; Ferreira, F. & Rosso, M.(2009). Successful treatment of Stenotrophomonas maltophilia meningitis in a preterm baby boy: a case report. *Journal of Medical Case Reports,* Vol 3, pp.7389.

Rosso, M.; Rojas, P.; Garcia, E.; Marquez, J.; Losada, A. & Muñoz, M.(2007). Kluyvera meningitis in a newborn. *Pediatr Infect Dis J,* Vol 26, pp. 1070-1071.

Sarria, JC.; Vidal, AM. & Kimbrough, RC.(2001) Infections caused by *Kluyvera* species in humans. *Clin Infect Dis.* Vol. 33, pp E69-E74.

Simón, M.; Sabaté, S.; Osanz, AC.; Bartolomé, R. & Ferrer, MD. (2010).Investigation of a neonatal case of Enterobacter sakazakii infection associated with the use of powdered infant formula. *Enferm Infecc Microbiol Clin,* Vol. 28, 10, pp. 713-15

Smeets, LC.; Voss, A.; Muytjens, H L.; Meis, J F G M. & Melchers, W J G. (1998). Genetische karakterisatie van Enterobacter sakazakii-isolaten van Nederlandse patiënten met neonatale meningitis. *Nederlands Tijdschrift voor Medische Microbiologie,* Vol.6, pp. 113–15.

Smith, PB.; Carges, HP.; Cotton, CM.; Walsh, TJ.; Clark, RH. & Benjamin, DK.Jr.(2008). Meningitis in preterm neonates: importance of cerebrospinal fluid parameters. *Am J Perinatol,* Aug; Vol.25(7):421-6. Epub 2008 Aug 22

Stoll, BJ.; Hansen, NI., Adams-Chapman, I.; Fanaroff, AA.; Hintz, SR.; Vohr, B. & Higgins, RD.(2004). Neurodevelopmental and growth impairment among extremely low-birth-weight infants with neonatal infection. *JAMA,* Vol.292, pp.2357–65

Strunk, T.; Gardiner, K.; Simmer, K.; Altlas, D. & Keli AD.(2007) Rhodoccocus equi meningitis after ventriculoperitoneal shunt insertion in a preterm infant. *Pediatr Infect Dis J.* nov; Vol.26(11), pp.1076-7.

Tiskumara, R.; Fakharee, SH.; Liu, C-Q.; Nuntnarumit, P.; Lui, K-M.; Hammoud, M.; Lee, JKF.; Chow, CB.; Shenoi, A.; Halliday, R. & Isaaes, D.(2009). Neonatal infections in Asia. *Arch Dis Child Fetal Neonatal Ed.* Vol. 94, pp.144-8.

Thaver, D. & Zaidi, AK.(2009). Burden of neonatal infections in developing countries: a review of evidence from community-based studies. *Pediatr Infect Dis J.* Jan; 28(1 Suppl), pp. S3-9.

Van den Oever, HL.; Versteegh, FG.; Thewessen, EA.; van den Anker, JN.; Mounton, JW. & Neijens HJ.(1998) Ciprofloxacin in preterm neonates: case report and review of the literature. *Eur J Pediatr,* Vol.157, pp.843-5.

Volpe JJ(2008b). Bacterial and fungal intracranial infections. In: *Neurology of the Newborn*. 5th. Philadelphia, Pa: Saunders Elsevier, pp.916-56.

Volpe JJ. (2008a).Viral, protozoal, and related intracranial infections. In: *Neurology of the Newborn*. 5th. Philadelphia, Pa: Saunders Elsevier, pp.851-915.

Wen-Tsung, L.; Chin-Chien, W.; Chuen-Ming, L. & Mong-Ling, C.(2002) Successful treatment of multi-resistant Stenotrophomonas maltophilia meningitis with ciprofloxacin in a pre-term infant. *Eur J Pediatr,* Vol.161, pp.680-2.

Yemisen, M.; Mete, B.; Tunali, Y.; Yentur, E. & Ozturk, R.(2008). A meningitis case due to Stenotrophomonas maltophilia and review of the literature. *Int J Infect Dis,* Vol. 23, pp.1-3.

3

Perspectives of Neonatal-Perinatal Bacterial Meningitis

Kareem Airede
University of Abuja
Nigeria

1. Introduction

Bacterial meningitis is generally a devastating infection of the leptomeninges and underlying subarachnoid cerebrospinal fluid with a high mortality rate, particularly in the perinatal and neonatal infant. This is more worrisome because despite the more available potent antimicrobials and variably effective vaccines, the disease remains a significant cause of morbidity and mortality. Mortality rates could be as high as between 25 - 50% depending on which series as well the area of practice, whilst morbidity, often neurologic, could be as elevated as 25 – 45%.

Many clinical and etiologic studies performed over the recent decades have demonstrated that different species of bacteria can precipitate Neonatal-Perinatal bacterial meningitis. *Streptococcus agalactiae, Staphyloccocus aureus,* Group B *β-Haemolytic streptococci* [GBS], Gram-negative bacilli, *Haemophilus influenzae* type *b, Neisseria meningitides, Listeria monocytogenes* and *Streptococcus pneumoniae* have all been implicated as etiologic pathogens. The ranking profile of the major causative organisms, however, depends majorly on the region of practice.

The major burden of Neonatal-Perinatal bacterial meningitis occurs in the developing world, however, most evidence derives from wealthy countries even though the spectrum of disease, etiology and prognosis may differ.

In this Chapter, we would dilate on the available evidence of Neonatal-Perinatal bacterial meningitis in developing countries; provide its detailed pathophysiologic process/pattern; describe the relevant clinical features at presentation; discuss its diagnosis and management strategy with particular highlights of adjuncts of steroids; indicate relevant differences from well-resourced settings; provide relevant lacunae in knowledge and comment on feasible preventive methods.

2. Incidence of disease

Bacterial meningitis is undoubtedly more common in the neonatal-perinatal period than at any other time in life. This newborn's gloomy feature of increased susceptibility to infection is due to its innate immature immune system that is deficient in humoral and cellular immune responses in phagocytic and in complement functions. In the developed\affluent world, mortality has dropped from nearly 50% in the 1970s to <10% currently, but morbidity, however, remains substantial, with 20–58% of survivors developing serious neurological sequelae, such as deafness.

Most worrisome is the fact that its incidence, mortality and morbidity in the developing world have remained unacceptably high; variably reported as between 40–58%. With a documented incidence of 6.5\1000 live births, the disease has shown a rising trend in Nigeria as against other more affluent regions maintaining relatively stable rates of less than 1\1000.

3. Etiopathogenesis

The chance of occurrence of bacterial meningitis becomes highly likely in the newly born baby with presence of adverse risk factors. These risk factors can generally be grouped into Prenatal, Intrapartum, Natal or Postnatal categories; or into Maternal, Obstetrics, or Postpartum divisions. These include low birth weight [LBW], very low birth weight [VLBW] and preterm gestation; maternal risk factors of premature ruptures of membranes, prolonged rupture of membranes (> 24 hours), maternal colonisation with Group B Streptococcus (GBS), maternal chorioamnionitis, maternal peripartum pyrexia and low socioeconomic status. These factors are universally important and well recognized. **Table 1** illustrates some of these factors.

Obstetric Factors	Intrapartum Factors
Antepartum haemorrhage	Preterm birth [no evidence of a non-infectious]
[1st and 2nd Trimester]	
Chronic hypertension in pregnancy	Prolonged rupture of membranes [>24hours]
Preeclampsia and Eclampsia	Peripartum maternal pyrexia
HELLP syndrome [Haemolysis, Elevated	Fetal distress or hypoxia
Liver enzymes, Low Platelets, Renal	Delivery requiring instrumentation
dysfunction]	
Maternal infections [Urinary tract infection,	Cerclage
Chorioamnionitis, Vaginal infection]	
Maternal age extremes [<18 and >40yrs]	Unexplained fetal tachycardia
Isoimmunization	

Table 1. Some well known predisposal risk factors to the occurrence of Neonatal-Perinatal meningitis.

4. The main pathogens of disease

The commonly involved pathogens of Neonatal-Perinatal bacterial meningitis often differ from community to community, region to region and continent to continent. The pathogens also frequently correlate with the degree of development, advancement and environmental hygiene, and thus what we encounter in the developing world differs from that of the developed\affluent world. In developed countries, the predominant pathogens identified from cerebrospinal fluid [CSF] are GBS, *Escherichia coli, Listeria monocytogenes,* other

Area	Refs*	Site	Yr	Pts, n	Age, days	Study-design	Organisms, %	Morta-lity, %	Comments
Multi-Centre	WHO; 1999a, 1999b, 1999c.	Gambia, Ethiopia, Philippines, Papua New Guinea	1998	40	0 -90	Prospective, Descriptive	*S. pneumonia* 43, *E. coli* 13, *Acinetobacter* spp .10, *H. influenzae* 10.	N.A.	Inter-site variation Noted
Middle East	El-Said, *et al;* 2002	Doha, Qatar	1998 - 2000	13	<30	Retro-spective	*S. agalactae* 31, *S. epidermidis* 31, *Pseudomonas* spp 15.	0	Complications; 23
	Koutouby & Habibillah, 1995	Dubai, UAE	1987 - 1992	10	0 - 30	Retro-spective	*S. agalactae* 70, *S. epidermidis* 10, *Pseudomonas* spp 10, *Klebsiella* spp. 10.	30	Study of Sepsis, & Cohort of a subset with Meningitis. VLBW & Premature Neonates Included.
	Daoud, *et al,* 1999	Irbid, Jordan	1993 - 1995	52	Full-term 0 - 28	RCT	*Klebsiella* spp. 48, *Enterobacter* spp 17, *S. aureus* 8, *E. coli* 8	25 [In Control]	Clinical trial studied steroids as adjuncts. Used CSF culture & Latex agglutination
Asia	Chotpitaya-sunondh, 1994	Bankok, Thailand	1982 - 1990	77	0 - ≤30	Retro-spective	*Pseudomonas* spp 17, *Klebsiella* spp 13, *S. agalactae* 12	46	Used Lat ex Agglutination & Counter - Immimmunoelectrop horesis.

Area	Refs*	Site	Yr	Pts, n	Age, days	Study-design	Organisms, %	Morta-lity, %	Comments
Sub-Saharan Africa	Molyneux, et al, 1998	Blantyre, Malawi	1996 - 1997	61	0 - ≤30	Prospective	*S. agalactae* 23 *S. typhimurium* 15, *S. pneumoniae* 11.5, Gram negative rods (other) 11.5.	34	Mixed Cohorts of 0-14yr Age-groups.
	Milledge, et al 2005	Blantyre, Malawi	1996 - 2001	202	0 - ≤30	Retro-spective	*S. agalactae* 30, *S. pneumoniae* 23, *Salmonella* spp. 16.	43	Gra+ve Gram Stain or >20WCC/μL but no Growth (n = 140) Cases (Mortality 21)
	Campagne, 1999	Niamey, Niger	1981 - 1996	101	0 - ≤30	Retro-spective	*S. pneumoniae 34,* *Salmonella spp. 15, N. meningitidis 11.*	58	Part of larger study
	Longe, *et al*, 1984	Benin-City, Nigeria	1974 - 1982	53	0 - ≤28	Prospective	*S. aureus* 29, *E. coli* 20, *Klebsiella* spp. 8, *S. pneumoniae* 8.	38	Studied all categories of Neonates
	Airede, 1993 (Author)	Plateau state, Nigeria	1988 - 1990	36	0 - ≤28	Prospective	*S. aureus* 31, *Klebsiella* spp. 11, *E. coli* 8, *S. pneumoniae* 8	33	Nine CSFs Suggestive of Meningitis *vis-à-vis a* sterile pattern but 5 grew *S. aureus* on Blood culture
	Nel, 2000	Western Cape, South Africa	1981 - 1992	88	0 - ≤28	Retro-spective	*S. agalactae* 30, *E. coli* 23, *Klebsiella pneumoniae* 15	34	

**Abbreviations:* Refs – References, Yr – Year, Pts – Patients, WHO – World Health Organization, N.A. – Not Available, FT – Full Term, RCT – Randomized Control Trial, +ve – Positive, WCC – White cell count, CSFs – Cerebrospinal fluids.

Table 2. Etiology of neonatal bacterial meningitis in developing countries

Gram-negative enteric bacteria and *Streptococcus pneumoniae*. Infections in the neonatal period are frequently divided into 'early onset', (first 5–7 days, implying vertical transmission) when frequently isolated bacteria include GBS, *E. coli* and *Listeria monocytogenes,* and 'late onset', (after the first week of life, implying nosocomial or community acquired infection), when common organisms include Gram negative organisms, *staphylococci* and GBS.

However, in the developing world, the pathogen profile appears different with most studies isolating *Staphylococcus aureus* and other gram negative organisms as leading culprits. Although the rate of isolates of *Escherichia coli* and *Klebsiella aeruginosa* are similar between the developed and developing regions of the world, however, there remains a very significant less encounter with GBS in the latter.

The speculated reasons for this difference are multi-factorial, and could include cultural difference in modes of genital care, population differences in colonisation, genetic differences in immune response and possibly geographic differences in laboratory techniques for pathogen isolation and reporting. **Table 2** highlights the pathogen profile and pattern of Neonatal-Perinatal meningitis in developing countries.

A good evaluation was a WHO-supported multi-centre study [covering Ethiopia, The Gambia, Papua New Guinea and the Philippines], but it only attempted to determine etiological agents responsible for serious infections in young infants [≤90 days]. However, this study was limited by identifying only 40 cases of neonatal meningitis, and the findings varied immensely between centres, which narrowed the conclusions that could be drawn. It is pertinent that unusual pathogens were identified in some other studies, e.g. *Neiseria Meningitidis, Haemophilus Influenzae* type *b,* and *Salmonella typhimurium.* **Table 2** is particularly worthwhile as it demonstrates the geographic differences of causal pathogens of Neonatal-Perinatal meningitis, which could serve as good guide to empirical antibiotic therapy.

5. Pathophysiology

Method of acquisition: Meningitis is basically an infection of the meninges (membranes that surround the brain and spinal cord) that enters through the bloodstream from other parts of the body. Meningococcal disease was first described as early as 1805, when an outbreak spread through Geneva, Switzerland. However, it was not until 1887 that a causative agent of meningococcal meningitis was identified. The pathogens that cause bacterial meningitis are very common and live naturally in the back of the nose and throat.At any given time, 10% of the populations are carriers of the disease but never actually become sick. In fact, most cases of meningitis are acquired through exposure to asymptomatic carriers.

Meningitis can be spread via nose and throat secretions [e.g. coughing, sneezing]. However, meningitis is not considered to be a highly contagious disease. Casual contact or breathing in the air where a person with meningitis has been normally would not expose someone to meningitis because the causative organisms cannot live outside the body for much long to allow their survival.

Acute bacterial meningitis usually develops from an invasion of bacterial pathogens from mucosal surfaces in nasopharynx, sinus cavities, and middle ear space into the blood stream. It can also result from head injuries, penetrating wounds, or neurologic surgeries.

In neonatal-perinatal infants, mother-to-infant transmission and aspiration of intestinal and genital tract secretions during labour and delivery are common modes of transmission.

However, the most implicated mode of acquisition of infection is via the haematogenous route in preponderant cases worldwide.

Pneumococcal meningitis usually arises in the setting of sustained bacteraemia that permits bacterial penetration across the blood-brain barrier and into the subarachnoid space. Once present in the central nervous system, bacterial multiplication incites host cell toxicity and release of a broad range of cytokines [e.g., Interleukin-1, Interleukin-6, and Tumour Necrosis Factor-α] that increase inflammation and vascular permeability. This is the same pattern with the other meningitis-causing pathogens. The resulting injury to the cerebral microvasculature causes brain edema that in turn leads to intracranial hypertension. Unless treated, this process usually leads to mortality and\or increased morbidity, such as neural deafness.

The importance of *S. pneumoniae* as a cause of childhood meningitis has been well described. *S pneumoniae* is also by far the most common pathogen recovered from community-acquired recurrent meningitis, accounting for a majority of cases of recurrent meningitis, even in the newborn infant. The overall case-fatality rate is close to 30%.

H. influenzae type *b* meningitis, once the most prevalent form of meningitis in children, is now rarer in the developed world because of successful immunization practices [*H. influenzae* type *b* conjugates vaccine) in the past 2 decades. In fact, incorporation of this vaccine into the routine immunization schedule resulted in a 94% decline in the number of cases of meningitis caused by *H. influenzae* type *b* in developed countries.

5.1 Detection of cases

The meninges have no host defenses to fight off invading organisms. One of the most important things to determine when meningitis is suspected is whether it is bacterial or viral. If a bacterial pathogen is the culprit, it is essential to identify the specific causative agent so that the appropriate antibiotics can be prescribed immediately. If left untreated, bacterial meningitis can lead to severe complications such as brain damage, hearing loss, epilepsy and death. Viral meningitis on the other hand, is generally less severe and typically resolves on its own.

The specific diagnosis of Neonatal-Perinatal bacterial meningitis remains protean and problematic. Its identification generally depends on a high index of suspicion. Clinically, the disease is often subtle and indistinguishable from that a metabolic problem or any illness solely due to sepsis, and without meningitis. The symptoms commonly include, lethargy, fever – which is better described as temperature instability, excessive crying with difficulty at being consoled, irritability, poor feeding, apprehension, and subtle and\or frank neonatal seizures. Neck stiffness or nuchal rigidity is often not detectable because of relative immaturity of the cranio-spinal nerve bundles with deficient myelination, but may rarely be present. Other problems are bulging anterior fontanelle, opistothonic posturing and any other non-specific neurological features.

Positive culture of CSF remains the gold standard for diagnosis and should be performed on all neonates where sepsis is suspected unless a contraindication exists. However, in view of the anatomic immaturity of the blood-brain-barrier area, caution should be employed when interpreting CSF parameters in the premature neonate.

Gram stains of CSF may could also provide useful information, even if CSF culture is not available. Simultaneous blood cultures are often positive in 40–80% of cases. Furthermore, it is notable that Neonatal-Perinatal meningitis can be present even in the absence of CSF pleocytosis, and CSF protein and glucose levels are age related. The simultaneously assessed CSF:Blood glucose relationship should not be less than 50% in any neonate, and solely detected hypoglycorracia [CSF sugar of 0-<1.3mmol\L] is always diagnostic

5.2 Diagnostic methods

Early diagnosis of Neonatal-Perinatal bacterial meningitis is very crucial. Because the symptoms of meningitis can closely mimic other viral illnesses, many clinicians miss the diagnosis and prescribe inappropriate treatments. In many cases, a missed diagnosis can have fatal consequences. All healthcare givers should be aware that early recognition of the symptoms can be a matter of life and death, and they should become familiar with all possible signs and symptoms. A careful and thorough diagnostic work-up must be undertaken.

A detailed work-up line is shown in **Table 3.** The specific microbiological culture procedure of all major fluid areas of the body, i.e. blood, CSF and urine should be performed. This is often referred to as a 'Panculture Procedure', and has the value of identifying those neonates or perinates that could have a concomitant septicaemia and nephritis [UTI]. This is vital and highly needed since it has been well documented in several reports, that as highly as 30% of newborn infants with septicaemia also have concomitant meningitis.

The CSF must be examined for general appearance, consistency, and tendency to clot. CSF analysis should include cell counts (including a WBC differential), glucose and protein analysis, and Gram staining of the centrifuged sediment. The use of C-reactive protein [CRP] levels has been shown to play an important role in differentiating among the various types of meningitis. More recently, some workers recommended the use of serum procalcitonin level for better diagnostic and prognostic value than CRP or leukocyte count to distinguish between bacterial and viral meningitis. Their cases were, however, older children of 4months and above. It requires validation in the neonate and perinate.

Polymerase chain reaction has remained sensitivity and quick in detecting and differentiating between viral and bacterial meningitis.

The hands, ears, nose, throat and sinuses should be checked for the possible source of infection, and a latex agglutination test to detect bacterial antigens of *Staphylococcus aureus, Streptococcus pneumoniae, Neisseria meningitides, Haemophilus influenzae* type *b*, Group B Streptococcus, *Klebsiella* sps and *Escherichia coli* strains, can aid in the diagnosis of Neonatal-Perinatal bacterial meningitis. However, this test may lack sensitivity unless ultrasonic enhancement is used.

Newborn infants with suspected bacterial meningitis should also undergo testing for glucose, serum electrolytes and blood urea nitrogen, which could indicate the degree of dehydration and identify hyponatraemia and hypoglycaemia; common symptoms of meningitis.

Clinical clues signaling the presence of bacterial meningitis may include sinusitis, otitis, mastoiditis, infective endocarditis and characteristic skin infections [such as those seen in infections caused by herpes, simplex virus, varicella-zoster virus]. Cardiovascular instability or focal neurologic signs such as papillary changes, hemi-paresis, and ocular palsies are indicative of bacterial meningitis. Patechial and purpuric rashes usually indicate meningococcemia or *H. influenzae* meningitis. Presence of arthritis may suggest the presence of *H. influenza* and *N. meningitides*, and head trauma or a chronically draining ear usually signals pneumococcal meningitis.

Name of Test	Outcome	Indications
Pan-Cultures - Urine [Suprapubic] - Blood - Sputum - Lumbar Puncture	Presence of pathogens	Definitive isolation of aetiology
Grain stain	Presence of Bacteria	Useful in directing Empiric antimicrobial Therapy
Chest radiograph	Pulmonary infiltrates, oedema	Pneumonia
Arterial Blood Gas	Low PCO2, low arterial pH Low bicarbonate	Complications of Concomitant sepsis initially yielding respiratory Alkalosis and later Metabolic acidosis.
Neutrophils	Levels as low as 20% with Rebound to 80%	Infection and sepsis progression
WBC	Elevated or elevated Immature forms (left shift). Total WBC <4000/mm3	Infection
Immature-to-Total Ratio	>/0.2	Sepsis\Meningitis
C - reactive protein	In term or near-term infants 2 serial measurements (12-24 hrs after onset of Symptoms) >10ml/L	Sepsis
Platelets	<100,000/microliter	Complications of Sepsis\Meningitis (Coagulation Abnormality)
Glucose	Hypoglycaemia	Sepsis\Meningitis

Table 3. Tests commonly utilized in the diagnosis of Neonatal-Perinatal bacterial meningitis

Bacterial meningitis in the newborn can be difficult to distinguish from other infectious diseases. To aid in the differential diagnosis, physicians should take a complete epidemiologic history, including contact with sick persons; maternal dietary habits, and\or illicit drug use; medication history; exposure to insects, rodents, or arthropods; and recent travel history.

Major epidemic of meningitis frequently occur during the hot dry seasons. Sub-Saharan Africa is plagued by the highest meningitis [*N. meningitides*] disease burden, is usually referred to as the "meningitis belt".

5.3 Treatment intervention

It cannot be overemphasized that treatment must be started early in the course of the disease, especially as it is of bacterial aetiology. Prompt intervention can reduce the risk of death to below 15%. If not treated as a medical emergency, bacterial meningitis can lead to seizures, coma, increased intracranial pressure, nerve damage, stroke and even death.

By identifying the causative agent, the appropriate antibiotic can be administered. The baby's age, co-morbidities and the status of his or her immune system can aid in this identification. For example, immunocompromised patients are at particular risk for infection with *S. pneumoniae, N. meningitidis, Listeria monocytogenes*, and aerobic Gram-negative bacilli. In the developing countries, *S. aureus* remains a highly predominant organism in the neonatal age, whereas GBS is rarely encountered. Antibiotic intervention only improves the baby's prognosis if the antimicrobial therapy is administered before the patient's clinical condition has deteriorated. If antibiotics are started when the baby is already in an advanced stage of the disease, the chances of survival is poor.

Administration of antibiotics can also protect the development of the disease among children, or parents who have been exposed to another case of meningitis. According to some investigators, giving the appropriate antibiotics to household contacts of the patient with meningococcal disease can reduce their risk of infection by 89%. Antibiotic therapy must be effective against common causative pathogens and must achieve adequate bactericidal activity without toxicity in the CSF. Most often used antibiotics include; ampicillin or penicillin and an aminoglycoside [e.g. Gentamicin] or a third-generation cephalosporin, such as ceftriaxone or cefotaxime. The recommendation of ceftriaxone includes the awareness that it may cause billiary sludge leading to jaundice in the neonate. Such caution appears to be theoretical, as in practice, the problem rarely occurs. Penicillin and gentamicin are widely available, cheap and the first line antimicrobial therapy in many resource-poor settings. In developed countries, initial therapy often includes some combination of three agents: Penicillin, an aminoglycoside and a third-generation cephalosporin - considered by some school-of-thought to be over use and miss use of antibiotics.

First-line therapy is usually either ampicillin and gentamicin or ampicilin and cefotaxime, or ceftriaxone and gentamicin. The value of the cephalosporins is their widely spaced dosage regimen with satisfactory better compliance. The use of cephalosporins has coincided with a reduction in mortality from neonatal meningitis in developed countries but with no associated fall in morbidity.

Gentamicin remains an effective antimicrobial, despite its small therapeutic window. Despite the fears of its causing renal toxicity and deafness, there is no documented occurrence of these complications during clinical use.

Third-generation cephalosporins (cefotaxime and ceftriaxone) are active against the major pathogens of neonates worldwide, including aminoglycoside-resistant strains. They have good CSF penetration and achieve adequate therapeutic concentrations in the CSF. Third-generation cephalosporings were recommended in the multi-centre WHO study group of serious infections in young infants.

If available, vis-à-vis a resource-poor setting, cefotaxime and ceftriaxone are currently recommended for use in Neonatal-Perinatal bacterial meningitis in view of the added advantage of a longer half-life, allowing less frequent administration.

However, it is pertinent that empiric antibiotic choice should be tailored to local epidemiology, early versus late infections and whether the infection was nosocomially acquired.

5.4 Adjunctive therapy

The use of corticosteroids as an adjunct to antibiotic therapy has been shown to render treatment of bacterial meningitis more effective, especially in children by reducing CSF inflammation and hearing loss. This has been shown conclusively for disease caused by *H. influenzae* type b and *S. pneumoniae* and it is, therefore, now routinely used worldwide. Its efficacy is said to improve if administered before, or along with the antibiotics. Though few studies have documented the valuable effects of steroids [dexamathasone] as an adjunct in neonatal meningitis, more evaluation requires to be done without timidity or over anxiety by clinicians. **Table 4** elucidates the improved outcome with its use in Nigeria.

	Mortality %	Recovery with disability, %	Full recovery, %
Dexamethasone Use, n=21	48	19	76.2
No Dexamethasone Use, n=18	55.6	11.1	33.3

* The disabilities and handicaps were: hearing-defects, subdural effusion, hydrocephalus, hemiparesis and recurrent afebrile seizures.

Table 4. Value of steroids (dexamethasone) and quality of recovery from Neonatal-Perinatal bacterial meningitis.

There was significant less mortality and improved full recovery with adjunctive use of steroids, $p=0.006$.

5.5 The interplay of bacterial resistance

Penicillin resistance is mediated by alterations in penicillin binding proteins (PBPs). PBPs are membrane-bound enzymes that catalyze the terminal steps in the assembly of the bacterial cell wall. The key PBPs involved in penicillin susceptibility includes PBP 1a, 1b, 2a, 2b, and 3. Strains with reduced susceptibility to penicillin also exhibit reduced susceptibility to beta-lactam drugs such as cephalosporins. *S. pneumoniae* resistance to other antibiotic classes is also now widespread, and includes resistance to macrolides, trimethoprim-sulfamethoxazole, chloramphenicol, and quinolones. Multiple mechanisms mediate resistance and are briefly described in **Table 5**. Drug resistance to a single class of antibiotics may also be mediated by multiple mechanisms. Acquired resistance to a particular class of antibiotics increases the likelihood that the strain will be resistant to other classes of antibiotics. For example, 94% penicillin-susceptible strains of S. pneumoniae were recently found to be susceptible to azithromycin, but 17% of penicillin-resistant strains were azithromycin-susceptible.

Resistance to macrolides, and trimethoprim-sulfamethoxazole is also widespread. Macrolides resistance is mediated by either an efflux pump [low-level resistance] or a ribosomal methylase [high-level resistance].

Penicillin-resistant strains are often resistant to cephalosporins such as ceftriaxone and cefotaxime. Vancomycin is active against all strains of S. *pneumoniae* but vancomycin-tolerant strains have now been described. The individual members of the flouroquinolone class demonstrate differential activity against *S. pneumoniae.*

Antibiotic Class	Mechanism of Resistance
Penicillin	Target-site alteration: Altered penicillin-binding Proteins
Macrolides	Efflux-pump [low-level resistance]
Quinolones	Target-site alteration: Alteration of DNA gyrase or Topoisomerase IV
Trimethoprim-Sulfamethoxazole	Metabolic by-pass pathway
Chloramphenicol	Enzymatic destruction: Acetyltransferase
Rifampicin	Target-site alteration: Alteration of the beta-subunit of RNA polymerase

Table 5. Mechanisms of antibiotic resistance of *S. pneumoniae*

6. Conclusion

It is intriguing that Neonatal-Perinatal bacterial meningitis continues to be a major cause of morbidity and mortality in the developing world. It is vital that more efforts are required for its control rather the offer of appropriate diagnosis and treatment. It is majorly necessary that efforts must be directed to community health education, provision of regular information, and a versatile up-keep of hygiene and routine cleanliness. The importance of immune boosting through vaccinations and their acceptance is further worthy, as prevention is always better than cure. Important differences in aetiology have been noted but early and focused treatment of established disease, with the use of steroid adjunct, remains essential.

7. References

[1] Airede AI. Neonatal bacterial meningitis in the middle belt of Nigeria. *Developmental Medicine and Child Neurology* 1993; 35:424–430.

[2] Airede K, Adeyemi O, Ibrahim T. Neonatal bacterial meningitis and dexamethasone adjunctive usage in Nigeria. *Nigerian Journal of Clinical Practice* 2008; 11:235–245.

[3] Airede KI, Jalo I, Bello M, Adeyemi S. Observations on oral Sultamicillin/Unasyn CP45899 Therapy of neonatal infections. *International Journal of Antimicrobial Agents* 1997; 8: 103-107.

[4] Airede KI. Neonatal seizures and a two-year neurological outcome. *Journal of Tropical Pediatrics* 1991; 37: 313-317.

[5] Airede Ki. Prolonged rupture of membranes and neonatal outcome in a developing country. *Annals of Tropical Paediatrics* 1992; 12: 283-288.

[6] Airede KI. Urinary tract infections in African neonates. *Journal of Infections* 1992; 25: 55-62.

[7] American College of Chest Physicians/Siciety of Critical Care Medicine Consensus Conference. Definitions for sepsis and organ failure and guidelines for the use of innovative therapies in sepsis. *Critical Care Medicine* 1992; 20: 864-874.

[8] Aronin SI, Quaggliarello VJ. Clinical pearls: Bacterial meningitis. *Infectious Medicine* 2003; 20: 142-153.

[9] Al-Harthi A, Dagriri K, Asindi AA, Bello CS. Neonatal meningitis. *Saudi Medical Journal* 2000; 21:550–553.

[10] Smith PB, Garges HP, Cotton CM, Walsh TJ, Clark RH, Benjamin DK. Meningitis in preterm neonates: importance of cerebrospinal fluid parameters. *American Journal of Perinatology* 2008; 25(7):421-6.

[11] Delouvois J, Blackbourn J, Hurley R, et al. Infantile meningitis in England and Wales: a two year study. *Archives of Disease in Childhood* 1991; 66: 603–607.

[12] Doctor B, Newman N, Minich N, et al. Clinical outcomes of neonatal meningitis in very-low birth-weight infants. *Clinical Pediatrics* 2001 (Phila); 40: 473–480.

[13] El-Said MF, Bessisso MS, Janahi MA, Habob LH, El-Shafie SS. Epidemiology of neonatal meningitis in Qatar. *Neurosciences* 2002; 7: 163–166.

[14] Isacs D, Barfield CP, Grimwood K, Mcphee AJ, Minutillo C, Tudehope DI. Systemic bacterial and fungal infections in infants in Australian neonatal units. *Medical Journal of Australia* 1995; 162: 198–201.

[15] Koutouby A, Habibullah J. Neonatal sepsis in Dubai, United Arab Emirates. *Journal of Tropical Pediatrics* 1995; 43: 177–180.

[16] Laving AMR, Musoke RN, Wasunna AO, Revathi G. Neonatal bacterial meningitis at the newborn unit of Kenyatta national hospital. *East African Medical Journal* 2003; 80: 456–462.

[17] Longe C, Omene J, Okolo A. Neonatal meningitis in Nigerian infants. *Acta Padiatrica Scandinavica* 1984; 73: 477–481.

[18] McCracken GH Jr, Mize SG, Mize NT. Intraventricular gentamicin therapy in gram-negative bacillary meningitis of infancy. Report of the Second Neonatal Meningitis Cooperative Study Group. *Lancet* 1980; 1: 787–791.

[19] Usama M Alkholi, Nermin Abd Al-monem, Ayman A Abd El-Azim, Mohamed H Sultan. Serum procalcitonin in viral and bacterial meningitis. *Journal of Global Infectious Diseases* 2011; 3: 14-18.

[20] Weber MW, Carlin JB, Gatchalian S, *et al.* Predictors of neonatal sepsis in developing countries. *Pediatric Infectious Disease Journal* 2003; 22: 711–716.

[21] WHO. World Health Organization Young Infants Study Group. Clinical prediction of serious bacterial infections in young infants in developing countries. *Pediatric Infectious Disease Journal 1999a*; 18(Suppl. 10): S23–S31.

[22] WHO. World Health Organization Young Infants Study Group. Conclusions from the WHO multicenter study of serious infections in young infants. *Pediatric Infectious Disease Journal* 1999b; 18 (Suppl.): S32–S34.

[23] WHO. Bacterial etiology of serious infections in young infants in developing countries: results of a multicenter study. The WHO Young Infants Study Group. *Pediatric Infectious Disease Journal* 18 (Suppl 10): S17–S22.

[24] WHO. Pocket Book of Hospital Care for Children - Guidelines for the Management of Common Illnesses with Limited Resources. *World Health Organisation*, 2005, Geneva.

[25] Saez-Llorens X & McCracken GH Jr. Bacterial meningitis in children. *Lancet* 2003; 361: 2139–2148.

[26] Stoll B. The global impact of neonatal infection. *Clinics in Perinatology* 1997; 24: 1–21.

[27] Tunkel AR, Hartman BJ, Kaplan SL, *et al.* Practice guidelines for the management of bacterial meningitis. Clinical Infectious Diseases 2004; 39: 1267–1284.

[28] Vergnano S, Sharland M, Kazembe P, Mwansambo C, Heath P. Neonatal sepsis: aninternational perspective. *Archives of Disease in Childhood. Fetal and Neonatal Edition* 2005; 90: F220–F224.

[29] Gaschignard Jean, Levy Corinne, Romain Olivier, Cohen Robert, *et al.* Neonatal Bacterial Meningitis: 444 Cases in 7 Years. *Pediatric Infectious Disease Journal* 2011; 30: 212-217.

[30] Nel E. Neonatal meningitis: mortality, cerebrospinal fluid, and microbiological findings. *Journal of Tropical Pediatrics* 2000; 46: 237–239.

[31] Odio CM. Cefotaxime for treatment of neonatal sepsis and meningitis. *Diagnostic Microbiology and Infectious Disease* 1995, 111–117.

[32] Rahman S, Hameed A, Roghani M, Ullah Z. Multidrug resistant neonatal sepsis in Peshawar, Pakistan. *Archives of Disease in Childhood-Fetal and Neonatal Edition* 2002; 87: F52–F54.

[33] Chotpitayasunondh T. Bacterial meningitis in children: etiology and clinical features, an 11- year review of 618 cases. *Southeast Asian Journal of Tropical Medicine and Public Health* 1994; 25: 107–115.

[34] Milledge J, Calis JCJ, Graham S, *et al.* Aetiology of neonatal sepsis in Blantyre, Malawi: 1996– 2001. *Annals of Tropical Paediatrics* 2005; 25: 101–110.

[35] Molyneux E, Walsh A, Phiri A, Molyneux M. Acute bacterial meningitis in children admitted to the Queen Elizabeth Central Hospital, Blantyre, Malawi in 1996–97. *Tropical Medicine and International Health*1998; 3: 610–618.

[36] Molyneux E, Riordan F, Walsh A. Acute bacterial meningitis in children presenting to the Royal Liverpool Children's Hospital, Liverpool, UK and the Queen Elizabeth Central Hospital in Blantyre, Malawi: a world of difference. *Annals of Tropical Paediatrics* 2006; 26: 29–37.

4

Neurologic Complications of Bacterial Meningitis

Emad uddin Siddiqui
Aga Khan University Hospital
Pakistan

1. Introduction

Bacterial meningitis is a serious and potentially life threatening CNS infection. It often results in disabling or deaths in 170,000 patients each year worldwide. Younger children are predominantly at risk of bacterial meningitis, mainly because of their immature immune systems and malnutrition while lack of immunization practices also makes them more susceptible to significantly high morbidity & mortality. (Anderson, V. et al., 2004). Even with the provision of highly effective antibiotic therapy, death and long-term disabilities are the common but still seroius consequences of acute bacterial meningitis in developing countries. Common neurological complications in adult are hearing loss, motor deficit, cognition defect and speech problem, whereas sensorineural deafness, followed by seizure disorder and motor deficit are more common in children. Sixteen percent of pediatric patients from developed countries have neurological complications, while this figure rose 26 percent from developing countries. (Braff, LJ. et al., 1993). Two third of all pediatric deaths due to meningitis occur in low income countries and as many as 50% survivors of childhood meningitis experience some neurological sequel. (Mace, SE 2008)

Neurological complications of meningitis can occur at any time during the course of disease and even after the completion of therapy. Neurological complications may either be focal or generalized or it may be of sudden or gradual in onset. Patients either remain conscious or may present with altered consciousness or even coma. Usually the complications develop during the course of acute bacterial meningitis but some of them manifest or persist as the long-term sequel such as; hearing loss, epilepsy, hemiplegia, neuropsychological impairment, developmental and learning disabilities. Shock or disseminated intravascular coagulation, frequently is associated with meningococcal meningitis. Pneumococcal meningitis is associated with the highest case fatality rate. Apnea and respiratory failure may occur with any bacterial meningitis, especially in infants. Post meningitis complications may occur in almost half of all cases, 81% of them may present with neurological sequel. A part of this may present with systemic sequel, while a quarter of them have both neurological and systemic complications. (Pfister, HW. et al., 1993)

2. Risk factors for neurological complications

There are multiple risk factors either directly or indirectly related to any one or more of the neurological complications as listed in Table 1. Extremes of age is directly associated with the consequences and prognosis. Organism type, virulence and number of bacteria entered, portal of entry along with the susceptibility of host all count in the development of neurological complications. Duration and progression of illness before initiation of effective antibiotic therapy is also associated with neurological complication. On the other hand mode of presentation, and compliance to the appropriate treatment or any associated co-morbid may also have detrimental effect on patient neurological outcome and morbidity. Patients on immunosuppressive drug, chronic liver disorders, alcoholics, diabetics and patients with congenital or acquired immune deficiency disease, malignancy and HIV, are at increased risk of meningitis and its sequel as compare to general population. Streptococcus pneumoniae is associated with most of the sequel as compared to the other organisms.

Neurological	Systemic (Non Neurological)
Acute onset Altered mental status/ coma Cerebral edema and raised intracranial pressure Acute onset Seizures Subdural effusion or empyema Cranial nerve palsies Hydrocephalus Sensorineural deficit Hemiparesis or quadriparesis Blindness **Late onset** Late onset seizure (epilepsy) disorder Ataxia Cerebrovascular abnormalities Neuropsychological impairment Developmental disability Intellectual deficit	Prolong fever Septic shock and DIC Vasomotor collapse Loss of airway reflexes Respiratory arrest Pericardial effusion Hypothalamic and other endocrine dysfunction Hyponatremia Bilateral adrenal hemorrhage Death

Table 1. Complications of meningitis and its types

Several studies have been conducted to identify the clinical factors that are associated with adverse outcomes in children with bacterial meningitis. Unconsciousness early in the disease, multiple or prolong seizures (>72 hours), use of inotrops, and leucopenia are important predictors of adverse neurological outcome. It has been observed that patients with neurological symptoms lasted for >24hrs, focal neurological signs, ataxia, or deteriorating conscious level despite the commencement of adequate and appropriate therapy and serum sodium concentration <130 mmol/L are associated with adverse outcomes. Other clinical presentations of meningitis that are associated with increased risk of neurologic complications are low CSF glucose concentration, and CSF bacterial count of ≥10 cfu/ml. (Feldman, WE. 1997). Patients on ventilatory support and PRISM score of ≥20 in first 24 hours of admission are few other common clinical predictors associated with increased incidence of neurological complications. (Madagame, ET. et al., 1995)

3. Altered mental status

Inflammation of CNS is responsible for the hallmark presentation of CNS infection which including fever, meningismus, and altered mental status. Altered mental status is described as irritability or lethargy. However in pediatric patients altered mental status is highly variable. Increased intracranial pressure (ICP) is one of the major causes of altered mental status. In adults, the incidence of altered mental status ranged from 78 to 83 percent at presentation, (de Gans, J et al., 2002), most patients are either confused or lethargic, while a quarter may be responsive only to pain only, and 6 percent unresponsive to all stimuli. (Durand, ML. et al., 1993). In adult patients with pneumococcal meningitis, 29% were found semi comatose or comatose at the time of admission. Coma with GCS <8 at initial presentation may present in 14 percent. (Durand, 1993 & Aronin 1998). From a pediatric study (Roine, I. et al., 2008) with bacterial meningitis, approximately 78% were irritable or lethargic, 7% were somnolent, and 15% semi comatose or comatose at the time of admission. The level of consciousness at the time of admission has prognostic significance; patients who are obtunded, semi conscious, or comatose at the time of admission are significantly more likely to have an adverse outcome than those who are lethargic or somnolent.

4. Cerebral edema & raised intracranial pressure

Cerebral blood flow (CBF) normally is maintained at a relatively constant rate by an auto regulatory mechanism. This auto regulation adjusts the CBF according to the metabolic need and regulates the changes in cerebral vascular resistant (CVR). During fever or seizures activity there is increase in the metabolic activity in brain, this result in increased CBF.

$$CBF = (CAP - JVP) \div CVR \tag{1}$$

(CAP is carotid arterial pressure, JVP is jugular venous pressure, and CVR is cerebrovascular resistance).

Arterial PaO2 and PaCO2 also have well-defined effects on CBF. Arterial PaO2 ≤ 50 mmHg has its most significant effect on CBF, and it cause vasodilatation in order to maintain the necessary oxygen and nutrient supply to the brain. High arterial PaCO2 also causes cerebral vasodilatation and increased CBF, whereas hypocapnia reduces CBF. Regulating PaCO2 by hyperventilation is a useful tool in the acute management of increased ICP.

Increased ICP in patients with bacterial meningitis seems to be multi factorial in origin. Released cytotoxic mediators and interstitial edema with increased permeability of the blood-brain barrier are some of the main factors leading to increased ICP, although increased intracranial blood volume and disturbances in CSF flow are also important. Inflammation on the other hand itself increases the permeability of the blood-brain barrier, via vasogenic mechanism and edema formation. (Tunkel, AR. 1993).

Cerebral edema in the nonexpendable cranial vault increases intracranial pressure (>300cm of H_2O) and results in secondary injury from diminished (<50cm of H_2O) cerebral perfusion (MAP-ICP) and ischemia. Mild to moderate increase in ICP causes headache, confusion, irritability, nausea, and vomiting. More severe increases can produce coma, Cushing reflex (bradycardia with hypertension), papilledema, cranial nerve palsy, mostly the abducent (VI) nerve, and herniation of the cerebellar tonsils, which may lead to death. (Durand, 1993 & de Gans 2002). Hydrocephalus is hardly ever reported to be the cause of raised ICP at presentation. Raised intracranial pressure is reported to be an indicator of a more severe disease related with a much higher mortality than in simple uncomplicated cases of bacterial meningitis.Judicious fluid management, dexamethasone, mannitol, hypertonic saline and hyperventilation to keep $PaCO_2$ to 25- 35mmHg and 30° head elevation, are helpful in reducing the raised ICP and cerebral edema. (Lindval, P. et al., 2004).

5. Seizures

Little is known about the pathogenesis of seizures in bacterial meningitis. Other than fever in younger children, inflammatory exudates, bacterial toxins, chemical mediators and neurochemical changes within brain parenchyma are supposed to cause seizures in 15 - 30 percent of adults (Zoons, E. et al., 2008) and 20-30 percent of children (Feigin, RD. et al., 2009). Seizures in bacterial meningitis may develop at any time during the course of disease or later on. Seizures are either generalized or partial; those occurring early in the course are rather easily controllable by anticonvulsant drugs, and are rarely associated with permanent neurologic deficit. In contrast, prolonged and difficult to control seizures, or seizures that begin after 72 hours of hospitalization are more likely to be associated with permanent neurologic sequel. (Arditi, M. 1998). Prolonged & intractable seizures may also suggest that a cerebrovascular complication might have occurred. Pneumococcal meningitis has 5-fold increase risk of seizures activity. (Zoons, E. et al., 2008). Patients with other inter current illnesses and infections, low GCS, focal neurological deficit, low CSF leucocytes and high protein are associated with increased risk of seizure activity. Seizures during acute phase of illness are associated with increased risk of neurological complication and deaths. (Aronin, 1998 & Annegers, 1988).

6. Subdural effusions

Subdural effusion is the collection of fluids in subdural spaces. This is another common complication of meningitis and occurs in 50 percent of adult meningitis and 10-30 percent of children. (Agarwal, A. et al., 2007). It is usually asymptomatic in most of the cases and is benign or self limiting. Mild effusions mostly resolve spontaneously and do not require any intervention. Subdural tap is indicated if there is persistent or recurrent fever, signs of raised ICP, focal neurological sign and presence of subdural empyema. Subdural empyema is usually unilateral but has the potential to spread rapidly through the falx cerebri in to tentorium cerebella and can spread to the base of brain and in to the spinal column. H. Influenzae meningitis is commonly associated with effusion. Clinical manifestations of effusion are often subtle or absent. Bulging fontanelle and irritability may be the only sign in infants. Diastasis of sutures, enlarging head circumference in infant, recurrence or new onset seizures, emesis and fever, and abnormal cranial transillumination are other common clinical findings. In older children it can produce increased ICP, a focal neurological sign and a mid line shift of intracranial structures. CT or MRI confirms the presence of effusion. In pediatric patients, subdural effusions produce few symptoms and so require no treatment. However, development of subdural empyema or symptomatic effusion requires drainage. (Snedeker, JD. Et al., 1990)

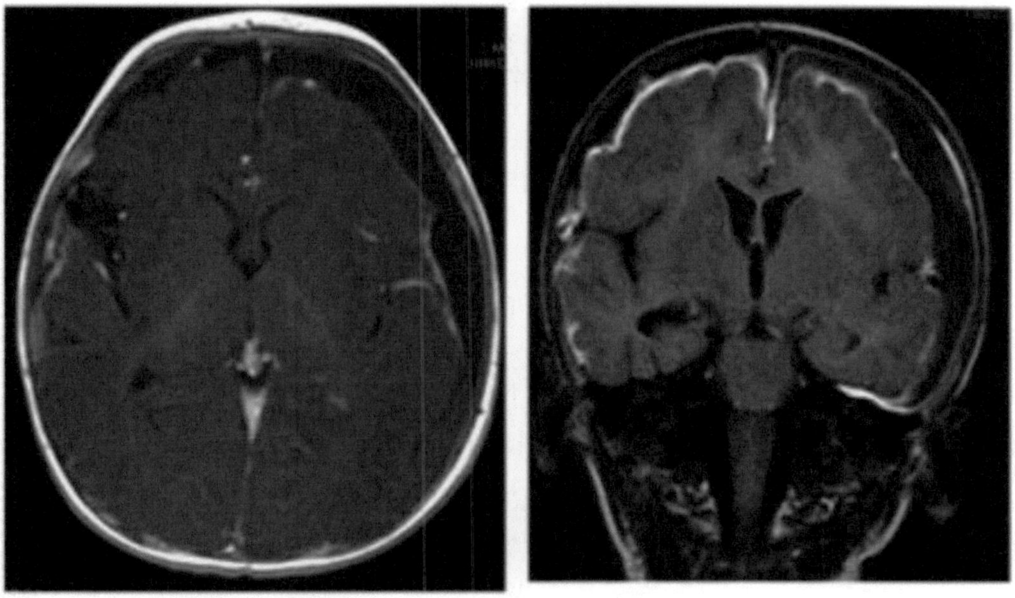

Fig. 1. MRI brain showing subdural fluid collection along the left cerebral convexity with ring enhancement in the contrast images

7. Cranial nerve palsies

Meningitis with basal exudate collection is often related with cranial nerves (CN) involvement. CN palsies likely to occur when the cranial nerve are sheathed by exudates (perineuritis) within the arachinoidal sheath. CN may also be affected by compressible pressure of brain in general. Abducent (VI) nerves with its longest intra cranial route adjacent to brain stem are more prone to raised ICP and exudates (perineuritis) related compression. Other CNs like III, IV, and VII may also be affected. CN involvement is more common in pediatric patients and is described in 5-11 percent of cases. Focal neurological sign may or may not be present. CN deficits related to meningitis are usually transient. Strabismus may be the presenting feature early in the course with only gaze towards the paralyzed side. Optic nerve involvement can lead to transient or permanent visual loss while optic nerve atrophy may result in irreversible total blindness, a rare complication of severe meningitis. Cranial nerve palsies may be the warning sign of raised intracranial pressure.

8. Hydrocephalus

Hydrocephalus is the complication of acute meningitis which usually manifest later as post meningitis sequel. It is commonly associated with untreated or partially treated pyogenic meningitis and tuberculous meningitis. Hydrocephalus more commonly occurs in infants and neonates especially with group B streptococcus type III. (de Louvois, J. 1994). Mild to moderate type can be treated pharmacologically while severe hydrocephalus compressing the brain parenchyma should be manage surgically with various types of shunt.

9. Focal neurological deficits

Focal neurological deficits account for most of the common complication of meningitis and it may account up to 50 percent of all neurological complication. (van de Beek, D. et al., 2004). This depends on the multiple factors like extremes of ages, duration of pretreatment illness, causative organism and efficacy of treatment. Pneumococcal and meningococcal in adults with the addition of H. Influenzae in children are associated with most of these complications. Majority of focal neurological complications tend to resolve with appropriate treatment but long term disability may persist.

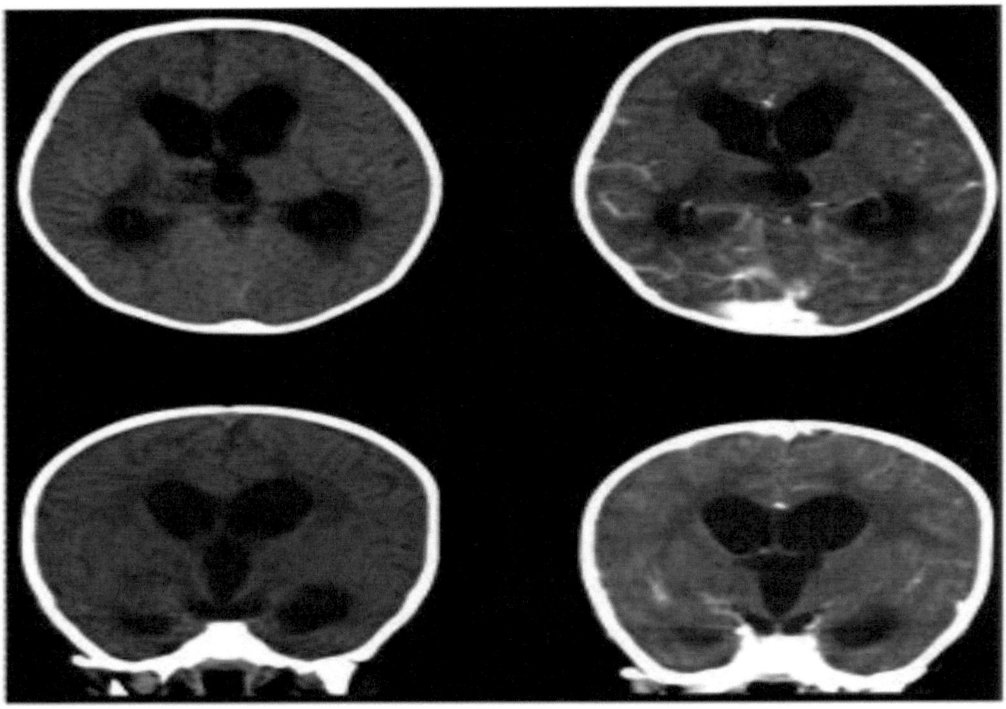

Fig. 2. CT scan brain with low attenuated areas and increase enhancements in right thalamus, posterior limb of internal capsule and right superior cerebellar peduncle with hydrocephalus.

9.1 Hemiparesis or quadriparesis

General weakness of the body following meningitis is usually generalized (quadriparesis) or on one side (Hemiparesis), rarely isolated monoparesis are also observed. This usually results from vasculitis, cortical vein or sagittal vein thrombosis, cerebral artery spasm, subdural effusion or empyema, hydrocephalus, cerebral infarct or abscess, or cerebral edema. Paresis generally improves with time.

9.2 Hearing loss

Hearing impairment after meningitis may have several reasons. Pneumococcus organism invading the cochlea through the internal auditory canal with exudative and inflammatory damage to the vestibulocochlear nerve, cochlea, and labyrinth, leads to sensorineural hearing loss. Animal studies and catastropic studies have shown that purulent material entering from the subarachnoid space to the perilymphatic space of the inner ear through the internal ear canal or aqueductus cochlearis of the temporal bone causes destruction of hair cells in the labyrinth following inflammation. The possibility of sterile labyrinthitis caused by toxic components (lipopolysaccharides) of the bacterial cell wall or perineuritis and damage of the eighth cranial nerve can also be there. (Bhatt, 1993 & Merchant, 1996). Thrombophlebitis and vascular occlusions with lesions and focal necrosis in peripheral and central auditory pathways may be the other possible mechanism. This may be transient or permanent. All of the children with hearing loss had either one or more of the risk factors which includes disease symptoms for ≥2 days before admission, CSF glucose concentration ≤10.8 mg/dL, streptococcus pneumoniae infection, and ataxia. Audiometry must be done in all patients with acute pyogenic meningitis before discharge. Delay response of brain stem evoked potential occurs within days and generally recovers in the initial two weeks of treatment. However major deficit may persist in 11 percent of children and 12-14 percent in adults with pyogenic meningitis.

Anti inflammatory agents like dexamethasone can reduce the neurologic complications of bacterial meningitis like sensorineural hearing loss by decreasing the intracranial pressure and modulating the production of cytokines particularly in H. Influenzae type b (grade 1A). However it does not reduce these post meningitis complications induced by other organisms. Similarly demographic studies support the use of dexamethasone in high income countries, while results are not promising from low income countries. (van de Beek, D. et al., 2004)

10. Cerebrovascular abnormalities

Brain tissues are extremely vulnerable to ischemic injury because of its relatively high oxygen consumption and near-total dependence on aerobic glucose metabolism. Interruption of cerebral perfusion, metabolic substrate (glucose) or severe hypoxemia rapidly results in functional impairment; reduced perfusion also impairs the clearance of potentially toxic substrates from brain. If oxygen tension, blood flow, and glucose supply are not reestablished to its normal range within 3–8 min, ATP stores start depleting and irreversible neuronal injury begins in most of cases. During ischemia, intracellular K^+ decreases and intracellular Na^+ increases. More important, intracellular Ca^{2+} increases because of failure of ATP-dependent pumps to either extrude the ion extracellularly or into intracellular cisterns, increased intracellular Na^+ concentration, and release of the excitatory neurotransmitter glutamate causes damage to neurons. Other than intracellular Ca^+, chemical mediators like prostaglandins and leukotrienes are potent cellular killers. Lastly, reperfusion of ischemic tissues can cause additional tissue damage due to the formation of oxygen-derived free radicals.

Other than ischemia thromboembolism, hemorrhage or infarction, and cerebral vessel anomalies like aneurysm and vasculitis may also lead to cerebrovascular complications of bacterial meningitis. Thrombosis of superior sagittal sinus is also evident in literature. Cerebral infarction in survivors of childhood bacterial meningitis emerges as a grave and moderately frequent complication. Factors associated with the development of cerebral infarction in childhood bacterial meningitis include age less than one year, infection with S pneumoniae, severe hypoglycorrachia, early inappropriate antibiotic therapy and male sex.

11. Brain abscess

Patient with meningitis induce intracranial abscess usually differs clinically from patients with meningitis or encephalitis. They are generally nontoxic with sub acute onset, but clinical condition rapidly deteriorates if brain abscess ruptures. Focal deficit and papilledema are usually present in most of these patients, while fever and neck stiffness are infrequent findings. Brain abscess is associated with high morbidity, seizures (80% of cases), persistent altered mental status, and focal motor deficits. Brain abscesses are common with rare pathogens like Enterobacter but are relatively rare in patients with S. pneumoniae, H. influenzae, and N. meningitides.

Mortality from a brain abscess has decreased to 20 percent, as a result of earlier diagnosis and appropriate treatment. CT scan with contrast is essential to make the diagnosis of brain abscess. The typical finding on CT scan is a hypodense area with a contrast ring enhancement. Lumber puncture is not recommended when cerebral abscess is suspected because of raised ICP and risk of herniation.

The management of brain abscess requires appropriate antibiotics and neurosurgical consultation. Broad spectrum antibiotics along with anaerobic coverage include third-generation cephalosporin and metronidazole. For penetrating trauma, surgical procedure or suspected staphlococcal add vancomycin.

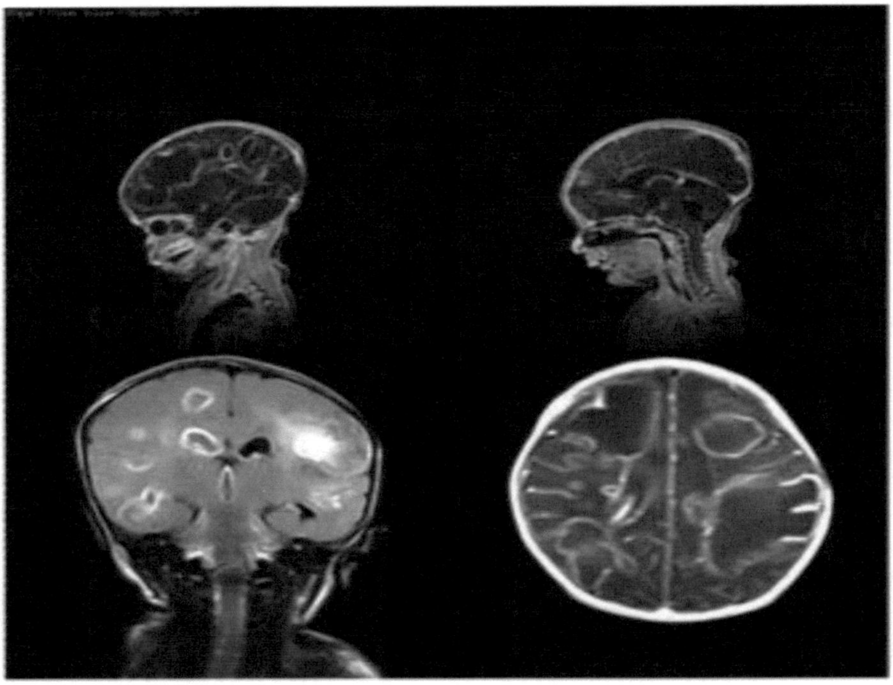

Fig. 3. MRI Brain showing multiple abscesses

12. Neuropsychological impairment

Neuropsychological impairment and cognitive dysfunction range from mild to severe disability and are well-recognized complication of bacterial meningitis. Neurobehavioral (50%) and neuro developmental (10-20%) sequel is more often found as residual long term defect in pediatric patients. A larger proportion of children with meningitis has IQ <70 and categorize as intellectual disability. (Braff, LJ et al., 1993). Meningitis in children under 12 months of age with high cellular count in CSF is significantly associated with impairment of language, learning, behavioral and cognitive skills. Cognitive impairment in adults is the commonest intellectual impairment in post meningitis patients. (Hogman, M. et al., 2007).

Other cognitive and somatic complaints, mood problems, social issues, thought and attention deficits, and delinquent behavior are amongst few rare complications, which need further research. (Halket, S. et al., 2003). Early identification and intervention may help to minimize the long-term impact of these problems, speech therapy.

13. Unusual complications

Severe permanent hydrocephalus, transverse myelitis, cortical visual impairment, aneurysm formation of focal intracranial vessels, aphasia and ataxia (Koomen, L et al., 2003) are rare neurological complications of meningitis. Reading and understanding the words and language deficit are other long term problems which should be anticipated and mange through special teaching modalities.

14. Acknowledgment

I would like to thanks Dr Yousuf Husen for his support in providing me the expert radiological assistant. I would also like to thank Ms Uzma Siddiqui who gave her enormous support and assistant in writing this book chapter.

15. References

Agrawal A, Timothy J, Pandit L, Shetty L, and J.P. Shetty, A Review of Subdural Empyema and Its Management. *Infect Dis Clin Pract* 2007;15:149–153

Anderson, V, Anderson, P, Grimwood, K, Nolan, T. Cognitive and executive function 12 years after childhood bacterial meningitis: effect of acute neurologic complications and age of onset. *J Pediatr Psychol* 2004; 29(2):67-81.

Annegers, JF, Hauser, WA, Beghi, E, Nicolosi, A. Kurland, LT. The risk of unprovoked seizures after encephalitis and meningitis. *Neurology* 1988; 38(9):1407-10.

Arditi, M, Mason EO Jr., Bradley, JS, Tan, TQ, Barson, WJ. Schutze, GE. Wald, ER. Givner, LB. Kim, KS. Yoqev, R. Kaplan, SL. Three-year multicenter surveillance of pneumococcal meningitis in children: clinical characteristics, and outcome related to penicillin susceptibility and dexamethasone use. *Pediatrics* 1998; 102(5):1087-97.

Baraff, LJ, Lee, SI, Schriger, DL. Outcomes of bacterial meningitis in children: a meta-analysis. Pediatr Infect Dis J 1993; 12(5):389-94.

Bhatt, SM. Lauretano, A. Cabellos, C. Halpin, C. Levine, RA. Xu, WZ. Nadol, JB Jr. Tuomanen, E. Progression of hearing loss in experimental pneumococcal meningitis: correlation with cerebrospinal fluid cytochemistry. *J Infect Dis* 1993; 167(3):675-83.

De Gans, J. van de Beek, D. European Dexamethasone in Adulthood Bacterial Meningitis Study Investigators. Dexamethasone in adults with bacterial meningitis. *N Engl J Med* 2002; 347(20):1549-56.

de Louvois, J. Acute bacterial meningitis in the newborn. J Antimicrob Chemother 1994; 34 Suppl A:61-73.

Durand, ML. Calderwood, SB. Weber, DJ. Miller, SI. Southwick, FS. Caviness, VS Jr. Swartz, MN. Acute bacterial meningitis in adults. A review of 493 episodes. *N Engl J Med* 1993; 328(1):21-8.

Feigin, RD. Cutrer,WB. Demmler-Harrison, GJ. Kaplan, SL. (2009). *Textbook of Pediatric Infectious Diseases, 6th ed,* chapter: Bacterial meningitis beyond the neonatal period. Saunders, Philadelphia, 2009. p.439.

Feldman, WE. Relation of concentrations of bacteria and bacterial antigen in cerebrospinal fluid to prognosis in patients with bacterial meningitis. *N Engl J Med* 1977; 296(8):433-35.

Halket, S. de Louvois, J. Holt, DE. Harvey, D. Long term follow up after meningitis in infancy: behaviour of teenagers. Arch Dis Child 2003; 88(5):395-98.

Hoogman, M. van de Beek, D. Weisfelt, M. de Gans, J. Schmand, B. Cognitive outcome in adults after bacterial meningitis. J Neurol Neurosurg Psychiatry 2007; 78(10):1092-96.

Koomen, I. Grobbee, DE. Roord, JJ. Donders, R. Fennekens-Schinkel, A. van Furth, AM. Hearing loss at school age in survivors of bacterial meningitis: assessment, incidence, and prediction. *Pediatrics* 2003; 112(5):1049-53.

Lindval, P. Ahlm, C. Ericsson, M. Gothefors, L. Naredi, S. Koskinen, LD. Reducing Intracranial Pressure May Increase Survival among Patients with Bacterial Meningitis. *Clinical Infectious Diseases* 2004; 38(3):384–90

Madagame, ET. Havens, PL. Bresnahan, JM. Babel, KL. Splaingard, ML. Survival and functional outcome of children requiring mechanical ventilation during therapy for acute bacterial meningitis. Crit Care Med 1995; 23(7):1279-83.

Merchant, SN. Gopen, Q. A human temporal bone study of acute bacterial meningogenic labyrinthitis. *Am J Otol* 1996; 17(3):375-85

Pfister, HW. Feiden, W. Einhaupl, KM. Spectrum of complications during bacterial meningitis in adults. Results of a prospective clinical study. *Arch Neurol.* 1993;50(6):575–581.

Roine, I. Peltola, H. Fernández, J. Zavala, I. González Mata, A. González Ayala, S. Arbo, A. Bologna, R. Miño, G. Goyo, J. López, E. Dourado de Andrade, S. Sarna, S. Influence of admission findings on death and neurological outcome from childhood bacterial meningitis. Clin Infect Dis 2008; 46(8):1248-52.

Mace, SE. Acute Bacterial Meningitis. Emerg Med Clin N Am 2008; 26(2):281–317

Snedeker, JD. Kaplan, SL. Dodge, PR. Holmens, SJ. Feigin, RD. Subdural effusion and its relationship with neurologic sequelae of bacterial meningitis in infancy: a prospective study. *Pediatrics* 1990; 86(2):163.

van de Beek, D. de Gans, J. Spanjaard, L. Weisfelt, M. Reitsma, JB. Vermeulen, M. Clinical features and prognostic factors in adults with bacterial meningitis. N Engl J Med 2004; 351(18):1849-59.

Zoons, E. Weisfelt, M. de Gans, J. Spanjaard, L. Koelman, JH. Reitsma, JB. Van de Beek, D. Seizures in adults with bacterial meningitis. Neurology 2008; 70:2109-15.

5

Early Neurologic Outcome and EEG of Infants with Bacterial Meningitis

Adrián Poblano and Carmina Arteaga
[1]*Laboratory of Cognitive Neurophysiology, National Institute of Rehabilitation, Mexico City,*
[2]*Clinic of Sleep Disorders, National University of Mexico, Mexico City, Mexico*

1. Introduction

Newborn infants (especially premature infants) are susceptible to bacterial infections and may develop primary meningitis or suffer a bacterial attack-associated neuroinfection.[1] Bacterial meningitis in newborns infants remains as a serious disease with significant long-term neurological morbidity.[2-5] Prediction of outcome is important in decision-making to provide information to parents, and for identification of subjects requiring close intervention and early follow-up. Clinical evaluation includes neurological examination, cerebrospinal fluid (CSF) culture, neuroimaging studies and neurophysiological studies, such as the electroencephalogram (EEG) and evoked potentials.

Neonatal bacterial meningitis continues to be a serious disease with an unchanging rate of adverse outcome of 20-60%, despite a worldwide decline in mortality. The 3 major pathogens in developed countries are: Group B *Streptococcus*, gram negative rods and *Lysteria monocytogenes*. Signs and symptoms of meningitis may be subtle, unspecific, vague, atypical or absent. In order to exclude neonatal meningitis, all infants with proven or suspected sepsis should undergo lumbar puncture. Positive culture of cerebrospinal fluid may be the only way to diagnose meningitis and to identify the pathogen, as CSF parameters smay be normal at early stages and meningitis may occur frequently (up to 30% of cases) in the absence of bacteraemia. When meningitis is suspected, treatment must be aggressive, as the goal is to achieve bactericidal concentration of antibiotics and to sterilize CSF as soon as possible. Antibiotics should be administered intravenously, at the highest clinically validated doses. Empiric antibiotic treatment should include agents active against all main pathogens; currently the recommended empiric treatment of meningitis is ampicillin, plus an aminoglycoside and a third-generation cephalosporin. Therapy should be reassessed after cultures and antibiotic susceptibility is available. Prevention of neonatal sepsis, early recognition of infants at risk, prompt treatment and future adjunctive therapies will improve prognosis.[6]

In the newborn, EEG provides an extremely useful non-invasive test for brain function. The degree of background activity abnormality has proved to be a predictor of long-term neurologic outcome.[7] Our goal, in this chapter was to show the contribution of neonatal EEG and its correlation with the neurological examination during the first year of life in clinical follow-up (at age 9 month) of newborns with bacterial neonatal meningitis.[8]

2. Neurologic assessment and follow-up

Twenty seven patients were studied: average maternal age at the birth of the infant was 27.59±5.41 years (range, 17-39 years). Fourteen mothers (50%) had one previous gestation, for seven mothers (25%) it was the first pregnancy, and the remaining mothers had two or more gestations (25%). Two infants (7%) were born vaginally and 25 (92%) by cesarean section.

Fifteen infants were male (55%) and 12 female (44%). Clinical characteristics of infants are shown in Table 1. Fourteen infants (51%) were born at age <32 weeks of gestation (wG), 10 between 32 and 36 wG (37%) and three with 37 or more wG (11%). Sixteen subjects (59%) had birthweight <1,500 g, eight were between 1501 and 2500 g (29%), and three (11%) infants weighed 2,501 g or more at birth. Height at birth ranged from 26 and 50 cm, while cephalic perimeter had a range of between 24 and 39.3 cm. Apgar score at 1 min (Apgar 1) ranged between 2 and 8, and 5-min Apgar (Apgar 5) score had a range of between 4 and 9, and Silverman-Andersen score ranged between 5 and 2.

Feature	**Average**	**SD**
Age at birth (weeks)	31.70	3.98
Weight at birth (g)	1504	722
Height at birth (cm)	39.12	5.81
Cephalic perimeter (cm)	29.20	4.01
Apgar 1	5.44	2.25
Apgar 5	8.03	1.40
Silverman-Andersen	3	1

SD. Standard deviation

Table 1. Clinical features of infants with neonatal bacterial meningitis

Bacterial cultures reported *Staphylococcus aureus* and *Staphylococcus* coagulase-negative in seven cases of each (25%). Group B *Streptococcus* was positive in four subjects (14%), Group D *Streptococcus* was positive in two cases (7%), and different bacteria in each of the seven remaining cases (3%). Antibiotic treatment included a combination of vancomycin-cephotaxim in 20 subjects (74%), vancomycine alone in four (14%) and an ampicillin-amikacin combination in three cases (11%). Average hospitalization days was 54.4±29.4 days with range of 10-120 days.

EEG recordings during neonatal period were normal in nine patients (one third of the sample, 9/27 of patients), while eight were mildly abnormal (8/27), nine were moderately abnormal (9/27), and one was markedly abnormal (1/27). Clinical characteristics comparison of infants by EEG alteration severity detected differences in Apgar 5 score between groups, and *post-hoc* analyses revealed that infants with moderately and markedly abnormality had significantly lower scores (p = 0.005). Amiel-Tison neurological examination[9] was performed in 26 infants at 3 and 6 months of age, and in 27 infants at age 9 months; results are show in Table 2.

Age (months)	**Cephalic perimeter** (n/ abn)	x (SD) cm	**Reflexes** (n/ abn)	**Passive tone** (n/ abn)	**Active tone** (n/ abn)
3 (26)	24/ 2	37.3 (1.4)	8/ 18	16/ 10	14/ 12
6 (26)	25/ 1	40.7 (1.6)	12/ 14	15/ 11	16/ 10
9 (27)	23/ 4	42.8 (1.7)	13/ 14	17/ 10	22/ 5

n = normal, abn = abnormal, x = average, SD = standard deviation, cm = centimeters

Table 2. Neurological examination results (in percentages) in infants with neonatal bacterial meningitis

No statistical differences were found when overall results were compared from both the Amiel-Tison neurologic examination and neonatal EEG (p = 0.08). Significant association was found between neonatal EEG result and cephalic perimeter alteration at 3, 6, and 9 months using normative data from our country[10] (Wald score = 11.40, 9.96, and 10.42; p = 0.001, 0.002, and 0.001 respectively) and active tone at 9 months (Wald score = 8.94; p = 0.003). EEG sensitivity and specificity for predicting change in neurologic examination at 9 months of age were 72% and 44% respectively.

CT was performed in two infants and both studies were abnormal. Magnetic resonance imaging (MRI) was performed in one patient who had abnormal result. US studies were abnormal in eight subjects (30%), abnormalities found included intraventricular hemorrhage in five patients (18%), and periventricular leukomalacia and hydrocephalous in three subjects each (11%).

3. Comments

We found that an EEG performed in the neonatal period during acute bacterial meningitis predicts adverse outcome early within the first year of life. Few studies have examined the value of neonatal EEG as a prognostic tool in patients with bacterial neuroinfection.

Watanabe et al.[11] studied EEG-polygraphically in 29 newborns with meningitis, and visual and auditory evoked potentials were also obtained in some infants: clinical findings correlated with outcomes. The authors commented that EEG background activity was a good prognostic tool but could not indicate complication type, although persistent abnormalities correlated with severe brain injury. Unfortunately, this study included infants without culture-proved meningitis.

Chequer et al.[12] retrospectively studied 29 infants with culture-proven meningitis. They found that degree of EEG background activity abnormality proved to be a good predictor of long-term neurologic outcome. Infants with normal or mildly abnormal EEG have normal outcomes, whereas those with markedly abnormal EEG died or manifested severe neurologic damage at follow-up.

Klinger et al.[13] studied 37 infants during the neonatal period and 21 had adverse outcomes; nine died and 12 infants had moderate to severe disability at 1 year of age. EEG background activity and overall EEG description were identified as predictors of adverse outcome; multivariate analysis indicated that the latter was a stronger predictor, with sensitivity of 88% and specificity of 90%. Infants with normal or mildly abnormal EEG had good outcomes, whereas those with moderate to markedly abnormal EEG died or survived with neurologic sequelae. Our data are in agreement with these latter results, although we found lower values of sensitivity and specificity.

Recently, ter Horst et al.,[14] carried-out Amplitude integrated EEG (aEEG), recordings in 22 infants with sepsis/meningitis, cases were retrospectively evaluated. Mean gestational age was 38 weeks (range: 34-42 weeks). Thirteen infants had meningitis. Survivors were seen for neurological follow-up. Four infants died, two were severely abnormal at 24 months. Amplitude integrated EEG background pattern, sleep-wake cycling (SWC) and electrographic seizure activity (EA) were analyzed. All infants with continuous low voltage or flat trace on aEEG (n = 4) had an adverse outcome. Low voltage aEEGs (n = 9) had a positive score for an adverse outcome at 6 h and at 24 h after admission. EA was more frequent in infants with adverse outcome and had a positive score for adverse outcome. SWC appeared more frequent in infants with good outcome. In conclusion, authors found that low voltage background pattern, SWC and EA on aEEG were helpful to predict neurological outcome in infants with neonatal sepsis or meningitis.

Etiologic agents found in our infants sample are in agreement and in partial agreement with those of other studies carried out at other NICUs in Mexico City,[15,16] but are not in total agreement with other studies performed elsewhere.[4,17] Thus any consideration with regard to differences in neurological outcomes related with specific bacterial agents must be performed carefully, more research is necessary in the future with larger number of patients and with multicenter samples with clinical, neurophysiological, neuroimaging and microbiological techniques to answer this question.

Correlation between EEG results and results concerning cephalic perimeter and active tone on the neurological examination were reported here and deserve greater attention. Correlation between Amiel-Tison examination and outcomes with other methods such as US, EEG, and cerebral function monitoring at 12-15 months of age was reported as good. The sensitivity to detect neurological abnormalities with various techniques is variable. Sensitivity for detecting infants with abnormal brain US was 0.97, whereas with EEG 0.89, and with cerebral function monitoring 0.88.[18] Thus combined EEG examination with the clinical Amiel-Tison neurological examination and other techniques augments probability of detection of early brain damage.

A significant relation between Apgar 5 with severity of EEG abnormalities was found. This finding underlines additive effects of early adverse conditions at birth in infants with central nervous system infection; this point has been observed in many diseases, such as post-hemorrhagic hydrocephalus, and apnea in infants.[19,20] We suggest that clinicians and investigators must perform a multivariate weighting of each risk-factor, neurological examination, neurophysiologic, and neuroimage studies, for prediction of neurological sequelae in infants with neonatal bacterial meningitis.

Our patients survived during the acute phase of neuroinfection and during the 9-month follow-up; therefore disease severity could be less than infants in the samples of Watanabe et al.[11], Chequer et al.[12], Klinger et al.[13], and ter Horst et al.[14] Infants with normal or mildly abnormal EEG survived without sequelae, and those with moderately and markedly abnormal activity were neurologically abnormal at follow-up. EEG abnormalities included an infant with burst-supression, and others with slowing of background activity, spikes and slow waves. Seizures occurred in some of these infants, others had intraventricular bleeding-related hydrocephalous in which ventriculo-peritoneal shunt placement was performed and were under control during follow-up period.

4. Conclusion

In conclusion, it is our recommendation that EEG recording be obtained early in acute phase of the neuroinfection, because neonatal EEG is useful for predicting abnormalities in cephalic perimeter and active tone at 9 months of age in infants with bacterial neonatal meningitis.

5. References

[1] Meade RH. Bacterial meningitis in the neonatal infant. Med Clin North Am 1985;69:257-267.

[2] Bedford H, de Louvois J, Halket S, Peckham C, Hurley R, Harvey D. Meningitis in infancy in England and Wales: follow-up at age 5 years. BMJ 2001;323:1-5.

[3] Jiang ZD, Liu XY, Wu YY, Zheng MS, Liu HC. Long-term impairments of brain and auditory functions of children recovered from purulent meningitis. Dev Med Child Neurol 1990;32:473-480.

[4] Stevens P, Eames M, Kent A, Halket S, Holt D, Harvey D. Long term outcomes of neonatal meningitis. Arch Dis Child Fetal. Neonatal Ed 2003;88:F179-F184.

[5] Wheater M, Rennie JM. Perinatal infection is an important risk factor for cerebral palsy in very-low-birthweight infants. Dev Med Child Neurol 2000;42:364-367.

[6] Berardi A, Lugli L, Rossi C, China MC, Vellani G, Contiero R, Calanca F, Camerlo F, Casula F, di Carlo C, Rossi MR, Chiarabini R, Ferrari M, Minniti S, Venturelli C, Silvestrini D, Dodi I, Zuchinni A, Ferrari F, Infezioni da Streptoccc B della regione Emilia Romagna. Neonatal bacterial meningitis. Minerva Pediatr 2010;62:51-54.

[7] Garza-Morales S, Poblano-Luna A. The abnormal electroencephalogram in the newborn (in Spanish). In: Gil-Nagel A, Parra J, Iriarte J, Kanner AM Handbook of electroencephalography. Madrid, McGraw Hill-Interamericana. 2002.pp.117-130.

[8] Poblano A, Gutiérrez R. Correlation between the neonatal EEG and the neurological examination in the first year of life in infants with bacterial meningitis. Arq Neuropsiquiatr 2007;65:576-580.

[9] Amiel-Tison C. Update of the Amiel-Tison neurologic assessment for the term neonate or at 40 weeks corrected age. Pediatr Neurol 2002;27:196-212.

[10] Ramos-Galván R. Pediatric somatometry. Follow-up study in infants and children from Mexico City (in Spanish). Arch Invest Med 1975;6, suppl 1:83-396.

[11] Watanabe K, Hara K, Hakamada S, Kuroyanagi M, Kuno K, Aso K. The prognostic value of EEG in neonatal meningitis. Clin Electroencephalogr 1983;14:67-77.

[12] Chequer RS, Tharp BS, Dreimane D, Hahn JS, Clancy RR, Coen RW. Prognostic value of EEG in neonatal meningitis: retrospective study of 29 infants. Pediatr Neurol 1992;8:417-422.

[13] Klinger G, Chin CN, Otsubo H, Beyene J, Perlman M. Prognostic value of EEG in neonatal bacterial meningitis. Pediatr Neurol 2001;24:28-31.

[14] ter Horst HJ, van Olffen M, Remmelts HJ, de Vries J, Boss AF. The prognostic value of amplitude integrated EEG in neonatal sepsis and/or meningitis. Acta Paediatr 2010;99:194-200.

[15] Reyna-Figueroa J, Ortiz-Ibarra FJ, Plazola-Camacho NG, Limón-Rojas AE. Bacterial meningitis in newborns. Experience of the National Institute of Perinatology from 1990-1999 (in Spanish). Bol Med Hosp Infant Mex 2004;61:402-411.

[16] Rios-Reategui E, Ruiz-Gonzalez L, Murguia-de-Sierra T. Neonatal bacterial meningitis in a third level care unit (in Spanish). Rev Invest Clin 1998;50:31-36.

[17] Harvey D, Holt DE, Bedford H. Bacterial meningitis in the newborn: a prospective study of mortality and morbidity. Sem Perinatol 1999;23:218-225.

[18] Paro-Panjan D, Neubauer D, Kodric J, Bratanic B. Amiel-Tison Neurological Assessment at term age: clinical application, correlation with other methods, and outcome at 12 to 15 months. Dev Med Child Neurol 2005;47:16-26.

[19] Robles P, Poblano A, Hernández G, Ibarra J, Guzmán I, Sosa J. Cortical, brainstem and autonomic nervous system dysfunction in infants with post-hemorrhagic hydrocephalous. Rev Invest Clin 2002;54:133-138.

[20] Poblano A, Márquez A, Hernández G. Apnea in infants. Ind J Pediat 2006;73:1085-1088.

6

Vaccines to Prevent Bacterial Meningitis in Children

Joseph Domachowske
Upstate Medical University, Department of Pediatrics, Syracuse NY, USA

1. Introduction

Vaccines are among the most effective public health interventions available. Global eradication of smallpox infection, the elimination of polio from the Western hemisphere, and dramatic reductions in diseases like diphtheria, tetanus, pertussis, measles, mumps, rubella, varicella, rotavirus, hepatitis A and B have all been achieved through immunization programs. The public health impact of well-structured immunization programs is well appreciated, but logistic and financial obstacles can interfere with vaccine availability and delivery. The frequency and severity of bacterial meningitis in children has also been favorable impacted by the widespread use of vaccines in all areas of the world where resources have allowed them to be implemented since the three most common causes of childhood meningitis, Haemophilus influenzae type B (HIB), pneumococcus, and meningococcus, are now, at least partially, vaccine preventable. In developed countries of the world, vaccines for all three of these bacterial infections are now considered the standard of care. Substantial progress is also being made in resource poor countries where, slowly and surely, the public health impact of immunization programs is being appreciated and international assistance to provide the money and knowledge needed for widespread vaccine delivery is being realized.

Bacterial meningitis is a life threatening infection that occurs in all age groups but disproportionately affects infants and young children. Most cases of bacterial meningitis result from hematogenous seeding of the meninges during a bloodstream infection. Direct extension of a bacterial infection from the sinuses, middle ear, or mastoid represent other routes of meningeal seeding. The most common microbiologic causes of bacterial meningitis differ based on the age of the affected patient. Common etiologic agents of bacterial meningitis in the first week of life include Streptococcus agalactiae (group B Streptococcus), Escherichia coli, and Listeria monocytogenes. Sadly, vaccines to prevent infections caused by these agents have remained elusive, although some progress has been made with experimental vaccines against group B streptococcus. Late-onset neonatal meningitis occurs after the first week of life and up to three months of age and may be caused by the agents listed above, other enteric gram negative bacilli, Pasteurella after animal exposure, pneumococci, meningococci, and staphylococci.

During later infancy and early childhood, S. pneumoniae and N. meningitidis, account for 80% of cases of bacterial meningitis in developed countries. Many of these infections are now vaccine preventable. The remaining 20% are caused by L. monocytogenes, Streptococcus pyogenes (group A strep) S. agalactiae (group B strep), H. influenzae (type B and nontypeable isolates), E. coli and other enteric gram negative rods (including salmonella species). Among these agents, only H. influenzae type B vaccines have been successful. Bacterial meningitis in adolescents and younger adults is usually caused by either S. pneumoniae or N. meningitides, however after the age of 50 years, L. monocytogenes becomes more prevalent. In elderly individuals, S. pneumoniae, N. meningitidis and L. monocytogenes remain the more common microbiologic etiologies, however a broad array of other pathogens have been described depending on the presence of co-morbidities, travel, and unusual exposures.

At present, bacterial meningitis is most common in children, particularly those living in under-developed countries of the world. In some parts of Africa, 1 in 250 children developing meningitis during their first year of life (Greenwood, 1987; Scarborough et al., 2007, Scarborough & Thwaites, 2008), and while epidemiologic surveys from the United States, Europe, Brazil, Israel and Canada show that bacterial meningitis is less common in developed parts of the world, infections are typically caused by the same bacterial species in all geographic areas. As noted, safe and effective vaccines have been developed to prevent infections caused by the three most common agents of bacterial meningitis in children—Haemophilus influenzae type B (HIB), Streptococcus pneumoniae, and Neisseria meningitidis. The introduction and implementation of these vaccines have had dramatic effects on the incidence of bacterial meningitis in all areas of the world where they have been successfully introduced, but challenges remain.

Obstacles to the prevention of bacterial meningitis in resource poor areas of the world relate to the cost of the vaccines, and the lack of solid infrastructure to store and deliver the vaccines to those most in need. A growing, and somewhat unanticipated barrier to vaccine coverage rates in developed countries has been a loss of public confidence in the safety of routine immunizations to the extent that immunization coverage rates are not as high as we have once achieved successfully. Even in countries where vaccine coverage remains excellent, cases of pneumococcal and/or meningococcal meningitis can still occur, as not all serotypes of these organisms are included in present day vaccines. For the most common causes of bacterial meningitis, vaccines are indeed available for the predominate serotypes, but since vaccines do not exist for every known serotype, cases will still be seen. This is especially important for Neisseria meningitidis serotype B, a common cause of meningitis in young infants. Moreover, the common etiologic agents affecting newborns (Escherichia coli and Streptococcus agalactiae, also commonly referred to as group B strep) and less common causes of bacterial meningitis in older children (Listeria monocytogenes, Staphylococcus aureus, Streptococcus pyogenes, and Salmonella species) are not currently preventable through licensed vaccines.

2. Available licensed vaccines for the prevention of bacterial meningitis

2.1 HIB vaccines

Haemophilus influenzae type B is an encapsulated pleiomorphic gram negative rod that causes bacteremia, sepsis, pneumonia, facial cellulitis, epiglottitis, and meningitis. Before the mid 1980's, HIB caused roughly 20,000 cases of invasive disease per year in the U.S. alone. Almost all of these infections occurred in children under five years of age, and half of these infections were meningitis, making HIB the most common cause of bacterial meningitis in children at the time, and identifying HIB disease as a logical target for vaccine development. Other capsular serotypes, and non-typeable strains of H. influenzae are less common causes of invasive infection, but non-type B cases of meningitis are still encountered on a regular basis.

2.1.1 Early HIB vaccine efforts

In 1985, the first HIB vaccines were licensed for use in the United States for children beginning at age two years. The original formulations of the vaccine were pure polysaccharide, had an efficacy of 55-92%, and was well tolerated. Three vaccines were licensed—Praxis introduced b-Capsa-1, Lederle introduced Hib-imune; and Connaught introduced Hibvax. At the time, this was a major advance in pediatric vaccination since HIB was the most common cause of meningitis in children under five years of age, and carried a significant morbidity and mortality. Many of the infected children developed profound sensorineural hearing loss as a complication of developing meningitis, others suffered developmental and cognitive deficits, and some died. In the early days of HIB vaccine, there was controversy regarding the overall value of routine immunization, especially since the early formulations of vaccines were not effective in infants. Although it was a start, the strategy that employed the use of pure polysaccharide vaccines was suboptimal for the prevention of invasive HIB infection for several additional reasons. First, polysaccharide vaccines are not immunogenic in patients under two years of age, the age group at highest risk for HIB disease. Second, polysaccharide immunogens are processed by the immune system in a T-cell independent manner. In the absence of T-cell engagement, immunity cannot be effectively boosted with subsequent doses of vaccine. B cells are certainly stimulated to produce antibodies, but the effect is relatively short lived, and antibody titers wane over the period of several years. An absence of T-cell help impairs the durability of the immune response. Five years following receipt of a polysaccharide vaccine, the humoral evidence of prior vaccination (and immunity), is reduced or no longer detected. Third, serial re-administration of polysaccharide vaccines to individuals at any age, particularly if done so at closely spaced intervals, leads to lower antibody titers than the first dose. This phenomenon, known as 'hypo-responsiveness' remains a major limitation for the use of any pure polysaccharide vaccine.

2.1.2 Solving the problems of polysaccharides vaccines

Clinical vaccine research suggested early on that the limitations associated with the use of polysaccharide immunogens could be overcome through the use of an elegant biochemical trick. The same polysaccharide antigens used in the original HIB vaccines were covalently linked to a simple peptide. Peptides that have been used successfully in this manner include tetanus and diphtheria toxoids, the outer membrane protein of Neisseria menigitidis, and CRM197 (cross reacting material 197, a protein similar to naturally occurring diphtheria toxin). The presence of such a peptide altered the manner in which the immune system processed the antigen, specifically with regard to T-cell engagement, and allowed the vaccine to induce a robust immune response in children as young as six weeks of age. Serial doses provide additional protection and higher antibody concentrations, and booster doses show clear evidence of immune memory. The technique whereby polysaccharide antigens are biochemically linked to a peptide produces a 'conjugate' vaccine. Table 1 shows examples of polysaccharide and conjugate vaccines made by different manufacturers, the conjugate protein used to develop them, and the year each was introduced in the United States. The successful development of conjugate HIB vaccines paved the way for the development of several other conjugate vaccines, including those currently in use for the prevention of both pneumococcal and meningococcal infections. Early pure polysaccharide, and later generation conjugate vaccines for all three types of infection are included in the Table.

Vaccine	Trade name	Manufacturer	Immunogens	Conjugate protein	Introduced in the U.S.
HIB	B-Caspa-1 Hib-Imune Hibvax	Praxis Lederle Connaught	PRP PRP PRP	None	1985, no longer used
	HIBTITER	Wyeth	HbOC	CRM197	1990, no longer used
	PedvaxHIB	Merck	PRP	OMP N. meningitidis	1989
	ActHIB	Sanofi Pasteur	PRP	Tetanus toxoid	1993
	OmniHIB	GlaxoSmithKline	PRP	Tetanus toxoid	1993, no longer used
	ProHIBIT	Connaught	PRP	Diphtheria toxoid	1987, no longer used
	Hiberix	GlaxoSmithKline	PRP	Tetanus toxoid	2010
Pneumococcal	Pneumovax	Merck	14 valent	None	1977, no longer used
	Pneumovax 23	Merck	23 valent*	None	1983
	Prevnar	Pfizer	4, 6B, 9V, 14, 18C, 19F, 23F	CRM197	2000
	Prevnar 13	Pfizer	1, 3, 4, 5, 6A, 6B, 7F, 9V, 14, 18C, 19A, 19F, 23F	CRM 197	2010
Memingococcal	Menomune	Sanofi Pasteur	A, C, Y, W135	None	1981
	Menactra	Sanofi Pasteur	A, C, Y, W135	Diphtheria toxoid	2005
	Menveo	Novartis	A, C, Y, W135	CRM197	2010

*1, 2, 3, 4, 5, 6B , 7F, 8, 9N, 9V, 10A, 11A, 12F, 14, 15B, 17F, 18C, 19A, 19F, 20, 22F, 23F, 33F
Abbreviations: PRP (polyribosylribitol phosphate), CRM (cross reacting material), OMP (outer membrane protein), HbOC (Haemophilus B oligosaccharide conjugate)

Table 1. Vaccines to Prevent HIB, Pneumococcal and Meningococcal Infections in the United States

With the introduction of conjugate HIB vaccine during the late 1980s throughout the U.S. and other developed countries, rates of all cause bacterial meningitis fell dramatically along with the observation that the mean age at presentation from any cause of bacterial meningitis went from 15 mos in 1986 to 25 years in 1995 (Schuchat et al., 1997; Berg et al., 1996; Giorgi Rossi et al., 2009; Mishal et al., 2008; Theodoridou et al., 2007; Urwin et al., 1994; Weiss et al., 2001; Schlech et al., 1985 Wenger et al., 1990). This age shift was a direct effect of near complete elimination of HIB meningitis in the under five-year old age group. This is perhaps the most notable recent, and publically under-recognized vaccine success story of recent years. Once a cause of approximately 10,000 cases of bacterial meningitis in children every year in the U.S. alone, there is currently an average of fewer than 100 cases of invasive HIB disease reported annually.

HIB vaccine programs are among the most effective modern public health interventions of the 20th century. Pediatric cases seen in the U.S. in the present day are almost always described in unvaccinated, under-vaccinated, or immune deficient patients. When invasive HIB disease is discovered in a vaccinated child, testing should always be performed to determine if that child has an immune deficiency. The HIB success story is mirrored across the globe in areas where resources have permitted widespread introduction of vaccine to children. These results are clear and impressive. In every area of the world where vaccine programs are initiated, HIB disease, including HIB meningitis, virtually disappears.

The public health benefits of HIB vaccination have not been realized in all corners of the globe, however. Delivery of HIB and other vaccines to resource challenged areas of the world remains suboptimal. Globally, it is estimated that about 38% of infants have HIB vaccine available to them, but progress in improving this percentage is steady. Even 38% of the worlds' children translates to roughly 130,000 lives saved annually from pneumonia and meningitis caused by HIB. In the last decade alone, combined efforts on the part of the World Health Organization, UNICEF, the Bill and Melinda Gates Foundation, and other international agencies have led to more vaccine availability in the areas of the world that still need it the most. In 1997, 29 countries were using conjugate HIB vaccine, but by 2009, 161 countries had introduced it. To date, 29 countries are still without access to HIB vaccine for infants, and the epidemiology of HIB infection in those areas remains similar to the problem seen in the U.S. prior to 1985. While there has been progress in Africa and some parts of Asia, significant effort, education, and resources are still needed in the underdeveloped world to prevent this form of meningitis.

2.2 Pneumococcal vaccines

Streptococcus pneumoniae are encapsulated gram positive diplococci that continue to cause invasive infections at all ages. Of the 92 different pneumococcal serotypes (grouped into 46 serogroups based on immunologic similarities) that have been identified based on antigenic differences in their capsular polysaccharides, ten serogroups account for most of the pediatric invasive pneumococcal infections worldwide with serogroups 1, 3, 6, 14, 19 and 23 being the most common. Pneumococci commonly infect the sinopulmonary tract causing otitis media, sinusitis, and pneumonia. Bacteremia with sepsis is not uncommon. Meningeal seeding, with a resulting bacterial meningitis can occur at any age, including previously healthy individuals, and patients with defined risk factors, including immune deficiency, HIV infection, asplenia, hemoglobinopathies, diabetes and alcoholism. Worldwide, S.

pneumoniae remains the most common cause of bacterial meningitis identifying it as an important target for vaccine development.

2.2.1 Early vaccine development

Vaccines designed to prevent invasive pneumococcal disease were available in the early 1900s, but early goals were focused primarily in the prevention of lower respiratory tract infection in adults. Two hexavalent vaccines were licensed for use in adults after World War II, but with the emerging availability of antibiotics, enthusiasm for the use of vaccines to prevent disease waned. In the absence of public demand, the vaccines were removed from the market. Interest in the prevention of pneumococcal infections re-emerged in the 1960s. A 14-valent pure polysaccharide vaccine was licensed for use in adults in 1977, ultimately being replaced by a new generation polysaccharide 23-valent vaccine in 1983. The 23-valent polysaccharide vaccine, which is still available, was FDA licensed in the United States in 1983 for use in adults and high-risk children older than 2 years. Its role has been primarily to prevent pneumococcal pneumonia in high-risk adults. Its major limitation as a pure polysaccharide vaccine (it is not a conjugate vaccine) is that it is poorly immunogenic in young children. Like other polysaccharide vaccines, it is processed by the immune system in a T-cell independent manner so the duration of immune protection is brief, and there is no potential for boosting with subsequent doses.

In 2000, a heptavalent pneumococcal vaccine, Prevnar, was added to the universal pediatric immunization schedule in the U.S. resulting in an almost immediate reduction in invasive pneumococcal infections, including a reduction in cases of meningitis. U.S. population-based data from the Active Bacterial Core Surveillance was published in 2003 showing a 59% decline in pneumococcal meningitis in young children (Whitney et al., 2003), and Nationwide Inpatient Service data showed that the incidence rate fell by 33% in children less than 5 years of age (from 0.8 to 0.55 cases per 100,000 population) (Tsai et al., 2008).

The power of national surveillance, coupled with the impressive efficacy of pneumococcal vaccine illustrated the public health benefits in just three years following vaccine introduction. When it is appreciated that Prevnar was in somewhat short supply during much of those early years, the dramatic beneficial effect becomes even more obvious. The majority of children in the U.S. during 2000-2002 received a 3-dose primary vaccine series, but an Advisory Committee on Immunization Practices recommendation to defer the booster fourth dose until supplies were available led to substantial delays in the timeliness of completing the four dose series. Despite this difficulty with timeliness to vaccine series completion, the public health impact of conjugate vaccine was almost immediately recognized through surveillance networks.

The heptavalent (7-valent) pneumococcal vaccine Prevnar included conjugated pneumococcal polysaccharide antigens against serotypes 4, 6B, 9V, 14, 18C, 19F, and 23F. At the time of licensure, these capsular types were the most likely to cause invasive infection in children in the Unites States. Serotype prevalence varies somewhat according to world geography, but for the most part, the same types are responsible for invasive infection in most of the world. As conjugate pneumococcal vaccine was being developed, another public health problem related to infections caused by S. pneumoniae had already become well recognized. Strains of S. pneumoniae had gradually emerged that were less and less susceptible to penicillin. Treatment of pneumococcal infections with penicillin or other beta-lactam antibiotics was no longer 'guaranteed' to eradicate infection. This problem impacted empiric management of mild to moderate infections such as otitis media and pneumonia, but also raised serious concerns about how to best manage empiric antibiotics in serious and life-threatening infections such as meningitis.

As antibiotic resistance increased in pneumococci, moderate and severe infections began to be managed with different antimicrobial regimens. Penicillin treatment of severe disease was used only after antimicrobial susceptibility profiles were confirmed. The problem was not isolated to the use of penicillin, as the mechanism of penicillin resistance in S. pneumoniae depends on a series of mutations in its penicillin binding proteins (PBPs) that also alter the antimicrobial susceptibility to all beta lactam antibiotics. It should be understood that this mechanism of antibiotic resistance does not depend on the production of a beta-lactamase enzyme, and that beta lactamase producing S. pneumoniae isolates have not ever been described. Instead, antibiotic pressure has led some strains of S. pneumoniae to alter their PBPs so that their affinity for penicillin is reduced. When this occurs, the penicillin can no longer bind to and inhibit the transpeptidase activity of the PBP, a function that is necessary for peptidoglycan cross linking. This biochemical alteration becomes obvious in the laboratory as gradual increases in the minimal inhibitory concentrations (MICs) of penicillin, and ultimately in the observation that the organism is 'intermediate' or 'resistant' to penicillin. As penicillin resistant strains gain additional mutations in these PBPs, the MICs to all beta lactam antibiotics begin to increase. MICs to first, then second, and then to third generation cephalosporins increase. Pneumococci that are resistant to advanced generation cephalosporins like cefotaxime and ceftriaxone are now encountered on a regular basis. The emergence of these resistant strains has led to a change in how bacterial meningitis is treated empirically, where a third generation cephalosporin (ceftriaxone or cefotaxime) in combination with vancomycin is typically used until antimicrobial susceptibility profiles are known. The rationale for incorporating vancomycin into the empiric regimen is to be sure that every patient with pneumococcal meningitis has effective antimicrobial therapy initiated at the time that meningitis is suspected. When the microbiology laboratory confirms that the infection is caused by S. pneumoniae, and that the infecting organism is susceptible to penicillin or a third generation cephalosporin, the treatment can be 'de-escalated' to the appropriate antibiotic.

One of the under-appreciated benefits of introducing the conjugate pneumococcal vaccine in the U.S. in 2000 was the observation that the original seven conjugate vaccine serotypes 4, 6B, 9V, 14, 18C, 19F, and 23F were among the most likely to be penicillin resistant. This offered the potential to reduce infection caused by the most prevalent pneumococci, while at the same time reduce the possibility that infections would be caused by antibiotic resistant strains. During the decade following introduction of the 7-valent conjugate vaccine, there was a substantial reduction in invasive pneumococcal infections reported in children, including meningitis, but a troubling pattern began to emerge in the form of nonvaccine replacement serotypes. Like early prevalent pneumococcal serotypes, several of these replacement types were resistant to beta lactam antibiotics.

In 2010, the heptavalent pneumococcal vaccine was replaced with a newly developed 13-valent vaccine (by the same manufacturer) to expand the number of covered serotypes. The new generation 13-valent vaccine became available in 2010, and was immediately recommended as a replacement for the 7-valent vaccine. The additional serotypes included 1, 3, 5, 6A, 7F, and 19A. The inclusion of serotypes 6A and 19A are of particular importance in this new generation vaccine as these capsular types were the ones that emerged as the most serious replacement serotypes during the successful decade following introduction of the heptavalent vaccine. Serotype 19A remains a serious threat. Some infections caused by this strain are highly resistant to all penicillins, cephalosporins, and carbapenems making treatment for infections of the central nervous system challenging. In such situations, treatment with vancomycin and/or lineazolid has been successful. As experience with and implementation of the 13 valent conjugate vaccine continues, an optimistic possibility is that infections caused by the most difficult-to-treat pneumococcal strains will diminish. The possibility that new serotypes could emerge as novel replacement serotypes remains a threat, highlighting the need for ongoing surveillance.

Like HIB vaccines, conjugate pneumococcal vaccines are not available in all parts of the world. In the developing world, invasive pneumococcal disease remains the 5th leading cause of childhood mortality with an estimated one million deaths annually in children under five years of age. It is the single most common cause of bacterial meningitis beyond the newborn period in all age groups. By the end of 2009, 44 countries worldwide had introduced conjugate pneumococcal vaccine representing approximately 11% of the global birth cohort.

The prevention of invasive pneumococcal infection in developing areas of the world has been identified as a priority of the Bill and Melinda Gates Foundation. Working with the Global Alliance for Vaccines and Immunizations (GAVI), a collaborative effort between the World Health Organization (WHO), UNICEF, the U.S. Center for Disease Control and Prevention, and the World Bank, the Bill and Melinda Gates Foundation and other civil organizations have initiated a long term strategy to bring conjugate pneumococcal vaccine to eligible countries. Through the efforts and resources of GAVI, conjugate pneumococcal 13-valent vaccines have recently been introduced in Kenya, Sierra Leone, Yemen, Guyana, Honduras and Nicaragua. A dozen more countries will be included in the effort by the end of 2011, and 40 GAVI eligible countries will have infant and childhood pneumococcal vaccination programs by the end of 2015. Data to track the impact of such vaccine programs on childhood morbidity and mortality will be collected and shared with all stakeholders to ensure that the programs develop sustainability over time. Reminiscent of programs such as the polio vaccination partnership with the March of Dimes in the 1940s, this ambitious initiative will save lives and bring education regarding the value of immunizations to areas of the world that need them most.

2.3 Meningococcal vaccines

N. meningitidis is a gram-negative diplococcus that is commonly carried in the human nasopharynx. The specific risk factors that lead to invasive disease are incompletely defined. When an individual acquires the organism from another person, the most common outcome is colonization for a period of time. Some individuals can carry N. meningitidis in their upper respiratory tract for prolonged periods of time. Presumably, such individuals develop mucosal immune responses, including secretory immunoglobulin A that prevents invasion. Specific risk factors for the development of invasive disease include new acquisition of a new serotype, recent or current upper respiratory tract infection, smoking, alcohol consumption, and age.

When N. meningitidis invades, it enters the bloodstream, causing septicemia. Meningococcemia is classically associated with a petechial rash that rapidly progresses to purpura. It the most violent form of infection, referred to as purpura fulminans, death can ensue within a few hours. Bacteria seed the meninges in approximately half of all cases. Less commonly, patients develop lobar pneumonia, epiglottitis, septic arthritis, or purulent pericarditis. Meningitis accounts for nearly half of all invasive meningococcal infections; more than half of survivors have long-term complications including cognitive defects, cranial nerve palsies, and sensorineural hearing loss.

The 12 serogroups of N. meningitidis known to infect humans are characterized by the polysaccharide expressed on their capsule: A, B, C, 29-E, H, I, K, L, W-135, X, Y and Z. Clinically, the most relevant, and most prevalent types are A, B, C, W135, and Y. While uncommon, outbreaks caused by other capsular types have been described. Nasopharyngeal carriage of the bacterium is relatively common. In the U.S., carrier prevalence in the general population is approximately 10%. During the teen years, carriage has been described to be as high as 35%, and in environments of close contact such as military barracks and college residence halls, carriage rates may approach 100% (vanDeuren et al., 2000). The balance between carriage and the development of infection is influenced by both host and environmental factors (Caugant et al., 2007; Dull et al., 2001). Social factors also increase risk, such as intimate contact with an infected person, or living or working under crowded conditions, smoking, and alcohol consumption (MacLennan et al., 2006; Imrey et al. 1995).

The proportion of cases of meningococcal disease caused by individual serogroups A, B, C, W-135, and Y vary by geographic region. In developed countries, serogroup distribution also differs within regions. In Great Britain, for example, serogroups B and C account for over 90% of cases, while in New Zealand, serogroup B alone causes 87% of all cases. In contrast, meningococcal meningitis diagnosed in the African "meningitis belt," is usually caused by serogroup A. Attack rates during epidemics in Africa approach 1% of the population (Pinner et al., Moore P.s., 1992; Moore et al., 1989). In Saudi Arabia, where serogroup W-135 predominates, attack rates have been described at 25 per 100,000 population during the Hajj (Rosenstein et al., 2001; Pollard AJ, 2004; Wilder-Smith et al., 2003; Wilder-Smith et al., 2003). The country of Niger has recently experienced the emergence of serogroup X where it caused half of 1,139 cases in 2006 (Boisier et al., 20007).

In the U.S. between 1200 and 3500 cases of meningococcal disease occur annually (0.9 to 1.5 cases per 100,000 population). Data for 2006 through 2008 show that serogroups B, Y and C account for most of the U.S. cases (http://www.cdc.gov/abcs/reports-findings/survreports/mening09.html). Unlike the African 'meningitis belt', and areas of Asia where meningococcus type A infections are endemic, disease caused by serogroup A has not been detected in the U.S. since the late 1970s. Serotyping of 843 strains isolated between 1964 and 1967 demonstrated that serogroup A accounted for 1.3% of infections during that time period (Evans et al., 1968). An outbreak among skid row occupants occurred between 1975 and 1977 (Centers for Disease Control and Prevention 2009). Since that time, there has been a shift in serogroup predominance. Based on serotyping of 261 isolates from patients with meningococcal disease between 1989 and 1991, serogroups B and C accounted for more than 90% of cases. Furthermore, between 1998 and 2000, the proportion of serogroup Y cases increased from 2% to 33% of the total. Data for 2006 through 2008 show that serogroups Y (33%) and C (29%) continue to account for a large proportion of U.S. cases.

Given the fulminant nature of the infection, with an overall mortality rate of ~10%, prevention has become a priority. Vaccines for the prevention of invasive meningococcal infection were first available in the United States in 1971, but for more than two decades targeted only higher risk individuals. The first available vaccine, a polysaccharide capsular type C vaccine, was used almost exclusively in military recruits to control outbreaks that were being seen in military barracks. The high attack rate of meningococcal infection in this cohort of individuals is not surprising. Otherwise young, healthy individuals from different geographical areas of the country, where different N. meningitidis serotypes are prevalent, are brought together in close proximity under stressful conditions. Acquisition of a new serotype is common under such condition, and invasive disease more likely during physiologic stress and other behavioral risk factors.

A quadrivalent, non-conjugated pure polysaccharide meningococcal vaccine containing serotypes A, C, Y and W135 (Menomune) became available for use in the U.S. in 1981, and was primarily used to protect military recruits, travelers going to endemic areas and immunocompromised individuals. By 1999, the U.S. Centers for Disease Control and Prevention (CDC) and American College Health Association (ACHA) recommended the vaccine for all incoming college freshmen given the increased risk of invasive disease described in this population. As with other pure polysaccharide vaccines, protective immunity is short-lived, but given the brief period of increased risk in college freshman and in military recruits, the vaccine was widely used. As with pure polysaccharide HIB and pneumococcal vaccines, lack of T-cell engagement leads to inability to boost prior responses. Similarly, no change in nasopharyngeal carriage was expected. Subsequent vaccine development allowed for emerging conjugate vaccines, and led to changes in how these vaccines are used currently.

Globally, the first large scale experience with conjugate meningococcal vaccines occurred in the 1990s. One of the best examples comes from the United Kingdom where an epidemic of group C meningoccocal infection was causing a serious public health problem. The epidemic peaked in 1999 with an estimated 1500 cases and 150 deaths in that country alone. In November 1999, the public health ministry introduced a monovalent group C meningococcal vaccine as a public health measure, focusing first on vaccinating teenagers. Population based surveillance was used to monitor the incidence of disease as the vaccination program was introduced. Within 12 months of vaccine delivery through public health efforts, a marked decline in the incidence of disease was observed, and the vaccine program was expanded to young children. Vaccine effectiveness was estimated to be 90% for vaccinated individuals, but a broader scale benefit was noted for the overall population, argued to be secondary to a reduction in nasopharyngeal carriage of the organism leading to reductions in disease transmission among the unvaccinated population as well. The observation that conjugate vaccines lead to reductions in nasopharyngeal carriage and provide a community immunity benefit that extends to those who are not vaccinated is unique to conjugate vaccines as pure polysaccharide formulations do not afford this benefit. In addition to the monovalent conjugate group C vaccine used to control the U.K. epidemic, several other mono and bivalent conjugate vaccines are currently available in the global market.

The first conjugate meningococcal vaccine (which includes immunogens targeting the same four serotypes in the polysaccharide vaccine Menomune-- A, C, Y and W135) became available in the U.S. in 2005, it was immediately recommended that it replace polysaccharide vaccine for most individuals. Since clinical vaccine trials demonstrated safety and efficacy up to age 55, but not beyond, the polysaccharide vaccine is still officially recommended for individuals 55 years and older. Conjugate meningococcal vaccines are recommended for use in high risk individuals including those with terminal complement deficiency, asplenia, HIV infection, and in those who travel to areas of the world endemic for meningococcal infection. In addition, given the epidemiology of invasive meningococcal infection during adolescence, conjugate meningococcal vaccine was added to the universal immunization schedule starting at 11-12 years of age in 2005. Because of concerns that vaccine effectiveness may drift over time, the U.S. Advisory Committee on Immunization Practices added a second dose recommendation at age 16 years (up to age 21) as a booster.

Recent clinical trials have also evaluated the conjugate vaccines for safety and efficacy in younger children, and by 2011, vaccine became available for use as early as 9 mos of age for high-risk individuals and travelers (Menactra). A combination HIB-Meningococcal C/Y vaccine that was studied in clinical trials in the U.S. is currently under review for licensure by the Food and Drug Administration. In the U.S., the ACIP has been reluctant to recommend universal use of meningococcal conjugate vaccines under the age of 11 years, since more than half of infant infections are currently caused by the non-vaccine serotype B meningococcus. Meningococcal vaccines designed to protect individuals against serogroup B illness are in phase 3 clinical vaccine efficacy trials.

2.3.1 Meningococcus serotype B and the unique challenges it presents

Given the epidemiology of invasive meningococcal disease, including a substantial contribution from N. meningitidis type B should not be capitalized, it is logical to question why it has been so difficult to develop a serotype B vaccine. The native group B polysaccharide is a poor vaccine candidate because it contains epitopes that cross-react with sialylated proteins in human brain. New strategies have emerged to use alternative components of the group B meningococcus as vaccine antigens since such residues have been identified that are not cross reacting with the same human tissues. Ultimately, the development of a safe and effective B vaccine will likely capitalize on these non-cross reacting group B antigens from genetically modified strains. Several such vaccine candidates are already undergoing clinical trials.

Reported cases of meningococcal meningitis in the U.S. are currently at historically low rates. It is premature to credit the introduction and implementation of conjugate meningococcal vaccines for this epidemiologic observation, but in the coming years it will become clear whether this promising trend continues. The obvious decline in both HIB and pneumococcal meningitis following the introduction of vaccines for those infections is already compelling. Vaccine programs are highly effective. A summary of the current Advisory Committee on Immunization Practices for use of HIB, pneumococcal and meningococcal vaccines in summarized in **Table 2.**

Vaccine	Age Given	Recommendation	High Risk Conditions
HIB conjugate	2, 4, 6, 12-15 mos*	Universal	Universal
Pneumococcal polysaccharide	After 23 mos	Following conjugate series, 2 doses 5 yrs apart	Sickle cell disease, asplenia, inherited or acquired immune deficiency, chronic cardiac and/or pulmonary disease, CSF leaks, renal insufficiency, diabetes
Pneumococcal conjugate	2, 4, 6, 12-15 mos	Universal	Universal
Meningococcal polysaccharide	56 yrs and older	High risk	See risk factors in conjugate box below. Meningococcal conjugate vaccine not approved for use after age 55 yrs.
Meningococcal conjugate	11-21 yrs 9 mos-55 yrs	Universal High Risk	Universal Terminal complement or properdin deficiency, asplenia, military recruits, college freshman living in catered halls, HIV infection, travel to endemic areas of the world

*6 mos dose not needed if PedvaxHIB is used

Table 2. Summary of recommendations from the Advisory Committee on Immunization Practices (ACIP) of the United States for the use of HIB, pneumococcal and meningococcal vaccines

3. References

Berg S, Trollfors B, Claesson BA, Alestig K, Gothefors L, Hugosson S, Lindquist L, Olcen P, Romanus V, Strangert K. Incidence and prognosis of meningitis due to Haemophilus influenzae, Streptococcus pneumoniae and Neisseria meningitides in Sweden. *Scand J Infect Dis.* 1996;28:247-252.

Boisier P, Nicolas P, Djibo S, Taha MK, Jeanne I, Mainassara HB, Tenebray B, Kairo KK, Giorgini D, Chanteau S. Meningococcal meningitis:unprecedented incidence of serogroup X-related cases in 2006 in Niger. *Clin Infect Dis* 2007;44:657-663.

Caugant DA, Tzanakaki G, Kriz P. Lessons from meningococcal carriage studies. *FEMS Microbiol Rev*. 2007;31(1):52-63.

Centers for Disease Control and Prevention. Notifiable diseases/deaths in selected cities weekly information. *MMWR*. 2009;58(16):440-451.

Dull PM, Abdelwahab J, Sacchi CT, et al. Neisseria menigitidis serogroup W-135 carriage among US travelers to the Hajj. *J Infect Dis*. 2005;191:33-39.

Evans JR, Artenstein MS, Hunter DH. Prevalence of meningococcal serogroup and description of 3 new groups. *Am J Epidemiol*. 1968;87:643-646.

Filice GA, Englender SJ, Jacobson JA, et al. Group A meningococcal disease in skid rows: epidemiology and implications for control *Am J Public Health*. 1984;74:253-254.

Giorgi Rossi P, Mantovani J, Ferroni E, Forcina A, Stranghellini E, Curtale F, Borgia P. Incidence of bacterial meningitis (2001-2005) in Lazio, Italy: the results of an intergrated surveillance system. *BMC Infect*. 2009;9:13.

Greenwood BM. 1987. The epidemiology of acute bacterial meningitis in tropical Africa, p.93-113. In JD Williams and J Burnie (ed), Bacterial meningitis. *Academic Press, London, UK*.

Imrey PB, Jackson LA, Ludwinski PH, et al. Meningococcal carriage, alcohol consumption, and campus bar patronage in a serogroup C meningococcal disease outbreak. *J Clin Microbiol*. 1995;33:3133-3137.

MacLennan J, Kafatos G, Neal K, et al. Social behavior and meningococcal carriage in British teenagers. *Emerg Infect Dis*. 2006;12:950-957.

Mishal J, Embon A, Darawshe A, Kidon M, Magen E. Community acquired acute bacterial meningitis in children and adults: an 11 year survey in a community hospital in Israel. *Eur J Intern Med*. 2008;19:421-426.

Moore PS, Reeves MW, Schwartz B, Gellin BG, Broome CV. Intercontinental spread of an epidemic group A Neisseria meningitides strain. 1989 *Lancet* ii:260-263.

Moore PS. Meningococcal meningitis in sub-Saharan Africa: a model for the epidemic process. *Clin Infect Dis* 1992;14:515-525.

Pinner RW, Gellin BG, Bibb WF, Baker CN, Weaver R, Hunter SB, Waterman SH, Mocca LF, Frasch CE, Broome CV. Meningococcal disease in the UNited States- 1986. Meningococcal Disease Study Group. *J Infect Dis* 1991;164:368-374.

Pollard AJ. Global epidemiology of meningococcal disease and vaccine efficacy. *Pediatr Infect Dis J*. 2004;23(12 suppl):S274-S279.

Rosenstein NE, Perkins BA, Stephens DS, et al. Meningococcal disease. *N Engl J Med*. 2001;344:1378-1388.

Scarborough M, Gordon SB, Whitty CJ, French N, Njalale Y, Chitani A, Peto TE, Lalloo DG, Zijlstra EE. Corticosteroids for bacterial meningitis in adults in sub-Saharan Africa. *N Engl J Med* 2007;357:2441-2450.

Scarborough M, Thwaites GE. The diagnosis and management of acute bacterial meningitis in resource-poor settings. *Lancet Neurol* 2008;7:637-648.

Schlech WF, Ward JI, Band JD, Hightower A, Fraser DW, Broome CV. Bacterial meningitis in the UNited States, 1978 through 1981. The national bacterial meningitis surveillance study. *JAMA* 1985;253:1749-1754.

Schuchat A, Robinson K, Wenger JD, Harrison LH, Farley M, Reingold AL, Lefkowitz L, Perkins BA. Bacterial meningitis in the United States in 1995. Active surveillance team. *N Engl J Med* 1997;337:970-976.

Theodoridou MN, Vasilopoulou VA, Atsali EE, PAngalis AM, Mostrou GJ, Syriopoulou VP, Hadjichristodoulou. Meningitis registry of hospitalized cases in children: epidemiological patterns of acute bacterial meningitis throughout a 32-year period. *BMC Infect Dis* 2007;7:101.

Tsai CJ, Griffen MR, Nuorti JP, Grijalva CG. Changinf epidemiology of pneumococcal meningitis after the introduction of pneumococcal conjgate vaccine in the United States. *Clin Infect Dis.* 2008;46:1664-1672.

Urwin G, Yuan MF, Feldman RA. Prospective study of bacterial meningitis in North East Thames region, 1991-3, during introduction of Haemophilus influenzae vaccine. *BMJ* 1994;308:1412-1414.

van Deuren M, Brandtzaeg P, van der Meer JW. Update on meningococcal disease with emphasis on pathogenesis and clinical management. *Clin Microbiol Rev.* 2000;13:144-166.

Weiss DP, Coplan P, Guess H. Epidemiology of bacterial meningitis among children in Brazil, 1997-1998. *Rev Saude Publica* 2001;35:249-255.

Wenger JD, Hightower AW, Facklam RR, Gaventa S, Broome CV. Bacterial meningitis in the Unites States, 1986: report of a multi-state surveillance study. The bacterial meningitis study group. *J Infect Dis* 1990;162:1316-1323.

Whitney CG, Farley MM, Hadler J, Harrison LH, Bennett NM, Lynfield R, Reingold A, Cieslak PR, Pilishvili T, Jackson D, Facklam RR, Jorgensen JH, Schuchat A. Decline in invasive pneumococcal disease after the introduction of protein-polysaccharide conjugate vaccine. *N Engl J Med* 2003;348:1737-1746.

Wilder-Smith A, Barkham TMS, Ravindran S, et al. Persistence of W135 *Neisseria meningitidis* Carriage in Returning Hajj Pilgrims: Risk for Early and Late Transmission to Household Contacts. *Emerg Infect Dis.* 2003;9:123-126.

Wilder-Smith A, Goh KT, Barkham T, Patoon NI. Hajj-associated outbreak strain of Neisseria meningitides serogroup W135: estimates of the attack rate in a defined population and the risk of invasive disease developing in carriers. *Cin Infect Dis* 2003;36:679-683.

http://www.cdc.gov/abcs/reports-findings/survreports/mening09.html
Accessed March 6, 2011

7

Tuberculous Meningitis

Maria Kechagia, Stavroula Mamoucha, Dimitra Adamou,
George Kanterakis, Aikaterini Velentza, Nicoletta Skarmoutsou,
Konstantinos Stamoulos and Eleni-Maria Fakiri
Sismanoglion General Hospital, Department of Microbiology,
Greece

1. Introduction

Tuberculosis (TB) was initially described during the fifth century B.C. by Hippocrates who reported patients with "consumption" (the Greek term is *phthisis*), a term used to describe wasting associated with chest pain, coughing and blood in the sputum. Since then it remains a devastating disease with more than 9 million new cases and over 1 million related deaths among human immunodeficiency syndrome (HIV) negative populations every year (Smith, 2003; Yasar et al., 2011). *Mycobacterium tuberculosis* complex, the causative agent of human TB is the most common pathogen of both pulmonary and non pulmonary tuberculosis cases, nevertheless as a result of their association with HIV infections nontuberculous *Mycobacteria* (NTM) species are encountered with increasing frequency. While pulmonary disease is the most common manifestation of TB, the involvement of the central nervous system (CNS) and associated tuberculous meningitis (TBM) represents its most severe form (Christensen et al., 2011; Puccioni-Sohler & Brandão, 2007; Venkataswamy et al., 2007). The case fatality rate of untreated TBM is almost 100% and a delay in treatment may lead to permanent neurological damage, therefore prompt diagnosis is needed for the timely initiation of antituberculous therapy in order to prevent secondary complications (Chandramuki et al., 2002). TBM may also involve children with the peak incidence during the first 4 years of life (van Well et al., 2009; Haldar et al., 2009).

2. Causative agents of tuberculous meningitis

Mycobacteria are aerobic, nonmotile, gram-positive rods ranging in appearance from spherical to short filaments, which may be branched. Their cell wall contains lipids, peptidoglycans, and arabinomannans. One distinct characteristic is their ability to retain dyes that are usually removed from other microorganisms by alcohols and dilute solutions of strong mineral acids such as hydrochloric acid. This ability is attributed to a waxlike layer composed of mycolic acids in their cell wall. As a result, they are termed acid-fast bacilli (AFB) after Ziehl-Neelsen (ZN) staining (Panicker et al., 2010; Rajni et al., 2011). The causative agents of TBM are mainly the members of *M. tuberculosis* complex and less commonly NTM. The incidence of CNS infection due to the latter has increased substantially since the onset of the HIV epidemic (Lai et al., 2008; Puccioni-Sohler &

Brandão, 2007). According to literature, although the NTM species involved in theaetiopathogenesis of meningitis include all four groups of the Runyon classification, those more commonly encountered are the *Mycobacterium avium* complex (MAC), *Mycobacterium kansasii, M. bovis, M. abscessus, M. fortuitum* and *Mycobacterium nonchromogenicum,* the latter being a nonpigmented, slow growing organism which belongs to Runyon group III and a part of the *Mycobacterium terrae* complex. It is reported that *M. avium* complex remains the most common organism causing systemic opportunistic bacterial infections in patients with HIV infection, carrying a higher mortality rate despite appropriate treatment, while *M. kansasii* meningitis is similar to *M. tuberculosis* meningitis. Therefore, when NTM are isolated in culture of cerebrospinal fluid (CSF), they should not routinely be dismissed as contaminants but considered a significant finding (Cegielski & Wallace, 1997; Flor et al., 1996; Jacob et al., 1993; Koirala, 2001; Lai et al., 2008; Maniu et al., 2001; Mayo et al., 1998; Puccioni-Sohler & Brandão, 2007; Wu et al., 2000).

3. Epidemiology

Tuberculosis of the central nervous system is the most severe manifestation of extrapulmonary TB and constitutes approximately 1% of all new cases annually, with TBM being the commonest form of the disease (Christensen et al., 2011). Several studies have attempted to assess its epidemiology with variable conclusions as the disease's incidence and mortality rates differ from country to country according to their individual socioeconomic and public health statuses. Mortality rates for instance have been described to range from 7 - 40% in developed countries, while the percentages from TB endemic countries as well as countries with high HIV prevalence have been found to be significantly higher, reaching a 69% in South Africa (Karstaedt et al., 1998; Kent et al., 1993). The key point in understanding the epidemiological pattern of the disease is the fact that TBM and tuberculosis infection are closely related in this aspect, so that it is generally accepted that occurrence of the former in a community is correlated with incidence of the latter and vice versa (Chakraborty, 2000). It is therefore considered safe to assume that at a global level these two entities share a common trend. According to the latest available data, in 2009 the global incidence of TB was 9.4 million cases which is equivalent to 137 cases per 100 000 population with most of them occurring in Asia and Africa and a smaller proportion occurring in Europe and the Region of the Americas. Developing countries in particular account for more than 80% of the active cases in the world. The global incidence rate after an initial fall during the 20th century rose due to the HIV epidemic with a peak in 2004 and a subsequent slow but steady decline that also involves the absolute number of TB related deaths. This impact of HIV on TB has accordingly influenced the pattern of TBM's incidence rates (Dye et al., 2009; Varaine et al., 2010; World Health Organization [WHO], 2010). In fact, HIV infection constitutes the most important determinant for the development of TBM followed by age. As far as the latter is concerned it is in turn determined by the socioeconomic status of a certain population. Therefore in populations with a low TB prevalence adults seem to be more affected than children. This is reversed in populations with a higher TB prevalence. Concerning childhood disease, TBM appears to affect mainly children under the age of 5 years with the mean age ranging from 23 to 49 months and according to literature close contact with a confirmed case of pulmonary tuberculosis is usually the culprit (van Well et al., 2009).

4. Pathophysiology

Since the first description of the disease in 1936 there has been undisputable progress in the understanding of the pathogenesis of TBM, with further ongoing research in the field. Nevertheless, the exact mechanism of establishment of this uncommon yet devastating manifestation of tuberculosis has not been fully elucidated. The disease develops as a result of a new infection or of reactivation of a latent one, but in both cases it constitutes a disseminated form of a primary extrameningeal focus rather than a primary localization of the tuberculous infection. According to recent evidence certain strains seem to be more capable of dissemination and might be more predominant in the development of CNS disease with the exact mechanisms of neurovirulence being uncertain (Arvanitakis et al., 1998; Nicolic, 1996). In this direction, studies have demonstrated the possible influence of the *M. tuberculosis* genotype in association with the host's genetic polymorphisms on the disease phenotype as different mycobacterial genotypes seem to induce separate patterns of host immune response (Dormans et al., 2004; Manca et al., 2004; Reed et al., 2004). For instance, there is evidence that some strains of *M. tuberculosis* commonly found in Europe and America are less likely to cause tuberculous meningitis in Vietnamese adults than strains predominantly found in Asia (Caws et al., 2008). The pathogenesis of TBM at a cellular level is incompletely understood. According to modern concepts the triad of macrophages, T helper lymphocytes and the host plays a central role and through interactions of its components the produced γ-interferon, interleukin 1-β and tumour necrosis factor promote granuloma formation in a manner similar to pulmonary disease. On a macroscopic level it is evident that the development of TBM is a two- step process, the onset of which is the entrance of the bacilli into the host with subsequent lung invasion and regional lymph node dissemination leading to the primary complex formation. In case of central nervous system involvement the characteristic lesions known as Rich's foci, first described in the early 1930s, which represent tuberculous subpial or subependymal foci about 1 mm in diameter, are formed through spread of the bacilli to the meninges or brain parenchyma (Be et al., 2009; Drevets at al., 2004). Although it is unclear whether *M. tuberculosis* crosses the blood brain barrier as an extra-cellular organism or via infected phagocytes (Chackerian et al., 2002), the spread takes place haematogenously. This transport occurs either during the short stage of bacteremia that accompanies the primary complex formation or as a result of a more prolonged bacteremia in those cases in which the primary compex fails to heal and which account for the 10% of all cases. If miliary TB develops, dissemination to the CNS is more probable and seems to be particularly involved in the pathogenesis of TBM in childhood (Donald et al., 2005). The infrequent possibility of direct spread from a site of tuberculous otitis or calvarial osteitis also exists. When mycobacteria are deposited in large numbers as part of primary tuberculosis in infants or young children, they form the characteristic lesions and cause TBM usually within six months of primary infection (Garg, 1999; Prince, 2002). However, in adults and older children deposited mycobacteria may not elicit any immune response and may cause latent disease until immune recognition or reactivation causes formation of the CNS lesions. The second step of the process involves the rupture of a Rich's focus and the release of bacilli into the subarachnoid space giving rise to a T cell dependent granulomatous inflammatory response resulting in the development of tuberculous meningitis (Burns, 1997). This inflammatory reaction can lead to adhesion formation due to the cell and fibrin rich basal meningeal exudates, to obliterative vasculitis mainly affecting the internal carotid artery, proximal middle cerebral artery and perforating vessels of the basal ganglia, or may even extend into the parenchyma leading to encephalitis. If the adhesions compromise the interpendicular fossa, cranial nerves (mainly II, IV and VI) are affected while in case of obstruction of the basal cisterns, the outflow of the forth ventricle or the cerebral aqueduct, hydrocephalus develops, the presence of which has been associated with poor prognosis and therapeutic failure (Lu et al., 2001). Vasculitis and parenchymal involvement lead to infarctions (most often involving the distribution of the middle cerebral artery and striate arteries) and encephalitis respectively, which account for the majority of the neurological deficits of the disease. Another entity of tuberculous meningitis is that affecting the spinal cord. Spinal meningitis can either develop due to direct extension from the vertebrae, secondary to downward extension of intracranial TBM or less commonly as a primary tuberculous lesion. In the fist case, tuberculous involvement of vertebral bodies known as Pott's disease is established through either haematogenous spread of the bacillus or less frequently through spread from involved contiguous para-aortic lymph nodes. In case of extension of intracranial disease, the most usual mechanism is the rupture of a Rich's focus into the spinal arachnoid space instead of the basal meninges (Dass et al., 2002; Garg, 1999; Harsha et al., 2006).

5. Clinical features

Tuberculosis of the central nervous system may take several forms, which cannot be easily classified (Table 1). Besides inflammation of the meninges, which is the most common form (Blaivas et al., 2005), it also includes space-occupying lesions in the brain parenchyma as well as focal disease of the spinal cord and its osseous structures.

Intracranial central nervous system tuberculosis	Tuberculous meningitis Tuberculous meningitis with miliary tuberculosis Tuberculous encephalopathy Tuberculous vasculopathy Central nervous system tuberculoma Tuberculous brain abscess
Spinal central nervous system tuberculosis	Pott's spine and paraplegia Tuberculous arachnoiditis Non osseous spinal tuberculoma Spinal meningitis

Table 1. Classification of central nervous system tuberculosis

Each of these variable entities may represent a distinct subset of the central nervous system tuberculous infection or severe sequelae of TBM. Due to the significant overlap that exists between the clinical features of TBM and those of its complications, in this section besides TBM we will also emphasize on those manifestations that are part of its continuum, without differentiating them from the disease's spectrum.

5.1 Intracranial tuberculous meningitis

TBM is characterized by a broad spectrum of manifestations, posing a diagnostic challenge and requiring a high index of clinical suspicion (Table 2). TBM tends to present subacutely, over a period of variable duration that ranges in literature from weeks to months (Christensen et al., 2011; Komolafe et al., 2008; Newton, 1994) but in the majority of patients there is a history of vague non specific symptoms of a duration of two to eight weeks prior to meningeal irritation. These prodromal symptoms are constitutional and include malaise, fatigue, anorexia, fever and headache. According to studies, 75% of individuals have a tuberculous infection at least twelve months before admission for meningitis and radiological evidence of active pulmonary tuberculosis is present at a 30-50% of the cases upon admission (Cherian & Thomas, 2011; D'Souza et al., 2002). At the time of examination adults usually present with altered mental status ranging from lethargy to coma, meningeal symptoms and focal neurological signs but studies have demonstrated that meningeal stiffness may be absent in as many as three quarters and headache and fever in as many as 25% of the patients (Christensen et al., 2011). In infants prodromal symptoms include irritability, drowsiness, poor feeding, and abdominal pain often associated with neck retraction and bulging fontanelles. As far as the elderly are concerned, headache and mental status changes are more common, on the other hand fever is frequently absent (Berger, 1995). Atypical presentations include a rapid progression mimicking pyogenic meningitis, dementia, and a predominant syndrome of encephalitis with frequent convulsions occurring at any stage (Christie et al, 2008; Golden & Vikram, 2005). Cranial nerve palsies occur in 20-30% of patients due to adhesions and may be the presenting manifestation of the disease or complicate its course. They most commonly involve cranial nerves II, III, IV, VI and VII, with VI being the one most commonly affected. Focal neurological deficits may also include hemiplegia, monoplegia and aphasia. Visual manifestations include visual impairment and opthalmoplegia and are attributed to optochiasmatic arachnoiditis, compression of optic chiasm in the setting of hydrocephalus, or optic nerve granulomas (Malik et al., 2002; Sinha et al., 2010). In case of tuberculomas or tuberculous brain abscess complicating meningitis the clinical features vary in accordance to their location. Tuberculous arachnoiditis is a rare complication of intracranial TBM, as a result of downward extension of the latter, that can lead to severe peripheral neurological deficit (Poon et al., 2003) often after an initial response to antituberculosis treatment, while syndrome of inappropriate antidiuretic hormone (SIADH) secretion is not an uncommon complication and is linked to a poor prognosis. As the inflammatory process progresses it might result in foci of encephalitis properly described as a diffuse meningoencephalitis with symptoms of cerebral disorder predominating and evolving from increasing lethargy to terminal illness coma (Drevets at al., 2004)

5.2 Spinal tuberculous meningitis

The clinical picture of spinal tuberculous meningitis is variable, depending on the stage of the disease and the mechanism involved in its pathogenesis. When secondary to a Rich's focus rupture, it may present acutely with fever, headache, radiating root pain and myelopathy, or progress gradually with symptoms of spinal cord compression dominating the picture which may lead to misdiagnosis of an intradural tumor. The clinical spectrum may also include paradoxical reaction after initiating antituberculous therapy, spinal arachnoiditis, and simultaneous or preceding manifestations of TBM. If Pott's disease is in the background, chronic manifestations of variable intensity reflecting the progressive destruction of the involved disc space and vertebral elements precede the meningeal involvement and should guide the diagnosis. In such cases spinal meningitis is associated with focal tenderness over the spinous processes, focal kyphosis and cord compression phenomena, depending on the level of the spine that is affected (Garg, 1999; Harsha et al., 2006; McLain & Isada, 2004).

Symptoms	Signs
Headache Vomiting Low grade fever Lassitude Depression Confusion Behavioural changes	Meningism Oculomotor palsies Papilloedema Depressed level of consciousness Focal hemisphere signs

Table 2. Most common clinical features of tuberculous meningitis (adapted from Allen & Lueck, 2002)

6. Staging

TBM tends to be classified according to its severity at presentation in an attempt to assess prognosis. The Medical Research Council staging system has been applied since 1948 to patients with TBM and uses three stages of increasing severity. Stage I refers to alert patients without focal neurological signs, stage II to non comatose patients with altered consciousness and focal neurological deficits and stage III to comatose patients and those with multiple cranial nerve palsies and hemiplegia or/and paraplegia (Prasad & Singh, 2008). Modifications of the above mentioned staging system have been adopted in recent literature (Heemskerk et al., 2011). The Acute Physiology and Chronic Health Evaluation II as well as the Glasgow Coma Scale have also been proposed for predicting the outcome of patients with TBM and are considered superior to the Medical Research Council scoring system by certain authors (Chou et al., 2010). Nevertheless, it is uniformly accepted that the stage of TBM at the onset of treatment seems to be the most crucial determinant of outcome, with mortality being highest if treatment started at Medical Research Council stage III.

7. Differential diagnosis

The diagnosis of TBM is challenging as it may mimic a wide range of medical conditions. It is generally based on clinical grounds and cerebrospinal fluid (CSF) examination (Table 3). The differential diagnosis of the disease is particularly wide and at a clinical basis includes:

1. Infections: bacterial (partially treated bacterial meningitis, brain abscess, listeriosis, *Neisseria* species infection, tularemia, brucellosis), spirochetal, viral (herpes, mumps, retrovirus, enterovirus), fungal (cryptococcal, histoplasmosis, actinomycetic, nocardiasis, candidiasis, coccidiosis) and parasitic (cysticercosis, acanthamoebiasis, strongyloidiasis, toxoplasmosis)
2. Non infective conditions: vasculitis, systemic lupus erythematosus, neoplastic, chemical meningitis, cardiovascular, Behçet disease, acute hemorrhagic leukoencephalopathy etc.

CONDITION	WHITE BLOOD CELLS	PROTEIN	GLUCOSE
TBM	Elevated, L > PMN	Increased	Decreased
Cryptococcal meningitis	Elevated, L > PMN	Increased	Decreased
Partially treated bacterial meningitis	Elevated	Increased	Decreased
Viral meningitis	Elevated, L > PMN	Increased	Normal or decreased
Acute syphilis	Elevated, L > PMN	Increased	Normal
Late stage trypanosomiasis	Elevated, L > PMN	Increased	Decreased
Malignancy	Elevated, L > PMN	Increased	Decreased
Leptospirosis	Elevated, L > PMN	Increased	Decreased
Amoebic	Elevated, L > PMN	Increased	Decreased

PMN: polymorphonuclear leucocytes, L: lymphocytes

Table 3. Differential diagnosis of TBM based on CSF findings (adapted from Harries et al., 2004)

From a radiological point of view, taking into consideration the fact that bacterial meningitis, therefore TBM as well, is not an imaging diagnosis, such investigations are carried out in order to exclude the presence of other conditions mimicking meningitis and to detect possible contraindications for lumbar puncture such as increased intracranial pressure. Based on radiological findings the differential diagnosis of TBM also includes other infectious agents as well as non-infectious inflammatory diseases affecting the leptomeninges and neoplastic meningeal involvement (meningiomatosis, neoplastic meningitis from a peripheral tumor source etc.) (Junewick, 2010).

8. Laboratory diagnosis

Taking into consideration the fact that the high mortality rate associated with TB meningitis is related to its late diagnosis as well as the difficulties not only in obtaining a precise history but also in collecting an adequate volume of CSF for laboratory investigation, lumbar puncture and the examination of CSF are key points in its diagnosis.

8.1 CSF parameters

Examination of CSF in TBM usually reveals an increase in pressure with the fluid's appearance ranging from clear to slightly turbid with, occasionally, a delicate web-like clot formation, due to the high protein level that is typical to the disease and a pleocytosis of 10–1000 leucocytes/ mm^3 with a lymphocytic predominance. The cell count rarely exceeds these values, on the contrary it is less than 500/ mm^3 in the majority of cases. CSF biochemistry reveals reduced glucose levels, increased lactate levels, while protein levels are increased, especially in cases in which there is a CSF flow obstruction and which are associated with a worse prognosis. Early in the course of the disease a polymorphonuclear reaction as well as normal biochemical parameters might be found complicating the differential diagnosis, particularly from bacterial meningitis. This polymorphonuclear predominance has been associated with a higher culture positivity and may even have a prognostic value, especially in HIV positive patients. In fact these patients occasionally exhibit a persistent polymorphonuclear predominance, which has been associated to higher survival rates, as it seems to have a protective role against *M. tuberculosis* (Hooker et al., 2003; Puccioni-Sohler & Brandão, 2007). For the performance of a total cell count of the CSF a fresh sample is loaded into an improved Neubauer chamber. A proportion of the fluid is centrifuged at 3000 g for 15 min and from the sediment obtained, a Giemsa stained smear must be examined for the differential cell count (Christensen et al., 2011; Hooker et al., 2003; Kashyap et al., 2010; Puccioni-Sohler & Brandão, 2007; Ramachandran, 2011; Thwaites et al., 2004).

8.2 Microscopy

As far as the direct microscopy of a Ziehl-Neelsen stained smear is concerned, it should be conducted in all cases despite the low sensitivity of the examination attributed to the paucibacillary nature of the CSF. Each slide must be examined under the oil immersion lens for about 30 min, with care being taken to view at least 300–500 high power fields. It is proposed for each slide to be re-examined by an independent examiner to ensure accuracy. The sensitivity of the method ranges from 10-87% depending on the volume and the number of the samples and might drop to 2% after 5-15 days following the onset of treatment (Puccioni-Sohler & Brandão, 2007; Thwaites et al., 2004). The Ziehl-Neelsen stain remains an important diagnostic tool in tuberculosis since its first introduction in 1882 by Robert Koch as it identifies the most infectious cases, it is rapid, inexpensive, technically simple, and specific for AFB. However, it is unable to discriminate between *M. tuberculosis* and other mycobacteria, lacks sensitivity, and cannot be applied in the monitoring of treatment, as it does not discriminate between viable and non–viable bacilli. Its sensitivity appears to be lower in non-respiratory specimens due to the lower bacterial load as well as for some NTM species due to poorer staining of their cell wall (Mamoucha et al., 2010).

8.3 Solid and liquid culture media

Mycobacterial culture is the microbiological Gold Standard method for the confirmation of TBM as the isolation of *M. tuberculosis* from CSF makes a definite diagnosis of the disease, although in the setting of a strong clinical suspicion the isolation of the agent from other specimens such as gastric aspirate, bronchial aspirate, sputum or lymph node also guides the diagnosis (Kashyap et al., 2010; van Well et al., 2009). There is a variety of culture media used for this purpose. These include egg-based (Lövenstein-Jensen-LJ, Petragnani, American Trudeau Society, and Ogawa), agar-based (Middlebrook 7H10 and 7H11) and liquid media (Middlebrook 7H9, Kirchner, BioFM and Dubos). Due to the slow growth of the organism (40 to 60 days), this exam is useful only from an epidemiological point of view. In order to shorten the time of detection, Centers for Disease Control and Prevention (CDC) have recommended the use of liquid media for primary culture. Liquid culture medium has been designed to significantly reduce incubation time to 12-15 days and has been reported in various studies. Liquid TB culture media and Middlebrook 7H10 agar-based media, have been shown to increase the yield of TB particularly from body fluids but the highest recovery rate has been obtained using a combination of both (Fadzilah et al., 2009; Kashyap et al., 2010; Khosravi et al., 2009; Mamoucha et al., 2010; Panicker et al. 2010;

Piersimoni & Scarparo, 2008; Sorlozano et al., 2009). This may be attributed to the fact that in liquid cultures a mix of growth supplements (OADC- Oleic acid, Albumin, Dextrose, Catalase) and antibiotics (PANTA- Polymyxin B, Amphotericin B, Nalidixic acid, Trimethoprim, Azlocillin) are used, which collectively prevent the growth of environmental bacteria. According to literature, the isolation rate on MGIT 960 has been found 7.4% (Tortoli et al., 1999), 18.36% (Rishi et al., 2007) or 11.6% (Selvakumar et al., 1996), while using LJ medium the isolation rate has been found 4.3-6.5% (Rishi et al., 2007; Venkataswamy et al., 2007). Growth on the surface of the LJ slope is indicated by the production of raised, dry, cream coloured colonies while on Kirchner media by the formation of a surface pellicle, which should then be subjected to ZN stain and subcultured onto LJ slopes for confirmation and further identification (Hooker et al., 2003; Panicker et al., 2010). A positive result must be confirmed by performing a ZN smear of the colonies, with AFB being demonstrated. Furthermore, owing to the paucibacillary nature of cerebrospinal fluid, some authors propose filtration of the sample and inoculation of the residue on the culture media in order to increase the sensitivity of the method (Kumar et al., 2008).

8.4 Adenosine deaminase levels and TBM

Adenosine deaminase (ADA) is an enzyme involved in the purine catabolism by catalyzing the deamination of adenosine to inosine and of deoxyadenosine to deoxyinosine and is found in all tissues, particularly those of the lymphoid system. High ADA levels in tuberculosis are related to the activated T lymphocytes and macrophages in response to the tuberculous antigens (Blake & Berman, 1982) and in our laboratory their determination in pleural fluid has been routinely used as an aid in the establishment of tuberculous or nontuberculous aetiology of pleural effusion in variable clinical settings. As far as its role in the diagnostic approach of TBM is concerned, although still controversial, it is considered to be an inexpensive, simple and rapid method that could be used routinely following a lumbar puncture. On this basis certain methods have been developed for the determination of ADA activity with the Giusti-Galanti one being the most commonly used (Laniado-Laborin, 2005; Oosthuizen et al., 1993). Moreover several studies have been conducted indicating that the ADA levels in CSF are higher in TBM than in nontuberculous meningitis. Depending on each study's selected cutoff values the sensitivity and specificity for ADA have exhibited slight heterogeneity. In fact, CFS ADA cutoff value of 6.5 IU/L showed a sensitivity of 95.83% and a specificity of 92.85% (Baheti et al., 2001), while cutoff of 10 IU/L has been associated with a sensitivity and a specificity of 94.73% and 90.47% respectively (Gupta et al., 2010). However a meta-analysis study that was conducted recently in order to evaluate its diagnostic use concluded that ADA, irrespectively of the cutoff levels adopted, cannot distinguish between TBM and nontuberculous meningitis, but suggested that the use of ranges of its CFS values could have a role in improving TBM diagnosis, especially after bacterial meningitis has been excluded (Tuon et al., 2010). Thus the role of ADA activity determination in the diagnosis of TBM is still questionable by many scientists with emphasis on the need of standardization of the methodology applied as well as of its cutoff values. Nevertheless, the enzyme's levels are still considered as an additional diagnostic tool.

8.5 Molecular diagnosis

The need of a rapid diagnosis in the case of TBM has made the use of molecular techniques essential. Although the majority of commercial tests are licensed for nonrespiratory specimens only, many of them have been in use along with in-house techniques and will be mentioned here, keeping in mind the fact that the data concerning their diagnostic value are based at large on the experience from studies emphasizing on respiratory samples. Even in such specimens, due to the need for further standardization between the different protocols and for implementation of solid guidelines concerning the evaluation of their results - attributed to the methods' innate disadvantages of practical nature as well as to the paucity of clinical data - their exact role remains controversial (Dora et al., 2008; Soini & Musser, 2001). Nucleic acid-based amplification (NAA) tests allow the direct detection of mycobacterial DNA or RNA and they include both in-house and commercial tests with the latter being more standardized and therefore more reliable. Post-amplification analysis includes electrophoresis, hybridization, restriction or sequencing of the products with hybridization being the most commonly used one. The Amplified *Mycobacterium tuberculosis* Direct Test (AMTD2, Gen-Probe, bioMerieux, Marcy, L'Etoile, France) which is based on the amplification of a *Mycobacterium tuberculosis* specific region of 16S rRNA using a reverse transcriptase was the first one to be approved by the Food and Drug Administration (FDA) in 1995, with its recommendations also including extrapulmonary samples, followed by the Amplicor *M. tuberculosis* test (Roche Diagnostic System Inc., Basel Switzerland) in 1996, which targets a segment of the same gene with the use of standard polymerase chain reaction (PCR). Other methods described include the BD ProbeTec ET Direct TB System (DTB, Becton Dickinson) which is a strand displacement amplification method targeting the IS6110 and 16S genes, the GenoType Mycobacteria Direct (Hain LifeScience, Nahren, Germany) and the INNO-LiPA Rif. TB kit (Innogenetics, Gent, Belgium), both using nucleic acid sequenced based amplification (NASBA) and offering the advantage of detecting not only members of the *M. tuberculosis* complex but certain common NTM as well. Newer techniques based on real-time PCR amplify simultaneously different DNA targets followed by fluorimetric detection and are considered promising. Among them the GeneXpertMTB/RIF (Cepheid, Summyvale, CA, USA and FIND Diagnostics, Geneva, Switzerland), which also offers the possibility for detection of RIF resistance, has recently been approved by the WHO (Alcaide & Coll, 2011; Dora et al., 2008; Soini & Musser, 2001). On the other hand, the in-house techniques use the PCR in order to amplify specific regions of *Mycobacterium tuberculosis* genome varying from one institution to another, with the IS6110 (Insertion sequence 6110) element and devR element (Haldar et al., 2009; Michael et al., 2002) being the ones most commonly used. Reported results of the molecular tests in CSF specimens vary in different studies with reported sensitivity and specificity ranging from 50%-87.6% and 92%-98.6% respectively (Dora et al., 2008; Haldar et al., 2009; Pai et al., 2003). This low sensitivity could be attributed to the volume of the sample, given the lower number of bacteria usually found in the CSF compared to other compartments, therefore the minimum suggested volume of the fluid is 2ml (Michael et al., 2002). In conclusion both commercial and in-house molecular techniques might have a role in confirming TBM, although their low sensitivity doesn't seem to allow them to exclude it with certainty.

9. Treatment of TBM

The most important determinant of TBM's prognosis is the stage of the disease at the time of initiation of appropriate treatment with evidence indicating that timely onset during the early phase of infection can significantly improve the outcome. Therefore, any patient suspected of having TBM based on the clinical symptoms and - when present - signs of increased intracranial pressure as well as CSF findings compatible with the disease should be started on anti-tuberculous chemotherapy without awaiting for the CSF laboratory results. The recommended first line treatment agents for all forms of CNS tuberculosis administered daily either individually or in a combination form are isoniazid (INH), rifampicin (RIF), pyrazinamide (PZA), streptomycin (SM), and ethambutol. Second-line therapy includes ethionamide, cycloserine, para-aminosalicylic acid (PAS), aminoglycosides, capreomycin, thiacetazone, while potential new agents include oxazolidinone, isepamicin and a new rifamycin called rifapentine. Fluoroquinolones that have a role in the treatment of TBM include ciprofloxacin, ofloxacin, and levofloxacin. Finally, because of the intensity of the inflammatory and fibrotic reactions at the meningeal site, adjunctive corticosteroids, in addition to standard antituberculous therapy, are recommended (Girgis et al., 1998; Ramachandran, 2011). Taking into consideration the fact that the same regimens are recommended for the treatment of pulmonary and extrapulmonary disease, isoniazid, rifampicin and pyrazinamide are considered mandatory at the beginning of TBM treatment and some centers use all three for the whole duration of therapy. There are no data from controlled trials to guide the choice of the fourth drug. Most authorities recommend either streptomycin or ethambutol, although neither penetrates the CSF in a satisfactory degree in the absence of inflammation, and both can produce significant adverse reactions. According to the guidelines recommended by the World Health Organisation (WHO) however, ethambutol should be replaced by streptomycin (Thwaites et al., 2009; WHO, 2010). The duration of therapy in tuberculous meningitis is controversial with considerable variation in recommendations by different expert groups on this issue (Prasad & Sahu, 2010). Some experts recommend 9-12 months of treatment for TB meningitis given the serious risk of disability and mortality (WHO, 2010). The Indian Academy of Paediatrics (Indian Academy of Paediatrics [IAP], 2011) recommends that the continuation phase of treatment in TB meningitis should last for 6-7 months, extending the total duration of treatment to 8-9 months. The recommended by the British Infection Society (Thwaites et al., 2009) first line treatment regimen for all forms of CNS tuberculosis is given in Table 4.

Drug	Daily dose		Route	Duration
	Children	Adults		
Isoniazid	10-20mg/kg (max 500mg)	300mg	oral	12 months
Rifampicin	10-20mg/kg (max 600mg)	450mg (<50 mg) 600mg (≥50 mg)	oral	12 months
Pyrazinamide	30-35mg/kg (max 2g)	1.5g (<50 mg) 2.0g (≥50 mg)	oral	2 months
Ethambutol	15-20mg/kg (max 1g)	15 mg/kg	oral	2 months

Table 4. Recommended treatment regimen for CNS tuberculosis caused by fully susceptible *M. tuberculosis* (adapted from Thwaites et al., 2009)

Among the bactericidal agents INH, RIF, and PZA, isoniazid has the best CSF pharmacokinetics with concentrations (Cmax), being only slightly less than in blood (Donald, 2010). It penetrates the CSF freely, has potent early bactericidal activity and at standard dosages it achieves CSF levels of 10-15 times the minimum inhibitory concentration of *M. tuberculosis*. Its main disadvantage is that resistance develops quite quickly when used as a monotherapy though this does not seem to happen when it is used for chemoprophylaxis (Cherian & Thomas, 2011). PZA also exhibits a good CSF penetration and in children receiving appropriate dosages the achieved Cmax exceeds the proposed minimal inhibitory concentration of 20 μg/ml. In this patient group rifampicin is more successful in reaching CSF concentrations above its minimum inhibitory concentration than in adult adjusted dosages but it can achieve optimal levels only when the meninges are inflamed. Streptomycin, other aminoglycosides and ethambutol have a poor CSF penetration and cannot be administered as first line agents (Ramachandran, 2011). Among the second line agents ethionamide, fluoroquinolones, with the exception of ciprofloxacin, and cycloserine display a relatively good CSF penetration and can be administered in TBM (Donald, 2010).

9.1 Use of steroids in TBM

The British Infection Society recommends that all patients with TBM should receive adjunctive corticosteroids regardless of disease severity at presentation. The value of adjuvant corticosteroids lies in reducing the harmful effects of inflammation while antibiotics kill the organisms and studies have demonstrated significant decrease in mortality and morbidity of patients receiving dexamethasone compared with those not receiving it (Girgis et al., 1998; Ramachandran, 2011; Thwaites et al., 2009).

9.2 Treatment of TBM and HIV infection

Determination of HIV status is mandatory in all patients with suspected CNS TB not only because TB may be the first indication of an underlying HIV infection and because of the increased frequency of extrapulmonary involvement in persons with immunosuppression, but also due to the impact that TB might have on the antiretroviral (ART) treatment decisions. In case of a positive HIV status the choice and duration of anti-TB therapy remains unaltered and patients should receive the drug regimen that is recommended for HIV negative individuals with rifampicin being administered when possible, taking into consideration the fact that this agent induces the metabolism of the protease inhibitors, delavirdine and nevirapine reducing their levels (Thwaites et al., 2009). According to WHO the recommended first line ART regimens for TB patients are those that contain efavirenz (EFV) since its interactions with anti-TB drugs are minimal. In individuals who require an ART regimen containing a boosted protease inhibitor (PI), it is recommended to give a rifabutin based TB treatment. If rifabutin is not available, the use of rifampicin and a boosted antiretroviral regimen containing lopinavir or saquinavir with additional ritonavir dosing is recommended but this regimen should be closely monitored. Adjunctive corticosteroids are also recommended (Cherian & Thomas, 2011; WHO, 2010).

9.3 Treatment of multi-drug resistant TBM

Despite the fact that multi-drug resistant (MDR) tuberculous meningitis is at present a worldwide reality, in contrast to MDR pulmonary TB, it has not been well described, with the exception of limited reports (Byrd & Davis, 2007; Daicos et al., 2003; Schutte, 2001). The low sensitivity of CSF smears and culture as well as the prolonged time required for culturing and susceptibility testing, which underestimate its true incidence, have contributed to this. The emergence of multi-drug resistant TB meningitis complicates the management of the disease, because the first line anti-TB regimen is inadequate. Second line agents with the exception of ethionamide, cross the blood-brain barrier poorly, resulting in suboptimal concentrations in CSF and since there are not enough pharmacokinetic data for drugs such as cycloserine and thiacetazone, the management of CNS disease caused by bacilli resistant to both INH and RIF is challenging (Daicos et al., 2003; Patel et al., 2004). Suspected isoniazid resistant disease, without rifampicin resistance, should be treated initially with conventional 4-drug first line therapy. If a low level resistance is proven or the cultures are uninformative, the British Infection Society recommends 12 months of treatment including rifampicin, isoniazid, and pyrazinamide and ethambutol, the latter being discontinued after 2 months. If a high level isoniazid resistance is proven, exchanging the agent for levofloxacin or moxifloxacin for at least 12 months in combination with rifampicin and pyrazinamide is recommended. For patients with suspected or proven MDR CNS tuberculosis the British Infection Society recommends initial therapy with at least a fluoroquinolone, pyrazinamide, ethionamide or prothionamide, and amikacin or capreomycin, unless there is resistance to any of these agents (Thwaites et al., 2009). The standard treatment regimens, which are designed according to the general principles of the therapeutic approach to MDR TB, should be changed to individualized ones once the results on drug susceptibility concerning other agents besides INH and PZA are available (WHO, 2010). As far as paediatric groups are concerned, further studies of the sensitivity patterns are required in order to standardise and optimise the second line treatment protocols (Padayatci et al., 2006).

9.4 Neurosurgery

Besides its diagnostic value and although it is used in the management of the late complications of the disease, neurosurgery plays a minor role in the treatment of TBM. Hydrocephalus, tuberculous brain abscess (TBA), and vertebral tuberculosis with cord compression, may be indications for urgent neurosurgical intervention, even though early hydrocephalus and tuberculous brain abscess can be successfully treated by drugs alone. So early recognition and timely treatment is critical in avoiding the surgery. The aim of surgical management of TBA is to reduce the size of the space-occupying lesion and subsequently diminish intracranial pressure. Anti-TB therapy prior to the surgery is considered mandatory and appears to reduce the risk of postoperative meningitis. Urgent surgical decompression should also be considered in all the cases with extradural lesions causing paraparesis (Cherian & Thomas, 2011).

10. Conclusion

Tuberculosis is a serious public health issue with tuberculous meningitis being the most severe extrapulmonary form as well as the most common manifestation of central nervous system disease. The causative agents are members of *M. tuberculosis* complex and NTM, which should be strongly considered as important CNS pathogens in patients with HIV infection. The three most commonly used laboratory methods of TBM diagnostics are smear microscopy, culture and molecular techniques but as the stage of the disease at the time of treatment onset is the most important determinant of prognosis, anti-TB therapy should be initiated even before their completion. Nevertheless, the disease's wide clinical spectrum combined with the significant overlap between its syndromes pose a diagnostic challenge, underlining the importance of a high index of clinical suspicion. We should keep in mind that rapid diagnosis of TBM besides its impact in the disease's outcome is also central to controlling primary tuberculosis, especially in the wake of the emergence of multi-drug resistant TB and its severe implications particularly for HIV infected patients.

11. References

Alcaide, F. & Coll, P. (2011). Advances in rapid diagnosis of tuberculosis disease and anti-tuberculous drug resistance. *Enferm Infecc Microbiol Clin,* Vol.29, No.1, pp. 34-40, ISSN 0213-005X

Allen, C. M. C. & Lueck, C. J. (2002). Neurological disease, In: *Davidson's principles and practice of medicine,* Haslett, C., Chilvers, E. R., Boon, N. A., Colledge, N. R., pp. 1103-1129, Churchill Livingstone, ISBN 0-443-07035-0, New Delhi

Arvanitakis, Z., Long, R. L., Hershfield, E. S., Manfreda, J., Kabani, A., Kunimoto, D. & Power, C. (1998). M. tuberculosis molecular variation in CNS infection: evidence for straindependent neurovirulence. *Neurology,* Vol.50, No.6, pp. 1827-1832, ISSN 0028-3878

Baheti, R., Laddha, P. & Gehlot, R. S. (2001). CSF - Adenosine Deaminase (ADA) Activity in Various Types of Meningitis. *J Indian Acad Clin Med,* Vol.2, No.4, pp.285-287, ISSN 0972-3560

Be, N. A., Kim, K. S., Bishai, W. R. & Jain, S. K. (2009). Pathogenesis of central nervous system tuberculosis. *Curr Mol Med,* Vol.9, No.2, pp. 94-99, ISSN 1566-5240

Berger, J. R. (1995). Tuberculosis of the CNS. In: *Medlink Neurology,* Johnson, R. T., Medlink Corporation, 10.06.2011, Available from http://www.medlink.com/CIP.ASP?UID =MLT002P9

Blaivas, A. J., Lardizabal, A. & Macdonald, R. (2005). Two unusual sequelae of tuberculous meningitis despite treatment. *South Med J,* Vol.98, No.10, pp. 1028-1030, ISSN 0038-4348

Blake, J. & Berman, P. (1982). The use of adenosine deaminase assays in the diagnosis of tuberculosis. *S Afr Med J,* Vol.62, No.1, pp.19-21, ISSN 0256-9574

Burns, D. K. (1997). The nervous system. In: *Basic Pathology,* Kumar, V., Cotran, R. S., S. Robbins, S., pp. 713-744, ISBN-10: 0721651224, USA

Byrd, T. F. & Davis, L. E. (2007). Multidrug-resistant tuberculous meningitis. *Curr Neurol Neurosci Rep,* Vol.7, No.6, pp. 470-475, ISSN 1528-4042

Caws, M., Thwaites, G., Dunstan, S., Hawn, T. R., Lan, N. T., Thuong, N. T., Stepniewska, K., Huyen, M. N., Bang, N. D., Loc, T. H., Gagneux, S., van Soolingen, D., Kremer, K., van der Sande, M., Small, P., Anh, P. T., Chinh, N. T., Quy, H. T., Duyen, N. T., Tho, D. Q., Hieu, N. T., Torok, E., Hien, T. T., Dung, N. H., Nhu, N. T., Duy, P. M., van Vinh Chau, N. & Farrar, J. (2008). The influence of host and bacterial genotype on the development of disseminated disease with *Mycobacterium tuberculosis. PLoS Pathogens,* Vol.4, No.3, pp. e1000034, ISSN 1553-7366

Cegielski, J. P. & Wallace, R. J. Jr. (1997). Central nervous system infections with nontuberculous mycobacteria. *Clin Infect Dis,* Vol.25, No.6, pp. 1496-1497, ISSN 1058-4838

Chackerian, A. A., Alt, J. M., Perera, T. V., Dascher, C. C. & Behar, S. M. (2002). Dissemination of *Mycobacterium tuberculosis* Is Influenced by Host Factors and Precedes the Initiation of T-Cell Immunity. *Infect Immun,* Vol.70, No.8, pp. 4501-4509, ISSN 0019-9567

Chakraborty, A. K. (2000). Estimating mortality from tuberculous meningitis in a community: use of available epidemiological parameters in the Indian context. *Indian J Tuberc,* Vol.47, No.1, pp. 9-13, ISSN 0019-5707

Chandramuki, A., Lyashchenko, K., Kumari, H. B., Khanna, N., Brusasca, P., Gourie-Devi, M., Satishchandra, P., Shankar, S. K., Ravi, V., Alcabes, P., Kanaujia, G. V. & Gennaro, M. L. (2002). Detection of antibody to *Mycobacterium tuberculosis* protein antigens in the cerebrospinal fluid of patients with tuberculous meningitis. *J Infect Dis,* Vol.186, No.5, pp. 678-683, ISSN 0022-1899

Cherian, A. & Thomas, S. V. (2011). Central nervous system tuberculosis. *Afr Health Sci,* Vol. 11, No.1, pp. 116-127, ISSN 1680-6905

Chou, C. H., Lin, G. M., Ku, C. H. & Chang, F. Y. (2010). Comparison of the APACHE II, GCS and MRC scores in predicting outcomes in patients with tuberculous meningitis. *Int J Tuberc Lung Dis,* Vol.14, No.1, pp. 86-92, ISSN 1027-3719

Christensen, A. S. H., Andersen, A. B., Thomsen, V. O., Andersen, P. H. & Johansen, I. S. (2011). Tuberculous meningitis in Denmark: a review of 50 cases. *BMC Infect Dis,* Vol.11, February, p.47, ISSN 1471-2334

Christie, L. J., Loefler, A. M., Honarmand, S., Flood, J. M., Baxter, R., Jacobson, S., Alexander, R. & Glaser, C. A. (2008). Diagnostic Challenges of Central Nervous System Tuberculosis. *Emerg Infect Dis,* Vol.14, No.9, pp. 1473–1475, ISSN 1080-6059

Daikos, G. L., Clearly, T., Rodriguez, A. & Fischl M. A. (2003). Multidrug-resistant tuberculous meningitis in patients with AIDS. *Int Tuberc Lung Dis,* Vol.7, No.4, pp. 394-398, ISSN 1027-3719

Dass, B., Puet, T. A. & Watanaknakorn, C. (2002). Tuberculosis of the spine (Pott's disease) presenting as 'compression fractures'. *Spinal Cord,* Vol.40, No.11, pp. 604-608 ISSN 1362-4393

Donald, P. R., Schaaf, H. S., Schoeman, J. F. (2005). Tuberculous meningitis and miliary tuberculosis: the Rich focus revisited. *J. Infect,* Vol.50, No.3, pp. 193-1955, ISSN 0163-4453

Donald, P. R. (2010). Cerebrospinal fluid concentrations of antituberculosis agents in adults and children. *Tuberculosis (Edinb),* Vol.90, No.5, pp. 279-292, ISSN 1472-9792

Dora, J. M., Geib, G., Chakr, R., Paris, F., Mombach, A. B., Lutz, L., Souza, C. F & Goldani, L. Z. (2008). Polymerase Chain Reaction as a Useful and Simple Tool for Rapid Diagnosis of Tuberculous Meningitis in a Brazilian Tertiary Care Hospital. *Braz J Infect Dis,* Vol.12, No.3, pp.245-247, ISSN 1413-8670

Dormans, J., Burger, M., Aguilar, D., Henrandez-Pando, R., Kremer, K., Roholl, P., Arend, S. M. & Van Soolingen, D. (2004). Correlation of virulence, lung pathology, bacterial load and delayed type hypersensitivity responses after infection with different *Mycobacterium tuberculosis* genotypes in a BALV/c mouse model. *Clin Exp Immunol,* Vol.137, No.3, pp. 460-468, ISSN 00099104

Drevets, D. A., Leenen, P. J. M. & Greenfield, R. A. (2004). Invasion of the Central Nervous System by Intracellular Bacteria. *Clin Microbiol Rev,* Vol.17, No.2, pp. 323-347, ISSN 0893-8512

D'Souza, R., Franklin, D., Simpson, J. & Kerr, F. (2002). Atypical presentation of tuberculosis meningitis. *Scot Med J*, Vol.47, No.1, pp. 14-15, ISSN 0036-9330

Dye, C., Lönnroth, K., Jaramillo, E., Williams, B. G. & Raviglione, M. (2009). Trends in tuberculosis incidence and their determinants in 134 countries. WHO Bulletin of the World Health Organization. Vol.87, No.9, pp. 683-691, ISSN 0042-9686

Fadzilah, M. N., Ng, K. P. & Ngeow, Y. F. (2009). The manual MGIT system for the detection of *M. tuberculosis* in respiratory specimens: an experience in the University Malaya Medical Centre. *Malays J Pathol*, Vol.31, No.2, pp. 93-97, ISSN 0126-8635

Flor, A., Capdevila, J. A.. Martin, N., Gavaldà, J. & Pahissa, A. (1996). Nontuberculous mycobacterial meningitis: report of two cases and review. *Clin Infect Dis*, Vol.25, No.6, pp. 1266-1273, ISSN 1058-4838

Garg, R. K. (1999). Tuberculosis of the central nervous system. *Postgrad Med J*, Vol.75, No.881, pp. 133-140, ISSN 0032-5473

Girgis, N. I, Sultan, Y., Farid, Z., Mansour, M. M., Erian, M. W., Hanna, L. S. & Mateczun, A. J. (1998). Tuberculus meningitis, Abbassia Fever Hospital-Naval Medical Research Unit No. 3-Cairo, Egypt, from 1976 to 1996. *Am J Trop Med Hyg*, Vol.58, No.1, pp. 28–34, ISSN 0002-9637

Golden, M. P., Vikram, H. R. (2005). Extrapulmonary Tyberculosis: An Overview. *Am Fam Physician*, Vol.72, No.9, pp. 1761-1768, ISSN 0002-838X

Gupta, B. K., Bharat, A., Debapriya, B. & Baruah, H. (2010). Adenosine Deaminase Levels in CSF of Tuberculous Meningitis Patients. *J Clin Med Res*, Vol.2, No.5, pp. 220-224, ISSN 1918-3003

Haldar, S., Sharma, N., Gupta, V. K. & Tyagi, J. S. (2009). Efficient diagnosis of tuberculous meningitis by detection of Mycobacterium tuberculosis DNA in cerebrospinal fluid filtrates using PCR. *J Med Microbiol*, Vol.58, No.5, pp. 616–624, ISSN 0022-2615

Harries, A., Maher, D. & Graham, S. (2004). *TB/HIV: A Clinical Manual*, WHO, Retrieved from whqlibdoc.who.int/publications/2004/9241546344.pdf

Harsha, C. K. S., Shetty, A. P. & Rajasekaran, S. (2006). Intradural spinal tuberculosis in the absence of vertebral or meningeal tuberculosis: a case report. *J Orthop Surg*, Vol.14, No.1, pp. 71 –75, ISSN 1022-5536

Heemskerk, D., Day, J., Chau, T. T., Dung, N. H., Yen, N. T., Bang, N. D., Merson, L., Olliaro, P., Pouplin, T., Caws, M., Wolbers, M. & Farrar, J. (2011). Intensified treatment with high dose rifampicin and levofloxacin compared to standard treatment for adult patients with tuberculous meningitis (TBM-IT): protocol for a randomized controlled trial. *Trials*, Vol.12, February, p. 25, ISSN 1745-6215

Hooker, J. A., Muhindi, D. W., Amayo, E. O., Mc'ligeyo, S. O., Bhatt, K. M. & Odhiambo, J. A. (2003). Diagnostic utility of cerebrospinal fluid studies in patients with clinically suspected tuberculous meningitis. *Int J Tuberc Lung Dis*, Vol.7, No.8, pp. 787–796, ISSN: 1027-3719

IAP Working Group on Tuberculosis. (2011). Task Force on Pneumonia. Consensus statement on childhood tuberculosis. *Indian Pediatr*, Vol.47, No.1, pp. 41-55, ISSN 0019-6061

Jacob, C. N., Henein, S. S., Heurich, A. E. & Kamholz, S. (1993). Nontuberculous mycobacterial infection of the central nervous system in patients with AIDS. *South Med J*, Vol.86, No.6, pp. 638-640, ISSN 0038-4348

Junewick, J. (2010). Tuberculous meningitis, In: *Advanced Radiology Services teaching*, 17.06.2011, Available from advancedradteaching.com/teachingfiles/382.pdf

Karstaedt, A. S., Valtchanova, S., Barriere, R. & Crewe-Brown, H. H. (1998). Tuberculous meningitis in South African urban adults. *QJM*, Vol.91, No.11, pp. 743-747, ISSN 1460-2725

Kashyap, R. S., Ramteke, S. S., Gaherwar, H. M., Deshpande, P. S., Purohit, H. J., Taori, G. M. & Daginawala, H. (2010). Evaluation of BioFM liquid medium for culture of cerebrospinal fluid in tuberculous meningitis to identify *Mycobacterium tuberculosis*. *Indian J Med Microbiol*, Vol.28, No.4, pp. 366-369, ISSN 0255-0857

Kent, S. J., Crowe, S. M., Yung, A., Lucas, C. R. & Mijch, A. M. (1993). Tuberculous meningitis: a 30-year review. *Clin Infect Dis*, Vol.17, No.6, pp. 987-994 ISSN 1058-4838

Khosravi, A. D., Seghatoleslami, S. & Hashemzadeh, M. (2009). Application of PCR-Based Fingerprinting for Detection of Nontuberculous Mycobacteria among Patients Referred to Tuberculosis Reference Center of Khuzestan Province, Iran. *Res J Microbiol*, Vol.4, No.4, pp. 143-149, ISSN 1816-4935

Koirala, J. (2001). Mycobacterium Kansasii. In: *Medscape Reference,*, 01.06 2011, Available from: http://www.emedicine.com/med/topic1537.htm

Komolafe, M. A., Sunmonu, T. A. & Esan, O. A. (2008). Tuberculous meningitis presenting with unusual clinical features in Nigerians: Two case reports. *Cases J*, Vol.1, No.1, p. 180, ISSN 1757-1626

Kumar, P., Srivatsava M. V., Singh, S. & Prasad, H. K. (2008). Filtration of Cerebrospinal Fluid Improves Isolation of Mycobacteria. *J Clin Microbiol*, Vol.46, No.8, pp. 2824–2825, ISSN 0095-1137

Lai, C. C., Chen, H. W., Liu, W. L., Ding, L. W., Lin, C. L., Lu, G. D. & Hsueh, P. R. (2008). Fatal meningitis caused by *Mycobacterium nonchromogenicum* in a patient with nasopharyngeal carcinoma. *Clin Infect Dis*, Vol.46, No.2, pp. 325–326, ISSN 1058-4838

Laniado-Laborin, R. (2005). Adenosine deaminase in the diagnosis of tuberculous pleural effusion: is it realty an ideal test? A word of caution. *Chest*, Vol.127, No.2, pp. 417-418, ISSN 0012-3692

Lu, C. H., Chang, W. N. & Chang, H. W. (2001). The prognostic factors of adult tuberculous meningitis. *Infection*, Vol.29, No.6, pp. 299-304, ISSN 0300-8126

Malik, Z. I., Ishtiaq, O., Shah, N. H., Anwer, F. & Baqai, H. Z. (2002). Analysis and outcome of 30 patients with Tuberculous Meningitis. *Pak J Med Res*, Vol.41, No.4, pp. 137-141, ISSN 0030-9842

Mamoucha, S., Velentza, A., Bassoulis, D., Bouza, K., Petrakis, G., Stamoulos, K., Pavlou, E., Papafrangas, E. & Fakiri, E. (2010). Laboratory approach to the mycobacterial infections in a tertiary hospital. Five year results. *Acta Microbiologica Hellenica*, Vol.55, No.2, pp. 133-141

Manca, C., Reed, M. B., Freeman, S., Mathema, B., Kreiswirth, B., Barry, C. E 3rd & Kaplan, G. (2004). Differential monocyte activation underlies strain-specific *Mycobacterium tuberculosis* pathogenesis. *Infect Immun, Vol.*72, No.9, pp. 5511–5514, ISSN 0019-9567

Maniu, C. V., Hellinger, W. C., Chu, S. Y., Palmer, R. & Alvarez-Elcoro S. (2001). Failure of Treatment for Chronic *Mycobacterium abscessus* Meningitis Despite Adequate

Clarithromycin Levels in Cerebrospinal Fluid. *Clin Infect Dis,* Vol.33, No.5, pp. 745–748, ISSN 1058-4838

Mayo, J., Collazos, J. & Martinez, E. (1998). Mycobacterium nonchromogenicum Bacteremia in an AIDS Patient. *Emerg Infect Dis,* Vol.4, No.1, pp. 124-125. ISSN 1080-6040

McLain, R. F., Isada, C. (2004). Spinal tuberculosis deserves a place on the radar screen. *Clev Clin J Med,* Vol.71, No.7, pp. 537-539, 543-549, ISSN 0891-1150

Michael, J. S., Lalitha, M. K., Cherian, T., Thomas, K., Mathai, D., Abraham, O. C. & Brahmadathan, K. N. (2002). Evaluation of Polymerase Chain Reaction for rapid diagnosis of Tuberculous Meningitis. *Indian J of Tuberc,* Vol.49, No.3, pp.133-137, ISSN 0019-5707

Newton, R. W. (1994). Tuberculous meningitis. *Arch Dis Child,* Vol.70, No.5, pp. 364-366, ISSN 0003-9888

Nicolic, S. (1996). Modern concepts on the pathogenesis and therapy of tuberculous meningitis. *Srp Arh Celok Lek,* Vol.124, No.1-2, pp. 24-28, ISSN 0370-8179

Oosthuizen, H. M., Ungerer, J. P. & Bissbort, S. H. (1993). Kinetic determination of serum adenosine deaminase. *Clin Chem,* Vol.39, No.10, pp. 2182-2185, ISSN 0009-9147

Padayatchi, N., Bamber, S., Dawood, H. & Robat, R. (2006). Multidrug-resistant tuberculous meningitis in children in Durban, South Africa. *Pediatr Infect Dis J,* Vol.25, No.2, pp. 147-150, ISSN 0891-3668

Pai, M., Flores, L. L., Pai, N., Hubbard, A., Riley, L. W. & Colford, J. M. Jr. (2003). Diagnostic accuracy of nucleic acid amplification tests for tuberculous meningitis: a systematic review and meta-analysis. *Lancet Infect Dis,* Vol.3, No.10, pp. 633-643, ISSN 1473-3099

Panicker, J. N., Nagaraja, D., Subbakrishna, D. K., Venkataswamy, M. M. & Chandramuki, A. (2010). Role of the BACTEC radiometric method in the evaluation of patients with clinically probable tuberculous meningitis. *Ann Indian Acad Neurol,* Vol.13, No.2, pp. 128–131, ISSN: 0972-2327

Patel, V. B., Padayatchi, N., Bhigjee, A. I., Allen, J., Bhagwan, B., Moodley, A. A. & Mthiyane, T. (2004). Multidrug-Resistant Tuberculous Meningitis in KwaZulu-Natal, South Africa. *Clin Infect Dis,* Vol.38, No.6, pp. 851-856, ISSN 1058-4838

Piersimoni, C. & Scarparo, C. (2008). Pulmonary infections associated with non-tuberculous mycobacteria in immunocompetent patients. *Lancet Infect Dis,* Vol.8, No.5, pp. 323-334, ISSN 1473-3099

Poon, T. L., Ho, W. S., Pang, K. Y. & Wong, C. K. (2003). Tuberculous meningitis with spinal tuberculous arachnoiditis. *Hong Kong Med J,* Vol.9, No.1, pp. 59-61, ISSN 1024-2708

Prasad, K., Singh, M. B. (2008). Corticosteroids for managing tuberculous meningitis. *Cochrane Database Syst Rev,* No. 1:CD002244

Prasad, K. & Sahu, J. K. (2010). Duration of anti-tubercular treatment in tuberculous meningitis: Challenges and opportunity. *Neurol India,* Vol.58, No.5, pp. 723-726, ISSN 0028-3886

Prince, A. (2002). Infectious Diseases, In: *Nelson Essentials of Pediatrics,* Behrman, R. E., Kliegman, R. M, pp. 359-468, W.B. Saunders company, ISBN 0-7216-9406-3, Philadelphia, Pennsylvania, USA

Puccioni-Sohler, M. & Brandão, C. O. (2007). Factors associated to the positive cerebrospinal fluid culture in the tuberculous meningitis. *ArqNeuropsiquiatr,* Vol.65, No.1, pp. 48-53, ISSN 0004-282X

Rajni, Rao, N. & Meena, L. S. (2011). Biosynthesis and Virulent Behavior of Lipids Produced by *Mycobacterium tuberculosis* : LAM and Cord Factor: An Overview. *Biotechnol Res Int,* Vol.2011, Article ID 274693, pp. 1-7, ISSN 2090-3146

Ramachandran, T. S. (2011). Tuberculous Meningitis. In: *Medscape Reference,* 12.06.2011, Available from: http://emedicine.medscape.com/article/1166190-overview

Reed M. B., Domenech P., Manca C., Su H., Barczak A. K., Kreiswirth, B. N., Kaplan, G. & Barry, C. E. 3rd (2004). A glycolipid of hypervirulent tuberculosis strains that inhibits the innate immune response. *Nature, Vol.*431, No.7004, pp. 84–87, ISSN 0028-0836

Rishi, S., Sinha, P., Malhotra, B. & Pal, N. (2007). A comparative study for the detection of Mycobacteria by BACTEC MGIT 960, Lowenstein Jensen media and direct AFB smear examination. *Indian J Med Microbiol,* Vol.25, No.4, pp. 383-386, ISSN 0255-0857

Schutte, C. M. (2001). Clinical, Cerebrospinal Fluid and Pathological Findings and Outcomes in HIV-Positive and HIV-Negative Patients with Tuberculous Meningitis. *Infection,* Vol.29, No.4, pp. 213-217, ISSN 0300-8126

Selvakumar, N. Vanajakumar, Thilothammal, N. &. Paramasivan, C. N. (1996). Isolation of *Mycobacterium tuberculosis* from cerebrospinal fluid by the centrifugation and filtration methods. *Indian l Med Res,* Vol.103, May, pp. 250–252, ISSN 0019-5340

Sinha, M. K., Garg, R. K., Anuradha, H. K., Agarwal, A., Singh, M. K., Verma, R. & Shukla, R. (2010). Vision impairment in tuberculous meningitis: predictors and prognosis. *J Neurol Sci,* Vol.290, No.1-2, pp. 27-32, ISSN 0022-510X

Smith, I. (2003). *Mycobacterium tuberculosis* Pathogenesis and Molecular Determinants of Virulence. *Clin Microbiol Rev,* Vol.16, No.3, pp. 463–496, ISSN 0983-8512

Soini, H. & Musser, J. M. (2001). Molecular Diagnosis of Mycobacteria. *Clin Chem,* Vol.47, No.5, pp. 809-814, ISSN 0009-9147

Sorlozano, A., Soria, I., Roman, J., Huertas, P., Soto, M. J., Piedrola, G. & Gutierrez, J. (2009). Comparative Evaluation of Three Culture Methods for the Isolation of Mycobacteria from Clinical Samples. *J. Microbiol Biotechnol,* Vol.19, No.10, pp. 1259-1264, ISSN: 1017-7825

Tortoli, E., Cichero, P., Piersimoni, C., Simonetti, M. T., Gesu, G. & Nista, D. (1999). Use of BACTEC MGIT 960 for recovery of mycobacteria from clinical specimens: multicenter study. *J Clin Microbiol,* Vol.37, No.11, pp. 3578– 3582, ISSN 0095-1137

Thwaites, G. E., Chau, T. T. & Farrar, J. J. (2004). Improving the bacteriological diagnosis of tuberculous meningitis. *J Clin Microbiol,* Vol.42, No.1, pp. 378-379, ISSN 0095-1137

Thwaites G., Fisher M., Hemingway C., Scott G., Solomon T. & Innes J (2009). British Infection Society guidelines for the diagnosis and treatment of tuberculosis of the central nervous system in adults and children. *J Infect,* Vol.59, No.3, pp. 167-187, ISSN 0163-4453

Tuon, F. F., Higashino, H. R., Lopes, M. I., Litvoc, M. N., Atomiyia, A. N., Antonangelo, L. & Leite, O. M. (2010). Adenosine deaminase and tuberculous meningitis—A systematic review with meta-analysis. *Scand J Infect Dis,* Vol.42, No.3, pp. 198–207, ISSN 0036-5548

van Well, G. T., Paes, B. F., Terwee, C. B., Springer, P., Roord, J. J., Donald, P. R., van Furth, A. M. & Schoeman, J. F. (2009). Twenty years of pediatric tuberculous meningitis: a retrospective cohort study in the western cape of South Africa. *Pediatrics*, Vol.123, No.1, pp. e1-8, ISSN: 0031-4005

Varaine, F., Henkens, M. & Grouzard, N. (2010). *Tuberculosis* (5th revised edition), Médecins Sans Frontières, ISBN 2-906498-75-0, Paris

Venkataswamy, M. M., Rafi, W., Nagarathna, S., Ravi, V. & Chandramuki, A. (2007). Comparative evaluation of BACTEC 460TB system and Lowenstein-Jensen medium for the isolation of *M. tuberculosis* from cerebrospinal fluid samples of tuberculous meningitis patients. *Indian J Med Microbiol*, Vol.25, No.3, pp. 236–240, ISSN 0255-0857

WHO. (2010). Treatment of Tuberculosis. Available from: http://www.whqlibdoc.who.int/publications/2010/9789241547833_eng.pdf

Wu, H. S., Kolonoski, P., Chang, Y. Y. & Bermudez L. E. (2000). Invasion of the Brain and Chronic Central Nervous System Infection after Systemic *Mycobacterium avium* Complex Infection in Mice. *Infect Immun*, Vol.68, No.5, pp. 2979-2984, pp. 2979-2984, ISSN 0019-9567

Yasar, K. K., Pehlivanoglu, F., Sengoz, G., Ince, E. R. & Sandikci, S. (2011). Tuberculous meningoencephalitis with severe neurological sequel in an immigrant child. *J Neurosci Rural Pract*, Vol.2, No.1, pp. 77-79, ISSN 0976-3147

Molecular Epidemiology and Drug Resistance of Tuberculous Meningitis

Kiatichai Faksri[1,3], Therdsak Prammananan[2,3], Manoon Leechawengwongs[3] and Angkana Chaiprasert[3,4*]
[1]*Department of Microbiology, Faculty of Medicine, Khon Kaen University,*
[2]*National Center for Genetic Engineering and Biotechnology, National Science and Technology Development Agency,*
[3]*Drug-Resistant Tuberculosis Research Fund, Siriraj Foundation,*
[4]*Department of Microbiology, Faculty of Medicine Siriraj Hospital, Mahidol University, Thailand*

1. Introduction

Tuberculosis (TB) continues to be one of the highest burdens and greatest challenges to public health. Annually, TB causes approximately 1.7 million deaths and 9.4 million incident cases worldwide. Although the incident rate of TB is slowly falling due to the expansion of the population, the absolute number of new TB cases is still increasing. It is estimated that two billion people (i.e., one-third of the global population) are infected with *Mycobacterium tuberculosis* (MTB), the causative agent of TB (World Health organization [WHO], 2009). MTB is one of the most successful human pathogens. Many efforts and resources have been invested to conquer this disease. Despite continuous efforts to generate effective strategies and approaches for prevention, control and treatment of TB, there has been little progress on developing vaccinations and drugs and increasing our understanding of the disease compared to the progression of the adaptability and pathogenicity of the pathogen, which is, even now, full of ambiguity regarding virulence factors and pathogenicity

Tuberculous meningitis (TBM), or TB meningitis, is the most devastating form of TB. The disease involves the infection of the meninges of the host, which is caused by MTB and other mycobacteria. This form of TB is of greatest concern due to its fatal outcome and neurological sequelae. The challenge is concentrated around rapid reliable diagnosis, treatment and understanding of its pathogenesis. The incidences of extrapulmonary TB and TBM are increasing (Kruijshaar *et al.*, 2009). Drug resistance and HIV infection are the complications that make the treatment and management of TBM patients more difficult, and there are still doubts regarding many aspects of the disease. The lack of knowledge regarding TBM is challenging for us and other researchers. This review assembles, summarizes and discusses information regarding the epidemiology and drug resistance of TBM and the associations between MTB lineages and disease drawn from previous studies, along with information from studies that have been performed in Thailand. The overview of pathogenesis and the possible mechanism of TBM development are also discussed.

1.1 Clinical features

The cardinal clinical features of TBM include fever, anorexia and headache. Confusion is a late feature, and coma is a sign of poor prognosis. However, these features are not specific for TBM. The clinical features and outcome may vary depending on the delay of treatment, underlying disease, host immunity and virulence or lineage of MTB. The duration of the symptoms may vary from 1 day to 9 months. The common symptoms of TBM in terms of proportions of patients affected are fever (60–95%), anorexia (60–80%), headache (50–80%), vomiting (30–60%) and photophobia (5–10%). The clinical signs in terms of proportions of patients affected are neck stiffness (40–80%), coma (30–60%), any cranial nerve palsy (30–50%), cranial nerve III palsy (5–15%), cranial nerve VI palsy (30–40%), cranial nerve VII palsy (10–20%), confusion (10–30%), hemiparesis (10–20%), paraparesis (5–10%) and seizures (children: 50%; adults: 5%) (Davis *et al.*, 1993; Farinha *et al.*, 2000; Girris *et al.*, 1998; Hosoglu *et al.*, 1998; Kent *et al.*, 1993; Verdon *et al*, 1996; Thwaites *et al.*, 2005a). The severity of TBM can be classified into three stages according to the patient's Glasgow coma score and the presence or absence of focal neurological signs by stage I: Alert and orientated without focal neurological deficit; stage II: Glasgow coma score (please see the following paragraph) 14–10 with or without focal neurological deficit or Glasgow coma score 15 with focal neurological deficit; and stage III: Glasgow coma score less than 10, with or without focal neurological deficit (British Medical Research Council, 1948; Teasdale *et al.*, 1974).

Notably, the Glasgow coma score is scaled between 3 and 15, where 3 is the worst and 15 is the best. Three factors are assessed: best eye response (1=no eye opening, 2=eye opening to pain, 3=eye opening to verbal command, 4=eyes open spontaneously), best verbal response (1=no verbal response, 2=incomprehensible sounds, 3=inappropriate words, 4=confused, 5=orientated), and best motor response (1=no motor response, 2=extension to pain, 3=flexion to pain, 4=withdrawal from pain, 5=localizing pain, 6=obeys commands) (British Medical Research Council, 1948).

1.2 Diagnosis

The diagnosis of TBM is difficult because there are no specific clinical features and no rapid reliable tests. The problem of misdiagnosis and the delay of diagnosis subsequently lead to the delay of treatment and the reduction of the cure rate. The clinical criteria for differentiating TBM are essential. However, the prodrome is usually nonspecific, and the diagnosis cannot rely only on clinical signs. Due to the difficulty of diagnosis of TBM and the lack of effective diagnosis tools, there have been efforts to generate diagnosis rules for differentiating TBM from other meningitis diseases (Kumar *et al*, 1999). Confusion with other meningitis diseases (e.g., viral meningitis and other bacterial meningitis) is a problem for the diagnosis of TBM. This form of TB should be considered when a patient presents with meningoencephalitis, especially with pre-diagnosed TB or is a member of any high-risk groups (Leonard *et al.*, 1990). For the TBM diagnostic test, it is important to perform a lumbar puncture; cerebrospinal fluid (CSF) can be examined by many tests (e.g., CSF AFB staining, CSF culture, CSF analysis of protein, glucose level, white blood cell count and detection of MTB complex nucleic acids and mycobacterium). The increase of protein and decrease of glucose with mononuclear cell pleocytosis are suspected indicators for TBM (Jeren & Beus, 1982). Radiographic assessments, such as computed tomography (CT) and magnetic resonance imaging (MRI), have vastly improved the identification of complications of TBM (Bhargava *et al.*, 1982; Bullock *et al.*, 1982). The ideal features of a diagnostic test for TBM would require good sensitivity, specificity and more rapidity. Acid-fast bacilli (AFB) staining from a direct specimen with careful and repeated searching for acid-fast bacilli (AFB) is still one of the most effective rapid diagnostic tests. However, AFB staining lacks sensitivity, though it is a common conventional detection method for pulmonary TB. The gold standard for definite diagnosis is based on the positive cultivation of mycobacteria from CSF. However, the culture results can be delayed and are often insufficient for aiding clinical diagnosis. There have been attempts to apply new rapid methods, such as molecular and immunological tests, to aid in the diagnosis of TBM (Kashyap *et al.*, 2002; 2000; Mathai *et al.*, 2001; Radhakrishnan *et al*, 1994; Robertson *et al.*, 1950; Srisaimanee *et al.*, 2002; Sumi *et al.*, 2002). Polymerase chain reaction is helpful for bacteriological confirmation. However, these new diagnostic methods have not been completely evaluated, and many tests require specific facilities and expertise. The diagnosis of TBM is still challenging and undoubtedly requires further approaches that are practical for use in all countries with improved reliability.

1.3 Treatments and management of TBM

Without appropriate treatment, TBM is a fatal disease with a high mortality rate. Many drugs used for the treatment of pulmonary TB have been used for the treatment of TBM as well. Nevertheless, there is much uncertainty regarding the treatment of TBM when compared to pulmonary TB (e.g., regimens, doses and the duration of chemotherapy). Streptomycin (SM) has been used for 60 years for TB treatment (Joint Tuberculosis Committee of the British Thoracic Society, 1998). The introductions of isoniazid (INH) and para-aminosalicylic acid (PAS) have provided further improvements in prognosis. A drug that can pass the blood-brain barrier (BBB) effectively can improve the efficacy of treatment. Rifampicin is 80% protein-bound in plasma; only 20% can penetrate the CSF in those with an intact BBB (Ellard *et al.*, 1993). Nevertheless, the slow penetration of rifampicin through the BBB could allow its concentration in the CSF above the minimum inhibitory concentrations for MTB (Ellard et al., 1993). In contrast, INH, which is non-protein-bound, rapidly penetrates through the BBB in both healthy and inflamed conditions, which can yield concentrations > 30 times the MIC for MTB (Fletcher, 1953). The excellent capacity of pyrazinamide (PZA) to penetrate the BBB and its sterilizing activity against MTB makes this drug as a potential treatment for TBM (Humphries, 1992). Ethionamide penetrates healthy and inflamed meninges, but it can cause severe nausea and vomiting (Donald *et al.*, 1989).

Presently, treatment of TBM involves a combination of several anti-tuberculous drugs, as does treatment for pulmonary TB. The appropriate regimen of treatment recommends starting with INH, RIF and PZA. The addition of a fourth drug depends on the decision of the clinicians. The British Thoracic Society (BTS), the Infectious Diseases Society of America and the American Thoracic Society (IDSA/ATS) recommend a short-course of chemotherapy for the treatment of TBM, as is used for the treatment of pulmonary TB, with variations in duration: an "intensive phase" (2 months) of treatment with four drugs, followed by a "continuation phase" (6-9 months) with two drugs (BTS, 1998; Thwaites *et al.*, 2009a). The 6-month duration of treatment, as is used in pulmonary TB, could be used for TBM if the likelihood of drug resistance is low (van Loenhout-Rooyackers *et al.*, 2001). Ethambutol and streptomycin are less effective for TBM treatment because of their poor penetrating capacities and the adverse effect of optic neuritis. However, the BTS still recommends the use of these drugs as a choice for the fourth drug in the intensive phase. In cases of multidrug-resistant TBM (MDR-TBM), there are still no standard guidelines for chemotherapy (BTS, 1998; Thwaites *et al.*, 2009a). Resistances to INH and RIF (MDR-TBM) are strong predictors of death (Thwaites *et al.*, 2005b). MDR-TB isolates in Thailand were evaluated by their *rpoB, katG* and *inhA* genes; the results revealed relatively high numbers of mutations in amino acids 531, 526 and 516 of the *rpoB* gene, amino acid 315 of the *katG* gene and the promoter region of *inhA* (Boonaiam *et al.*, 2010; Prammananan *et al.*, 2008). Ethionamide, cycloserine, ofloxacin, and PAS could be used as second-line drugs based on the susceptibility profile of the infected strain or the data available in each country. Susceptible rates for ethionamide, ofloxacin and PAS in MDR-TB isolates from Thailand were 78.8%, 90.9%, and 85.9%, respectively (Prammananan *et al.*, 2005; 2011). The molecular mechanism of ethionamide resistance in MDR-TB strains in Thailand was found to be partially related to a point mutation in the *ethA* gene in 54.1% of isolates (Boonaiam *et al.*, 2010). The appropriate duration of treatment for TBM is still controversial. The conventional duration for chemotherapy for TBM is 6-9 months (BTS, 1998; CDC, 2003). In young children, the 6-month duration can be used with high doses of anti-TB agents. Children must be treated for 12 months with a combination of antibiotic therapy and adjunctive corticosteroids.

Systemic steroids may also be used, but the roles of steroids for TBM treatment are also in doubt, especially in HIV-infected patients. A finding from a drug trial study suggested that all TBM patients who are not infected with HIV should be given dexamethasone, regardless of age or disease severity (Thwaites *et al.*, 2004). Adjuvant steroids may be used in the presence of increased intracranial pressure, altered consciousness, focal neurological findings, spinal block, and tuberculous encephalopathy. The benefit for using adjuvant corticosteroids for TBM patients involves reducing inflammation (Dooley *et al.*, 1997; Humphries *et al.*, 1992; Thwaites *et al.*, 2004). In patients with obstructive hydrocephalus and neurological deterioration, placement of a ventricular drain or ventriculoperitoneal or ventriculo-atrial shunt should be performed. Prompt shunting improves outcome, particularly in patients with minimal neurological deficits. Additionally, surgical therapy for TBM patients can also be used in some cases, depending on the physician's judgment.

BCG vaccination has been debated concerning its capacity to protect against TB. The severe forms of TB, such as milliary TB and TBM in children, can probably be prevented by the BCG (Bacillus Calmette-Guérin) vaccine. Several studies have indicated the protective effects of the BCG vaccine against TBM (Awasthi and Moin, 1999; Puvacic *et al.*, 2004; Mittal *et al.*, 1996; Trunz *et al.*, 2006; Xiong *et al.*, 2009). A protective efficacy of approximately 60-70% for the BCG vaccine against TBM has been reported (Thilothammal *et al.*, 1996; Chavalittamrong *et al.*, 1986). The study compared clinical presentations between BCG-vaccinated and unvaccinated children and revealed that vaccinated TBM patients showed better mentation and had superior disease outcomes (Kumar *et al.*, 2005). However, other studies have shown low protective effects of the BCG vaccine against TBM (Guler *et al.*, 1998; Tsenova *et al.*, 2007; Wunsch Filho *et al.*, 1990). More than 40% of TBM patients have been immunized with the BCG vaccine in Turkey (Hosoglu *et al.*, 2003). The protective effect of the BCG vaccine against TBM in Thailand has been shown; though Thai people who have been immunized with the BCG vaccine still develop TBM, infected individuals are in a very small proportion. Thailand has included mass immunization with the BCG vaccine for every newborn as the national public health policy since 1970. In Thailand, 76% of the protective effect of BCG against TB has been previously demonstrated, and a significantly lower extrapulmonary TB rate compared to pulmonary TB has also been demonstrated (Chavalittamrong *et al.*, 1986). However, clear evidence of BCG vaccine efficacy against TB and extrapulmonary TB by experimental study is still required.

2. Epidemiology of TBM

Information on the epidemiology of TBM is fundamental for the prevention, treatment and control of the disease. Nevertheless, due to the difficulty of the collection of specimens from patients and its low incidence rate, TBM is a relatively rare form of TB for study. A large collection of patient samples (e.g., more than 100 samples) is even less affordable for study. Therefore, gathering study information is an easy way to obtain an overview of the available knowledge of TBM epidemiology.

2.1 Incidence

Human migration and the availability of air travel are the major factors that have distorted the human population structure, geographic distribution and spread of MTB. Nevertheless, associations between the human race in certain regions and specific lineages of MTB have still been observed (Gagneux *et al.*, 2006). In 1997, TBM was the fifth most common form of extrapulmonary TB (WHO, 1997). From all TB cases, 90-95% of infected cases only have asymptomatic latent TB, whereas 5-10% of individuals (8-9 million people) have developed active disease, accounting for approximately 2 million deaths annually. The most common form of the disease is pulmonary TB, which has been estimated to represent 80% of all TB cases. Apart from the 20% of extrapulmonary TB cases, TBM has been calculated to represent 5.2% of extrapulmonary TB (WHO, 2009). The incidence of TBM from all reported TB cases is 0.7%. The incidence of central nervous system (CNS) TB is related to the prevalence of TB in the community. In countries with a high burden of pulmonary TB, the incidence of extrapulmonary TB and TBM are expected to be proportionately high. The incidence of TBM in the United States has been calculated to represent approximately 4.5% and 4.7% of total extrapulmonary TB cases in 1969-1973 and 1975-1990, respectively. From all samples that were sent to Siriraj Hospital in Bangkok, Thailand, for TB identification during 2000-2007, approximately 15% were CSF samples, 10% of which contained MTB and were identified as TBM.

2.2 Mortality rate

TBM is the most severe form of TB that involves the central nervous system. The mortality rate ranges from 20-60%, with an average of approximately 35% (table 1). Neurological sequelae can be found in approximately 25% of surviving patients (Hosoglu *et al.*, 2002). It is not clear whether HIV infection is associated with TBM outcome. The summarized data indicate that the high mortality rate of TBM in South Africa from both studies is associated with a high proportion of HIV-infected cases, whereas no such associations were found in Thailand or France (table 1). Conflicts of such associations have been found in previous studies (Katrak *et al.*, 2000; Thwaites *et al.*, 2005a). However, HIV infection seems to be the strongest factor that predisposes an individual to development of TBM. The mortality rate of TBM is different among countries, which may involve differences in medical personnel, management and facilities.

Authors	Countries of study	Year	Mean (range) age (yrs)	Gender (% M/F)	HIV-infected (number/%)	Mortality rate (%)
1. Faksri *et al.*, 2011a and Yorsangsukkamol *et al.*, 2009	Thailand (n=184)	1996-2007	33.6 (0.25-83)	64/36	48/72 (66.7%)	25
2. Roca *et al.*, 2008	Spain (n=29)	1991-2005	34 (17-78)	59/41	15/29 (52%)	41
3. Nagarathna *et al.*, 2007	Egypt (n=336)	2001-2005	NA (13-50)	68/32	48/107 (44.9%)	NA
4. Thwaites *et al.* 2005a	Vietnam (n=545)	2001-2003	33 (15-88)	72/28	96/528 (18.2%)	30
5. Patel *et al.*, 2004	South Africa (n=30)	1999-2002	25.7 (0.4-45)	30/70	18/30 (60%)	56
6. Sutlas *et al.*, 2003	Turkey (n=61)	1988-2000	34.5 (16-74)	64/36	NA	27.8
7. Kalita and Misra, 1999	India (n=58)	1992-1996	25.6 (1-64)	69/31	NA	20.6
8. Hosuglo *et al.*, 1998	Turkey (n=101)	1985-1996	30.6 (14-67)	60/40	NA	43.5
9. Karstaedt *et al.*, 1998	South Africa (n=56)	1994-1997	33.5 (18-59)	53/47	39/56 (69.6%)	69.6
10. Verdon *et al.*, 1996	France (n=48)	1982-1993	46 (18-83)	67/33	10/32 (31.25%)	64.5
11. Davis *et. al.*, 1993	United States (n=54)	1970-1990	NA (4-86)	NA	NA	23

Note: NA= data not available, M=male, F= Female, HIV=human immunodeficiency virus

Table 1. Epidemiological information of TBM patients from previous studies

2.3 Predisposing risk factors

The strongest risk factors for developing TBM are immunological status (e.g., HIV infection) and pre-diagnosed TB. Ages and genders of TBM patients also affect predisposition for TBM development. Prior to the predomination of HIV, the age of the patient was the most important factor leading to the development of TBM. The ages of TBM patients are different from pulmonary and other extrapulmonary TB diseases; TBM is commonly found in children ages 0-5 years (Farer and Meador, 1979). In populations with a low prevalence of TB, most cases of TBM occur in adults. In general, TBM is more common in children than in adults. Notably, the young ages of children are not always the most prevalent risk factors for TBM in all populations with high TB burdens, which might result from worldwide BCG vaccination. For instance, in the Thai population, the most predominant ages of TBM patients are 31-45 years (35.3%), and only 12% of TBM patients are less than 15 years old (Yorsangsukkamol *et al.*, 2009). With BCG vaccination, a significantly lower incidence of disseminated TB, such as TBM, was found in patients less than 12 years old compared to pulmonary TB (Chavalittamrong *et al.*, 1986). The average ages of TBM patients in particular regions, even on different continents, are around 30 years higher (table 1). This evidence supports the idea that the HIV epidemic has increased the risk for adult TBM in the last three decades. In general, young children are more likely to develop meningeal or disseminated TB, whereas adolescents more frequently present with pleural or peritoneal TB compared to adults.

Patient gender is also a predisposing factor for TBM development. Incidence is consistently higher for men than for women, with a ratio around 2:1. The proportion of affected females is slightly lower than that of males in the overall world population. However, the 2:1 ratio between male and female TBM patients has been found consistently in many countries. In children with TBM, the ratios between males and females are less affected. In Thailand, a male/female TBM patient ratio of 3:2 has been conserved over three periods of four-year intervals (Faksri *et al.*, 2011a). The effect of gender on TBM development may be explained by socio-economic or anatomical-physiological factors.

Co-infection with HIV and MTB, especially in AIDS patients, is also the strongest risk factor for progression to active TB. Compared to non-HIV-infected individuals, who have a 5-10% risk of developing active TB, HIV increases the risk of developing clinical TB post-infection to 1 in 3 individuals (Selwyn and Lewis, 1989). Furthermore, HIV also increases the possibility of developing extrapulmonary TB, especially TBM (Bishburg *et al.*, 1986). The increase in TBM incidence is most likely due to an increased incidence of CNS-TB among patients with HIV/AIDS and to the increasing incidence of TB among infants, children and young adults. Cell-mediated immunity is the most important defense against TB infection, and a decline of CD4 T cells is associated with the development of TBM (De Cock *et al.*, 1992). Although patients who have HIV infection and TB are at increased risk for TBM, the effects of HIV infection on the clinical features and outcomes of TB are still disputed (Berenguer *et al.*, 1992). Several studies that have assessed the effects of HIV infection on the clinical presentation of TBM have identified conflicting findings. HIV-infected patients may have altered clinical presentations, such as in pathological features, CSF parameters, frequency of infection with MDR-TB and mortality. Hospital-associated mortality was significantly higher in HIV-infected patients (Cecchini *et al.*, 2009; van der Weert *et al.*, 2006; Katrak *et al.*, 2000; Bandyopadhyay *et al.*, 2009). Other studies have found that HIV infection was not associated with mortality rate or altered neurological presentation in TBM, though additional extrapulmonary TB was more likely to occur in HIV-infected patients and may have also affected the survival rate (Faksri *et al.*, 2011a; Thwaites *et al.*, 2005a)

Another important risk factor is pre-diagnosed TB. The most often associated form is milliary TB on chest x-rays, which presents as a disseminated form of TB with small 1- to 2-mm lesions spreading in a large area of the lung and/or other organs. The development of TBM can consist of either the primary infection with a short incubation or a secondary reactivation of pulmonary TB with a long latent period.

Previous studies using the tuberculin conversion rate have shown that black-skinned people are more susceptible to TB infection than are white-skinned people (Stead *et al.*, 1990).

Consequently, the development of TBM may associate with certain host groups. The most striking study of host variation and TB is from Gagneux *et al.*, which showed that the lineages of MTB are associated with certain geographical regions and ethnic groups from the patients' countries of origin: the East Asian (Beijing) lineage predominates in patients from East Asia, whereas the Euro-American lineage mostly infects European people (Gagneux *et al.*, 2006). Certain lineages of MTB are predominant in certain geographical regions and ethnic groups that are associated with TBM. Therefore, environmental factors (i.e., geographical region and race) also predispose individuals to develop TBM. More discussion on host variation and predisposing factors follows in sub-topic 5.2: "Host variation and development of TBM".

Other risk factors that may be involved in TBM development include: diabetes mellitus (Bernard-Griffiths *et al.*, 1959; Pablos-Mendez and Knirsch, 1997), malignancy, malnutrition, alcoholism, head trauma (Davis and Lambert, 1993) and recent corticosteroid use (Mori and Welty, 1992).

3. Overview of the pathogenesis of TBM

A pathological view of TBM was first described in 1836 (Green, 1836). Then, in 1882, Robert Koch demonstrated that TB was caused by MTB (Koch, 1882). In 1912, a pathological experimental infection of TBM in an animal model was demonstrated (Manwaring, 1912). Subsequently, there have been several studies focused on the pathogenesis of TBM using animal experiments, in which a rabbit model is commonly used, as mice do not provide similar pathological characteristics to human TBM (Behar *et al.*, 1963; Matsubara, 1956; Sidel'Nikova and Rozina, 1956; Tsenova *et al.* 2005; 2007; van Well *et al.*, 2007).

For an overview of pathogenesis (Figure 1), MTB infection occurs through the inhalation of aerosol droplets containing the bacilli. Only small droplets (1-5 μm in diameter) can reach and eventually deposit in the alveoli of the lungs. Inside the alveoli, the bacilli are engulfed by alveolar macrophages. Because MTB can survive in this hostile environment, the bacteria can infect and grow inside the macrophages *ex vivo*. Once these immune cells are triggered, numerous cytokines and chemokines are released. The activation of a Th1 cell-mediated immune response, the critical defense mechanism that plays a major role against MTB infection, occurs; ultimately, a granuloma, mainly composed of macrophage-derived giant cells and lymphocytes, is formed. In latent tuberculosis cases, the granuloma functions to contain the bacilli and is maintained depending on the strength of the host cellular immune response. Furthermore, the interaction between immune factors in the host and virulence factors in the pathogen may determine whether the infection will be restricted or disseminated and progressed into the next stage of the disease. Before the bacilli can gain access to the brain, spreading outside of the lung into the blood circulation is the critical step for extrapulmonary TB, a step that is poorly understood. The transportation of infected alveolar macrophages into the blood circulation is a current hypothesis for extrapulmonary spread. However, the discovery that MTB hematogenous dissemination is dependent on heparin-binding hemagglutinin adhesin, a bacterial virulence factor that interacts with epithelial cells, has suggested that other trafficking pathways may be important (Pethe *et al.*, 2001). The failure of immune responses from the host, along with virulence factors from the pathogen that promote a high capacity for evading immune responses (which may determine by lineages), are the factors that promote extrapulmonary spreading.

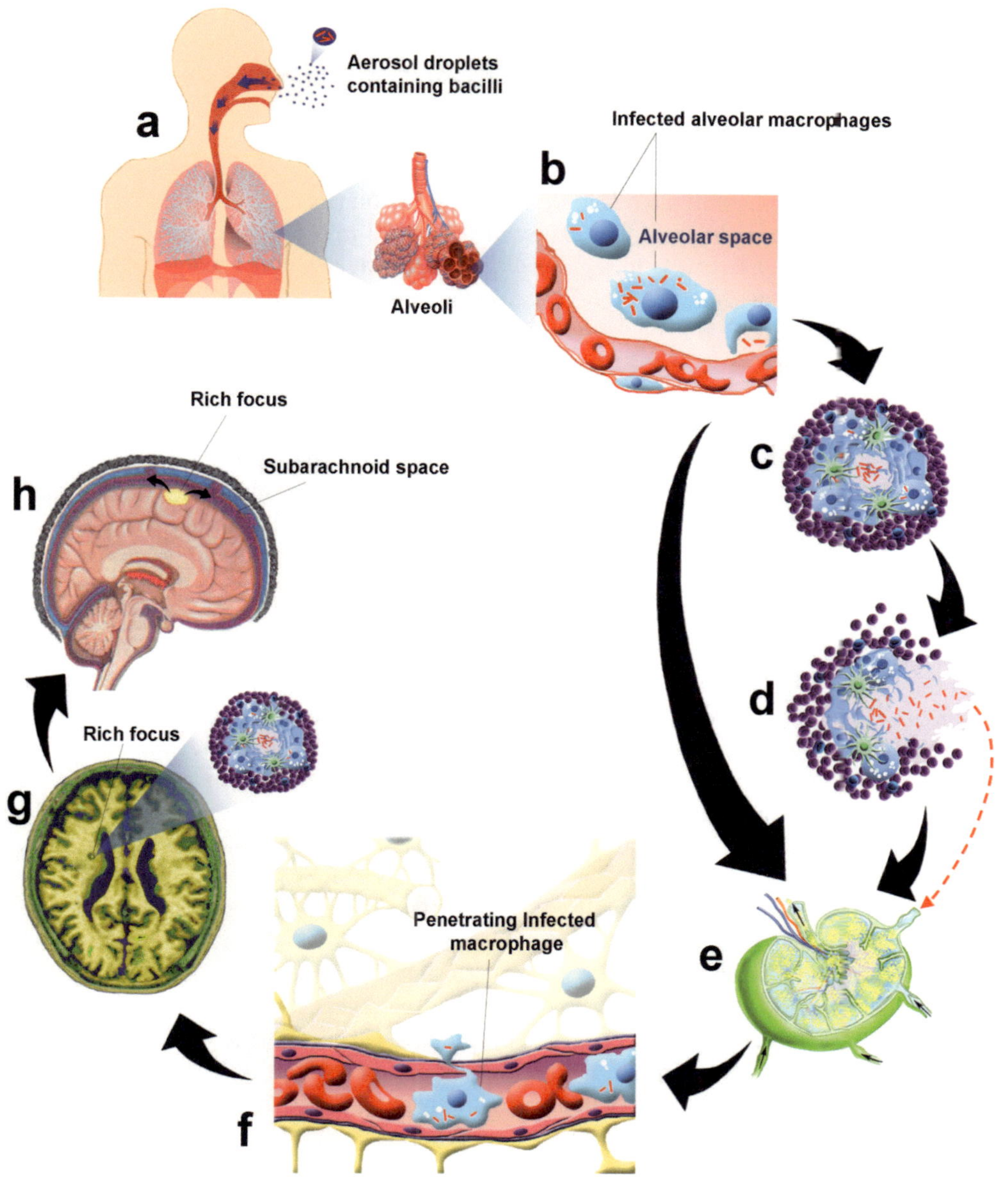

Fig. 1. Pathogenesis of TBM and postulation of the formation of Rich foci. (a) Aerosol transmission of MTB, (http://www.graphicshunt.com/health/ images/alveoli-268.htm) (b) Phagocytosis of MTB by alveolar macrophages inside alveoli. (c) Granuloma formation in the lung, which subsequently occurs due to cellular and cytokine network responses; 90% of hosts with granulomas maintain them stably over the course of their lives. (d) MTB escapes from the granuloma, which occurs in 10% of latent TB patients. (e) MTB can cause TBM by escalating from the lung or by secondary reactivation from a "leaked granuloma", which is then filtered into a regional lymph node. (http://www.graphicshunt.com/health/ images/alveoli-268.htm) (f) After spreading through the blood circulation, MTB can enter the CNS through the BBB, likely by a Trojan horse mechanism. (g) Bacilli seed to the meninges or the brain parenchyma, forming subpial or sub-ependymal primary complexes,

termed "Rich foci". (h) Rich foci increase in size, rupture and discharge into the subarachnoid space, which indicates the onset of TBM. (http://digitalunion.osu.edu/r2/summer08/dzeleznikar/anatomy.html). Some part of figures (a, e, h) were modified from online sources as described.

For TBM, the process of pathogenesis can be divided into two steps (Rich, 1993). First, the bacilli are filtered and disseminated into the draining lymph nodes. During this stage, there is a short but significant bacteremia that can seed the bacilli into other organs. Hematogenous spreading occurs most frequently in regions of the body that are highly oxygenated, including the brain. The pathogenesis of TBM might occur from a primary infection of MTB and develop into TBM directly or might be derived from the reactivation of pulmonary TB that subsequently develops into TBM (figure 1). Like other bacterial meningitis diseases, a prerequisite step of the pathological mechanism of TBM is the movement of the bacilli through the BBB (Kim *et al.*, 2008). The factors that contribute to this movement remain unknown. The process may be a multifactorial process involving host–pathogen interactions. The bacilli can cross the BBB using both transcellular and paracellular mechanisms; alternatively, infected phagocytes may transmigrate via a so-called Trojan horse mechanism (Kim *et al.*, 2008). Consequently, the pathogen can cause BBB dysfunction by inducing injury to the endothelium, resulting in an increase in permeability, pleocytosis and encephalopathy. For TBM, the Trojan horse mechanism seems to be the most possible strategy for traversal, as MTB is an intracellular pathogen and primarily infects macrophages; including a mechanism in which the bacilli, by themselves, evade the host immune responses and reach the brain would be difficult. However, transcellular penetration of the BBB has also been demonstrated for this pathogen (Jain *et al.*, 2007). In addition, the factors that determine the fate of bacilli for hematogenous dissemination and development of TBM include the capacity to survive and replicate inside macrophages. Furthermore, the capacity of bacilli to reduce the occurrence of programmed cell death, which would reduce the viability of bacilli, may also be involved in the process of TBM pathogenesis. In those who develop TBM, bacilli seed to the meninges or the brain parenchyma, forming subpial or sub-ependymal primary complexes, termed "Rich foci" (Rich, 1993). This step, which has not yet been defined, may also determine the progress of the disease by both pathogen and host factors. In the second step, in approximately 10% of the cases that develop such complexes, particularly in children and immunocompromised hosts, the primary complex does not heal but progresses. This event can occur months or years after the formation of Rich foci (Rich, 1993; Thwaites and Schoeman, 2008). The location of the Rich foci determines the type of CNS involvement. In TBM, the Rich foci increase in size until they rupture and discharge into the subarachnoid space, which indicates the onset of TBM. The following processes can also take place: adhesions around the interpeduncular fossa can lead to CN palsies; adhesive exudates can obstruct CSF, leading to hydrocephalus; and obliterative vasculitis can lead to infarction. Encephalitis and tuberculomas can also occur. Rich foci located deeper in the brain or the spinal cord parenchyma can cause tuberculomas or abscesses. Notably, abscesses or hematomas can rupture into the ventricle, but not in the case of Rich foci (Rich, 1993). After the rupture of Rich foci, the bacilli and numerous leukocytes are released into the subarachnoid space. Then, the local T-cell-dependent response is activated. The subsequent necrotizing granulomatous and inflammatory responses are the result of the pathological events of TBM.

On the cellular scale of TBM pathogenesis, the cytokines and chemokines that are consequently released from the host cellular response are thought to be important factors of pathogenesis. Most of the symptoms, signs, and sequelae of TBM are the result of an immunological inflammatory reaction to the infection. Tumor necrosis factor-alpha TNF-α) is the key cytokine in the inflammatory response and is the critical cytokine in the neuropathogenesis of MTB (Mastroianni *et al.,* 1997; Tsenova *et al.,* 1999). Evidence has indicated a direct correlation between the level of this cytokine in the CSF and the progression of the pathogenesis of TBM (Tsenova *et al.,* 1999). Also, TNF-α is a major determinant of disease in a rabbit model of meningitis (Tsenova *et al.,* 2005). TNF-α also benefits the host by playing an important role in granuloma formation (Kaneko *et al.,* 1999). These conflicting roles of TNF-α might depend on which polarity of cytokine responses (i.e., Th1 or Th2) dominate. Metalloproteinase-9 (MMP-9) is another cytokine that may play an important role in TBM pathogenesis by increasing the degradation of the BBB, which results in an increase in its permeability. Evidence has demonstrated that different genotypes of MTB can induce different host immune responses (Chaves *et al.,* 1997, Yorsangsukkamol *et al.,* 2011).

Alternatively, host genetic polymorphisms can also affect their susceptibility for developing disease. Some cytokines and proteins that are released from host cells, such as TNF-α, are related to the development and pathogenesis of TBM. In TB, a strong Th1-like immunity is considered important for containment of mycobacteria. The major immune effector mechanism involved in the activation of infected macrophages is stimulated by Th1-type cytokines (Seth and Sharma, 2002). The protective effects of Th1-type cytokines can be antagonized by Th2-type cytokines (Manca *et al.,* 2001), and increased production of Th2-type cytokines may be responsible for the characteristic immunopathology of the disease. A balance between the Th1- and Th2-type cytokine responses in TB may influence mycobacterial growth, immunopathology and the fate of the disease (Seth and Sharma, 2002). In addition, regarding the cytokine response, inflammatory cytokines are also determinants of immunopathology. The pathogenesis and virulence of the pathogen can also be determined by the balance between pro-inflammatory and anti-inflammatory cytokines.

It remains unclear why only some individuals develop disseminated TB that spreads to the meninges and then the central nervous system, while most people suffer only localized disease in the lung. Important factors include HIV infection and younger patient age. This may indicate that the host immune response is a major factor that plays a role in the development of TBM. Apart from socio-economic and environmental factors, pathogen and host factors are considered to be more important in the development of TBM. However, it is not yet known which factors are the most important. Although it seems to be a multifactorial process, a number of studies have recently demonstrated that not only pathogen factors but also host factors could influence the development of TBM (Takahashi *et al.,* 2005; Thuong *et al.,* 2007; 2008). Studies have demonstrated that genetic polymorphism of Toll-interleukin 1 receptor domain-containing adaptive protein (TRAP-MAL) and Toll-like receptor 2 (TLR2) are associated with the susceptibility for developing TBM (Hawn *et al.,* 2006; Thuong *et al.,* 2007). Gene expression profiles of human monocyte-derived macrophages (MDMs) have demonstrated that certain genetic variations, especially chemokine (C-C motif) ligand 1 (CCL1), could predispose an individual to develop a particular disease phenotype (i.e., pulmonary or latent TB, or TBM) (Thuong *et al.,* 2008). Furthermore, Caws *et al.* demonstrated that particular mycobacterial genotypes (East Asian and Euro-American lineage) identified by large sequence polymorphisms (LSPs) and host genetic polymorphisms in TLR2 influence the development of TBM (Caws *et al.,* 2008). A study of the capacity of the HN878 Beijing strain to cause TB meningitis in a rabbit model revealed that a disruption of the *pks15/1* gene that encodes a polyketide synthase-derived phenolic glycolipid (PGL) reduced virulence (Tsenova *et al.*, 2005). However, *pks15/1* is not a unique property of the Beijing lineage of MTB (Chaiprasert *et al.*, 2006). Despite these findings, however, the pathogen virulence and host genetic polymorphism factors governing the development of TBM are still unclear.

4. Anti-tuberculous drug resistance in TBM

Many decades ago, TB was considered an incurable, deadly disease. With the availability of effective treatments, TB can now be cured. However, the complete treatment requires several months to stabilize the patient's condition and to prevent the reoccurrence of disease. Pan-drug-resistant (PDR) TB strains are now a new emerging and serious public health problem. Although the incidence of PDR-TB is not yet high, we cannot underestimate the adaptability of MTB, a highly successful human pathogen. In addition, the TB burden dominates in low- and middle-income countries (LMIC) where the drug susceptibility test is not fully available. The real prevalence of drug-resistant TB may therefore be markedly higher than the estimation. Furthermore, extensively drug-resistant (XDR) TB, which is more expensive and more difficult to treat than multidrug-resistant (MDR) TB, has more serious adverse effects, and the outcomes for patients are much worse. Despite the fact that there are several novel anti-tuberculous drugs that have been developed and discovered recently, the levels of drug-resistant TB, especially MDR- and XDR-TB (and PDR-TB), are still increasing. It is very threatening to consider the imbalance between the effective anti-tuberculous drugs and drug-resistant TB, especially with the outbreak of MDR-TB in large areas. The most effective way to eradicate TB is with effective vaccination and control of latent TB. However, we are still struggling to find ways to beat this pathogen. For now, treatments for drug-resistant TB are still where we must focus. Yet, PDR-TB and TB with resistance to new drugs should be surveyed and monitored worldwide (Prammananan et al., 2006). The real hope lies with continuing to develop novel, effective anti-tuberculous drugs and vaccines.

In TBM, drug resistance and HIV infection constitute additional conditions that make the treatment of patients become more complex and difficult. The diagnosis, treatment and management of these patients are major challenges. The delay of diagnosis and treatment of TBM can cause the subsequent deaths of patients. Therefore, drug-resistant TBM is a major issue of concern for the treatment and management of TBM.

From data collected on TB cases from 81 countries between 2002 and 2006, the WHO reported that the incidence of pulmonary MDR-TB was approximately 4.8%. The highest numbers of MDR-TB were found in China, India, and the Russian Federation (WHO, 2008). In 2009, 3.3% of all new TB cases had MDR-TB (WHO, 2009). Unfortunately, information on the drug resistance of TBM from these countries was not available for this review. Studies on the drug resistance of TBM are relatively rare. From the data available, the drug-resistance patterns for TBM were obtained from four countries: Thailand, Egypt, Vietnam and South Africa. Information gathered from previous studies found that the average incidence of TBM that was resistant to any drug was approximately 21.5% (with a range of 12-31%). MDR-TBM was found in 2.2 to 8.6% of cases, with an average of approximately 3.3% (table 2). The incidence of MDR-TBM was up to 18% in pediatric cases, with a mortality rate of 100%. Nevertheless, the sample size from this study was only 20 cases

(Chander, 2008). Resistance to particular anti-tuberculous drugs, such as isoniazid, represented the most resistant MTB strains in four out of five studies in the available data (table 2). Isoniazid resistance in TBM has been suggested to correlate with HIV co-infection (Thwaites *et al.*, 2002). The second most-resistant drug is streptomycin. TBM showed minimal resistance to rifampicin (which can partially penetrate an intact BBB) and ethambutol. There was no evidence to support an increase in penetration capacity through the BBB for rifampicin after inflammation (Nau *et al.*, 1992). The information in this review may support the idea that rifampicin is a good drug for effective treatment of TBM, with a lower chance of development of drug-resistant TBM, compared to isoniazid and streptomycin. Ethambutol has been called a poor choice for a first-line treatment for TBM due to its poor penetration capacity and the adverse effect of optic neuritis (Donald *et al.*, 1998). The summarized information shows that ethambutol resistance is less likely to occur when it is used as a first-line agent for TBM treatment. However, the low resistance level may be a result of poor exposure between the drug and the pathogen.

Compared to other countries, Thailand has the second-highest drug-resistance rate for TBM (table 2). The trend for drug-resistant TBM in Thailand has been previously analyzed; it was found that a 3% incidence of MDR-TBM in the first period increased into a 12% incidence in the third period (Faksri *et al.*, 2011a). Information regarding the trends of drug resistance in other regions is unknown. Nevertheless, it is more likely that drug resistance is underestimated, which indicates that the incidence of drug-resistant TBM may be increasing. Patel *et al.* reviewed the medical records of TBM patients from South Africa and found that MDR–TBM is a serious problem that has increased the mortality rate up to 57%, with the majority of the patients having been treated with anti-tuberculous drugs (Patel *et al.*, 2004). Whether or not HIV co-infection and AIDS are involved in the development of MDR-TBM, these combined factors result in a marked increase in the difficulty of treatment and the mortality rate (Daikos *et al.*, 2003; Patel *et al.*, 2004). This information has raised our concerns regarding proper treatment and drug-resistance surveillance for TB and TBM.

Authors	Geographical regions	Year of collection	Drug resistant profiles (%)					
			H	R	S	E	MDR	Suscep
1. Yorsangsukkamol *et al.*, 2009 and Faksri *et al.*, 2011a	Thailand (n=184)	1996-2007	20.4	6.1	17.0	5.4	6.1	75.5
2. Nagarathna *et al.*, 2008	Egypt (n=336)	2001-2005	13	0	0.3	0.2	2.4	82.2
3. Caws *et. al.*, 2006	Vietnam (n=198)	2000-2003	18.7	3	24.2	0.5	2.5	68.7
4. Patel *et al.*, 2004	South Africa (n=350)	1999-2002	NA	NA	NA	NA	8.6	NA
5. Cooksey *et al.*, 2002	Egypt (n=67)	1998-2000	10.4	1.5	7.5	1.5	0	76.1
6. Padayatchi *et al.*, 2006	South Africa (n=362)	1992-2003	NA	NA	NA	NA	2.2	88.4
7. Girgis *et al.*, 1998	Egypt (n=857)	1976-1996	10	3	0	7	0	80
8. Karstaedt *et al.*, 1998	South Africa (n=56)	1994-1997	NA	NA	NA	NA	4.3	NA

Note: H: isoniazid, R; rifampicin, S: streptomycin, E; ethambutol, MDR: multidrug-resistant, Suscep; susceptible to all drugs

Table 2. Summary of drug-resistant profiles in TBM patients from previous studies

5. MTB lineages, TBM and evolution

The most common pathogen of TB and TBM is MTB. There are a few reports of TBM caused by *M. bovis* (Cooksey *et al.*, 2002; Tardieu *et al.*, 1988). Meningitis can also be caused by nontuberculous mycobacteria (NTM) (Huempener *et al.*, 1966). Interestingly, several studies have shown different pathogenicities, determined by clinical analysis among MTB lineages (Ganiem *et al.*, 2009; Lan *et al.*, 2003; Kong *et al.*, 2007). Studies in animal models (Manca *et al.*, 2001; Reed *at el.*, 2004) and macrophage cell lines (Li *et al.*, 2002; Lopez *et al.*, 2003) have also indicated that the Beijing genotype of MTB is the most virulent genotype. Furthermore, this genotype is also associated with drug resistance, especially MDR (Drobniewski *et al.*, 2005). It has been hypothesized that this genotype is an escape mutant of the BCG vaccine (van Soolingen *et al.*, 1995). Six lineages of MTB have defined names according to specific markers based on large sequence polymorphisms (i.e., regions of difference) and geographical regions: East Asian (Beijing), Euro American (EuA), East African Indian (EAI), Indo-Oceanic (IO), West African I (WA I) and West African II (WA II).

5.1 TBM and the variation of MTB lineages

For TBM, the Beijing lineage is also suggested to be the most neurovirulent genotype. The most predominant genotype of TBM in Thailand is the Beijing (East Asian) genotype, with an incidence of 58%. The Indo-Oceanic (34%) and Euro-American lineages (10%) are the second most and least predominant genotypes (Faksri *et al.*, 2011a). MTB lineages found in TBM may associate with the lineages that are found in pulmonary TB. However, the proportions of lineages may not be the same. More than half of MTB from TBM patients were the Beijing genotype (Yorsangsukkamol *et al.*, 2009), whereas only approximately 20% of MTB from pulmonary TB were the Beijing genotype (Rienthong *et al.*, 2005). The proportion of MTB lineages in TBM patients in Thailand is roughly concordant with TBM strains from Vietnam, in which the Beijing (42%) and Indo-Oceanic lineages (44%) are in higher proportions; the Euro-American lineage (14%) is the least prevalent. Studies conducted in Vietnam suggest that Beijing MTB is the most virulent genotype that causes TBM, based on correlation analysis with clinical features. They found that the Beijing lineage showed associations with a shorter duration of illness before presentation and drug resistance (i.e., the influence of disease progression, intracerebral alteration of inflammatory responses and difficulty of treatment) (Thwaites *et al.*, 2008). In Thailand, the predominance of the Beijing lineage revealed associations with MDR-TB, a trend that is increasing in proportion; additionally, it had the highest clustered rate, supporting its virulence for causing TBM. Inversely, the Euro-American lineage has been thought to be the attenuated lineage, causing the lowest proportions of TBM, with a decreasing trend of proportion and lacking cluster formation (Faksri *et al.*, 2011a). RFLP pattern analysis of CNS–MTB strains also suggested that the occurrence of CNS TB might be strain-dependent (Cooksey *et al.*, 2002; Arvanitakis *et al.*, 1998). Nevertheless, the absence of an association between MTB genotypes and the clinical presentation and outcome of TBM has also been described. The most predominant strain in this study was not the Beijing genotype (principal genetic group 1, or PGG 1) of MTB. They found that all 3 PGGs were represented (group 1, 27.1%; group 2, 59.3%; group 3, 13.6%) (Maree *et al.*, 2007). This information may indicate the variations in capacities for causing neurovirulence and TBM among MTB lineages.

In addition, variations in virulence within the Beijing family of MTB have been proposed (Alonso *et al.*, 2010; Faksri *et al.*, 2011b; Hanekom *et al.*, 2007; Iwamoto *et al.*, 2009; Kong et al., 2007; Theus *et al.*, 2007). Particular sublineages of the Beijing family of MTB seem to be more virulent based on associations with drug resistance and MDR (Twamoto *et al.*, 2008; Mokrousov *et al.*, 2006) and exhibit greater transmissibility (Wada *et al.*, 2009). The genetic analysis of the Beijing family of MTB isolates based on SNPs, LSPs, IS*6110* and VNTR profiles from Thailand revealed interesting genetic polymorphisms among Beijing strains. While the SNPs showed good correlations with other genetic markers, such as LSPs and IS*6110*, some SNPs may not be irreversible genetic events (i.e., they may occur repeatedly in phylogeny). A determination of the variation of virulence of the Beijing sublineages based on a combination of genetic markers has been conducted. The results demonstrated associations between Beijing sublineages based on phylogeny and virulence, with the modern Beijing lineage being more virulent than the ancestral strain (Kaksri *et al.* unpublished). The modern Beijing strain has an increasing trend toward causing TBM in Thailand than the ancestral Beijing strain in Thailand (Faksri *et al.*, 2011b). The differences in transmissibility based on cluster analysis and the increasing trend of proportion in TBM patients compared to the ancestral Beijing sublineage support this hypothesis.

5.2 Host variation and development of TBM

Certain host groups seem to be susceptible to TB infection. There are several studies that indicate the association of host genetic vitiation and pulmonary TB. For instance, the polymorphisms of genes that are involved with cytokines and chemokines showed associations with the susceptibility of TB, such as IFN-gamma (Hashemi *et al.*, 2011), TNF-alpha (Fan *et al.*, 2010), CXCL-10 (Tang *et al.*, 2009), CCL5 (Sanchez-Castanon *et al.*, 2009) and SLC11A1 or NRAMP1 (Bellamy *et al.*, 1998). Genome-wide SNP-based linkage analysis in TB cases in Thailand showed particular regions, such as 5q, 17p and 20p, on chromosomes associated with TB susceptibility (Mahasirimongkol *et al.*, 2009). Other examples of genetic polymorphisms and susceptibility to TB are the MC3R promoter, the CTSZ 3 UTR (Adams *et al.*, 2011), P2X7 (Xiao *et al.*, 2010) and MMP-9 (Lee *et al.*, 2009). Notably, MMP-9 is the enzyme that may be involved in BBB permeability. The variation in MMP-9 encoding gene may also be associated with the development of TBM. The origin countries of patients are associated with the development of TBM (Bidstrup *et al*, 2002). The association between host genetic variations and susceptibility to the development of TBM has been proposed. SNPs at genes encoding Toll-interleukin 1 receptor domain containing adaptor protein (TIRAP) (Dissanayeke *et al.*, 2009) and Toll-like receptor-2 (TLR-2) have been shown to be associated with TB caused by the East Asian (Beijing) lineage of MTB (Thuong *et al.*, 2007), which indicates an association between host variation, the preference of certain strains of MTB and the development of certain disease types.

5.3 Co-evolution between MTB and the host in TBM

In terms of evolution, MTB is regarded as a young pathogen, which means that its evolutionary process has occurred relatively recently. MTB underwent an evolutionary bottleneck and was derived from the most recent common ancestor (MRCA) approximately 15,000-30,000 years ago (Gibbons, 2008; Kapur, 1994; Hughes *et al.*, 2002; Wirth *et al.*, 2008). Inversely, MTB may have infected humans for hundreds of thousands of years, or longer, before the MRCA appeared (Smith *et al.*, 2009). The nature of this pathogen includes an intracellular lifestyle. Humans are always a definite host of MTB. Nevertheless, infection caused by MTB can also be found in some animals, such as non-human primates (Corcoran and Thoen, 1991) and elephants (Angkawanish *et al.*, 2010; Murphree *et al.*, 2009). Although the natural defense mechanism of the host is the elimination of pathogens and foreign agents mediated by immune responses, co-adaptation between host and pathogen also occurs in nature. A good classical model of co-evolution between humans and bacteria involves the hypothesis that mitochondria used to be bacteria that co-adapted to live within eukaryotic cells as organelles (Henze and Martin, 2003). A similar model has been posited involving chloroplasts or plastids of plant cells (Patrick, 2004). A more obvious co-adaptation of bacteria to human hosts is the *Escherichia coli* found in the human gastrointestinal tract. The co-evolution between MTB and human hosts may have occurred several hundreds of thousands of years ago. However, the pathogens try to survive within the host by avoiding or suppressing the host immune response. Latent TB may be the result of a co-adaptation between MTB and host immune responses.

Regarding TBM, MTB is an obligate aerobe and prefers oxygen for growth. The underlying reason for this may reflect a preference of MTB to spread to other tissues that contain a high oxygen content, including the brain. As evidence of this, lung lesions usually occur in the right upper lobe. The altered capacity to pass the BBB may an evolutionary response for better growing conditions. Unlike other body tissues, the CNS and the CSF are parts of the body in which the immune system is less strict. The adaptation of the pathogen by escaping from the host immune system and passing the BBB for more oxygen may explain the variation of virulence and the evolution of MTB-associated TBM. However, TBM is a severe from of TB, and the evolution of MTB toward a better capacity to enter the CNS, eventually causing the death of the host, in turn causing its own death, seems to conflict with an adaptive evolutionary response. Further studies are certainly needed to explore this possibility.

6. Future research topics for TBM

The neurovirulence of MTB is still unknown. The virulence determinants of the causative agent of TBM can contribute to clinical intervention. The lineage-dependent virulence of MTB is also interesting to study, especially when applied to the consequences of treatment and vaccination. It is worthwhile to note that certain MTB strains may have specific properties that facilitate meningeal involvement and result in neurotropism, as found in *M. leprae,* which predispose it to infect peripheral nerves. Information in our unpublished study shows that certain MTB strains that vary in the copy numbers of variable number tandem repeats (VNTR2163A and 2163B) are associated with TBM rather than pulmonary TB. Further studies are needed to confirm this finding.

The pathogenesis of TBM is mainly based on studies that were performed many decades ago. The use of animal models, which are mostly based on rabbits and mice, limit the validity of the results. There is a need for appropriate animal models, such as non-human primates, for experiments that better reflect human TBM and that may reveal novel knowledge regarding pathogenesis and treatment for TBM and TB. Cynomolgus monkeys (Walsh *et al.*, 1996) and pigs (Bolin *et al.*, 1997) developed TBM with similar pathologic characteristics to human TBM following intratracheal or intravenous inoculation of mycobacteria. The mouse model is not a good animal model for TBM study due to its immunological response against infection and granuloma formation. However, because of its ease of use and the availability of facilities, mouse models are still practical to use as animal models for studying TBM. An attempt to modify the mouse model to provide the immunological inflammatory response of TBM is an applicable approach (van Well *et al.*, 2007). Other aspects of the pathogenesis of TBM can help identify novel interventions. The mechanism by which the pathogen spreads hematogenously from the lung or other infected organs into the CNS is unknown. The roles of some cytokines, such as MMP-9, vascular endothelial growth factor (VEGF) and TNF-α, for controlling the breakdown and permeability of the BBB and the role of cell death mechanisms in the pathogenesis of TBM, such as apoptosis and autophagy, are included in the list of unanswered questions. The implications of the findings from these studies will help to improve the treatment and intervention of not only TBM but also other extrapulmonary TB diseases.

The improvement of molecular methods and strategies to gain more sensitivity and specificity can largely aid the diagnosis of TBM. The development of a rapid diagnostic method with high sensitivity and specificity that is appropriate for LMIC is also a challenge. Furthermore, the rapid diagnosis of drug-resistant TB and TBM will facilitate the treatment and management of TBM patients and drug resistance surveillance.

The development of new effective treatments and novel drugs, especially drugs that can effectively penetrate the BBB, is challenging. The role of adjunctive corticosteroids in TBM patients co-infected with HIV and the effects or relationships involved in HIV-MTB co-infection, particularly the aspects of promoting effects of HIV infection and the development of MDR-TBM, are also important to study. Developing a rapid method for detection of drug-resistant strains (especially for MDR- and XDR-TB) in TBM can promote good prognoses and positive outcomes. A few studies have shown that bacteriophages can increase the sensitivity of detecting MTB in the CSF by using a fluorescent signal that can be detected within a few days rather than weeks, as in conventional culture techniques (Jacobs 1993; Drobniewski 1997). The improvement of the reliability and the standardization of these diagnosis methods may improve the phenotypic-based drug susceptibility testing of MTB. Whether there is a protective effect against the severe form of TB (i.e., TBM) and determining the immunological role of BCG vaccination against TBM are also important topics to address.

7. Acknowledgments

We would like to thank the Drug-Resistant Tuberculosis Research Fund, Siriraj Foundation, for financial support and information on drug-resistant TB. AC is supported by the Chalermprakiat grant from the Faculty of Medicine at Siriraj Hospital, Mahidol University. We thank the Department of Microbiology, Faculty of Medicine, Siriraj Hospital, Mahidol University, for providing information from patient medical records. This work is dedicated to the late HRH Princess Galyani Vadhana KromLaung Narathiwas Rajnakarindth, the Patronage of the Drug-Resistant Tuberculosis Fund, Siriraj Foundation, on the occasion of HRH's 86th birthday.

8. References

Adams, LA.; Moller, M.; Nebel, A.; Schreiber, S.; van der Merwe, L.; van Helden, PD.; & Hoal, EG. (2011). Polymorphisms in MC3R promoter and CTSZ 3'UTR are associated with tuberculosis susceptibility. *Eur J Hum Genet*, Vol. 19, No. 6, pp. 676-81.

Alonso, M.; Rodriguez, NA.; Garzelli, C.; Lirola, MM.; Herranz, M.; Samper, S.; Herranz, M.; Samper, S. & Cabrera, P. (2010). Characterization of *Mycobacterium tuberculosis* Beijing isolates from the Mediterranean area. *BMC Microbiol*, Vol. 10, pp. 151.

Angkawanish, T.; Wajjwalku, W.; Sirimalaisuwan, A.; Mahasawangkul, S.; Kaewsakhorn, T.; Boonsri, K. & Rutten, VP (2010). *Mycobacterium tuberculosis* infection of domesticated Asian elephants, Thailand . *Emerg Infect Dis,* Vol. 16, pp 1949-51.

Arvanitakis, Z.; Long, RL.; Hershfield, ES.; Manfreda, J.; Kabani, A.; Kunimoto, D.; & Power, C. (1998). *M. tuberculosis* molecular variation in CNS infection: evidence for strain-dependent neurovirulence. *Neurology*, Vol. 50, No. 6, pp 1827-32.

Awasthi, S. & Moin, S. (1999). Effectiveness of BCG vaccination against tuberculous meningitis. *Indian Pediatr*, Vol. 36, No. 5, pp 455-60.

Bandyopadhyay, SK.; Bandyopadhyay, R. & Dutta, A. (2009). Profile of tuberculous meningitis with or without HIV infection and the predicators of adverse outcome. *West Indian Med J*, Vol. 58, No. 6, pp 589-92.

Behar ,AJ.; Feldman, S. & Weber, D. (1963). Experimental Tuberculous Meningitis in Rabbits. 3. Sequence of Histological Changes Following Intracisternal Infection in Sensitized and Non-Sensitized Animals. *Acta Neuropathol*, Vol. 2, No. 3, pp 40-7.

Bellamy, R.; Ruwende, C.; Corrah, T.; McAdam, KP.; Whittle, HC. & Hill, AV. (1998) Variations in the NRAMP1 gene and susceptibility to tuberculosis in West Africans. *N Engl J Med*. Vol. 338, No. 10, pp. 640-4.

Berenguer, J.; Moreno, S.; Laguna, F; Vicente, T.; Adrados, M.; Ortega, A.; Gonzalez-LaHoz, J. & Bouza, E. (1992). Tuberculous meningitis in patients infected with the human immunodeficiency virus. *N Engl J Med*, Vol. 326, No. 10, pp 668-72.

Bernard-Griffiths, C.; Dagneaux, M.; Pastre, A.; Belin, J. & Journet, JC. (1959). Diabetes mellitus and diabetes insipidus during the evolution of tuberculous meningitis. *Sem Hop*, Vol. 35, No. 11, pp 772-5.

Bhargava, S, Gupta, AK & Tandon, PN. (1982). Tuberculous meningitis: a CT study. Br J Radiol. Vol. 55, PP. 189–96.

Bidstrup, C.; Andersen, PH.; Skinhoj, P. & Andersen, AB. Tuberculous meningitis in a country with a low incidence of tuberculosis: still a serious disease and a diagnostic challenge. *Scand J Infect Dis*, Vol. 34, No. 11, pp 811-4.

Bishburg, E.; Sunderam, G.; Reichman, LB. & Kapila, R. (1986). Central nervous system tuberculosis with the acquired immunodeficiency syndrome and its related complex. *Ann Intern Med*, Vol. 105, No. 2, pp 210-3.

Bolin, CA.; Whipple, DL.; Khanna, KV.; Risdahl, JM.; Peterson, PK. & Molitor, TW. (1997). Infection of swine with Mycobacterium bovis as a model of human tuberculosis. *J Infect Dis*, Vol. 176, No. 6, pp 1559-66.

Boonaiam, S.; Chaiprasert, A.; Prammananan, T. & Leechawengwongs, M. (2010). Genotypic analysis of genes associated with isoniazid and ethionamide resistance in MDR-TB isolates from Thailand. Clin Microbiol Infect, Vol. 16, pp. 396-9.

British Medical Research Council. Streptomycin treatment of tuberculous meningitis. (1948). BMJ, Vol. 1, pp. 582–97.

Bullock, MRR & Welchman, JM. (1982). Diagnostic and prognostic features of tuberculous meningitis on CT scanning. J Neurol Neurosurg Psychiatry, Vol. 45, pp. 1098–101.

British Thoracic Society. (1998). Chemotherapy and management of tuberculosis in the United Kingdom: recommendations 1998. Thorax, Vol. 53, pp. 536–48

Caws, M.; Thwaites, G.; Stepniewska, K.; Nguyen, TN.; Nguyen, TH.; Nguyen, TP.; Mai, NT.; Phan, MD.; Tran, HL.; Tran, TH.; van Soolingen, D.; Kremer, K.; Nguyen, VV.; Nguyen, TC. & Farrar, J. (2006). Beijing genotype of *Mycobacterium tuberculosis* is significantly associated with human immunodeficiency virus infection and multidrug resistance in cases of tuberculous meningitis. *J Clin Microbiol*. Vol. 44, No. 11, pp 3934-9.

Caws, M.; Thwaites, G.; Dunstan, S.; Hawn, TR.; Lan, NT.; Thuong, NT. Stepniewska, K.; Huyen, MN.; Bang, ND.; Loc, TH.; Gagneux, S.; van Soolingen, D.; Kremer, K.; van der Sande, M.; Small, P.; Anh, PT.; Chinh, NT.; Quy, HT.; Duyen, NT.; Tho, DQ.; Hieu, NT.; Torok, E.; Hien, TT.; Dung, NH.; Nhu, NT.; Duy, PM.; van Vinh Chau, N. & Farrar, J. (2008).The influence of host and bacterial genotype on the development of disseminated disease with *Mycobacterium tuberculosis. PLoS Pathog*, Vol. 4, No. 3: ISBN 1000034.

Cecchini, D.; Ambrosioni, J.; Brezzo, C.; Corti, M.; Rybko, A.; Perez, M. Poggi, S. & Ambroggi, M. (2009). Tuberculous meningitis in HIV-infected and non-infected patients: comparison of cerebrospinal fluid findings. *Int J Tuberc Lung Dis*, Vol. 13, No. 2, pp. 269-71.

Centers for Disease Control. Treatment of tuberculosis. (2003). MMWR Recomm Rep, Vol. 52, pp. 1–77.

Chander, PB. (2008). Multi Drug Resistant Tuberculous Meningitis in Pediatric Age Group. *Iran J Pediatr*, Vol. 18, No. 4, pp 309-14.

Chaiprasert, A.; Yorsangsukkamol, J.; Prammananan, T.; Palittapongarnpim, P.; Leechawengwong, M. & Dhiraputra, C. (2006). Intact pks15/1 in non-W-Beijing *Mycobacterium tuberculosis* isolates. Emerg Infect Dis, Vol. 12, No. 5, pp. 772-4.

Chavalittamrong, B.; Chearskul, S. & Tuchinda M. (1986). Protective value of BCG vaccination in children in Bangkok, Thailand. *Pediatr Pulmonol*. Vol. 2, No. 4, pp. 202-5.

Chaves, F.; Dronda, F.; Cave, MD.; Alonso-Sanz, M.; Gonzalez-Lopez, A/; Eisenach, KD.; Ortega, A.; Lopez-Cubero, L.

Fernandez-Martin, I.; Catalan, S. & Bates, JH. (1997). A longitudinal study of transmission of tuberculosis in a large prison population. *Am J Respir Crit Care Med*, Vol. 155, No. 2, pp. 719-25.

Cooksey, RC.; Abbadi, SH.; Woodley, CL.; Sikes, D.; Wasfy, M.; Crawford, JT.; & Mahoney, F. (2002). Characterization of *Mycobacterium tuberculosis* complex isolates from the cerebrospinal fluid of meningitis patients at six fever hospitals in Egypt. *J Clin Microbiol*, Vol. 40, No. 5, pp. 1651-5.

Corcoran, KD. & Thoen, CO. (1991). Application of an enzyme immunoassay for detecting antibodies in sera of Macaca fascicularis naturally exposed to *Mycobacterium tuberculosis. J Med Primatol*, Vol. 20, No. 8, pp. 404-408.

Daikos, GL.; Cleary, T.; Rodriguez, A. & Fischl, MA. (2003). Multidrug-resistant tuberculous meningitis in patients with AIDS. *Int J Tuberc Lung Dis*, Vol. 7, No. 4, 394-8.

Davis, LE.; Rastogi, KR.; Lambert, LC.; & Skipper, BJ. (1993). Tuberculous meningitis in the southwest United States: a community-based study. *Neurology*, Vol. 43, No. 9, pp. 1775–8.

De Cock, KM.; Soro, B.; Coulibaly, IM. & Lucas, SB. (1992). Tuberculosis and HIV infection in sub-Saharan Africa. *Jama. Vol.* 268, No. 12, pp. 1581-7.

Dissanayeke, SR.; Levin, S.; Pienaar, S.; Wood, K.; Eley, B.; Beatty, D.; Henderson, H. Anderson, S. & Levin, M. (2009). Polymorphic variation in TIRAP is not associated with susceptibility to childhood TB but may determine susceptibility to TBM in some ethnic groups. *PLoS One*, Vol. 4, No. 8, ISBN e6698.

Donald, PR.; Schoeman, JF.; Van Zyl, LE.; De Villiers, JN.; Pretorius, M. & Springer, P. (1998). Intensive short course chemotherapy in the management of tuberculous meningitis. *Int J Tuberc Lung Dis*. Vol. 2, No. 9, pp. 704-11.

Donald, PR. & Seifart, HI. (1989). Cerebrospinal fluid concentrations of ethionamide in children with tuberculous meningitis. J Pediatr, Vol. 115, pp. 483–6.

Dooley, D.; Carpenter, JL. & Rademacher S. (1997). Adjunctive corticosteroid therapy for tuberculosis: a critical reappraisal of the literature. Clin Infect Dis, Vol. 25, pp. 872–87.

Drobniewski, F.; Balabanova, Y.; Nikolayevsky, V.; Ruddy, M.; Kuznetzov, S.; Zakharova, S.; Melentyev, A. & Fedorin, I. (2005). Drug-resistant tuberculosis, clinical virulence, and the dominance of the Beijing strain family in Russia. *JAMA*, Vol. 293, No. 22, pp. 2726-31.

Drobniewski, FA. & Wilson, SM. (1997). The rapid diagnosis of isoniazid and rifampicin drug resistance in Mycobacterium tuberculosis: a molecular story. J Med Microbiol, Vol. 47, pp. 189–96.

Ellard, GA.; Humphries, MJ. & Allen, BW. (1993). Cerebrospinal fluid drug concentrations and the treatment of tuberculous meningitis. *Am Rev Respir Dis*, Vol. 148, No. 3, pp. 650-5.

Fan, HM.; Wang, Z.; Feng, FM.; Zhang, KL.; Yuan, JX.; Sui, H.; Qiu, HY.;.Liu, LH.; Deng, XJ. & Ren, JX. (2010). Association of TNF-alpha-238G/A and 308 G/A gene polymorphisms with pulmonary tuberculosis among patients with coal worker's pneumoconiosis. *Biomed Environ Sci*, Vol. 23, No. 2, pp. 137-45.

Faksri, K.; Drobniewski, F.; Nikolayevskyy, V.; Brown, T.; Prammananan, T.; Palittapongarnpim, P.; Prayoonwiwat N. & Chiprasert, A. (2011). Epidemiological trends and clinical comparisons of *M. tuberculosis* lineages in Thai TB meningitis. Tuberculosis *(Edinb)*, Vol 91, No 6, pp. 594-600.

Faksri, K.; Drobniewski, F.; Nikolayevskyy, V.; Brown, T.; Prammananan, T.; Palittapongarnpim, P.; Prayoonwiwat N & Chiprasert, A. (2011). Genetic diversity of the *Mycobacterium tuberculosis* Beijing family based on IS*6110*, SNP, LSP and VNTR profiles from Thailand. *Infect Genet Evol*, Vol. 11, No. 5, pp. 1142-9.

Farer, LS. & Meador, MP. (1979). Extrapulmonary tuberculosis in the United States. *Am J Epidemiology*, 109, pp. 205–17.

Farinha, NJ.; Razali, KA.; Holzel, H.; Morgan, G. & Novelli, VM. (2000). Tuberculosis of the central nervous system in children: a 20-year survey, *J Infect Vol.* 41, pp. 61–68.

Fletcher, AP. (1953) C.S.F.--isoniazid levels in tuberculous meningitis. *Lancet*, Vol. 265, No. 6788, pp. 694-6.

Ganiem, AR.; Parwati, I.; Wisaksana, R.; van der Zanden, A.; van de Beek, D.; Sturm, P.; van der Ven, A.; Alisjahbana, B.; Brouwer, AM.; Kurniani, N.; de Gans, J. & van Crevel, R. (2009). The effect of HIV infection on adult meningitis in Indonesia: a prospective cohort study. *Aids*, Vol. 23, No. 17, pp. 2309-16.

Gagneux, S.; DeRiemer, K.; Van, T.; Kato-Maeda, M.; de Jong, BC.; Narayanan, S.; Nicol, M.; Niemann, S.; Kremer, K.;' Gutierrez, MC.; Hilty, M.; Hopewell, PC. & Small, PM. (2006). Variable host-pathogen compatibility in Mycobacterium tuberculosis. *Proc Natl Acad Sci U S A*, Vol. 103, No. 8, pp. 2869-73.

Gibbons, A. (2008). American Association of Physical Anthropologists meeting. Tuberculosis jumped from humans to cows, not vice versa. *Science*. Vol. 320, ISSN 608.

Girgis, NI.; Sultan, Y.; Farid, Z.; Mansour, MM.; Erian, MW.; Hanna, LS.; & Mateczun, AJ. (1998). Tuberculosis meningitis, Abbassia Fever Hospital-Naval Medical Research Unit No. 3-Cairo, Egypt, from 1976 to 1996. *Am J Trop Med Hyg*, Vol. 58, No. 1, pp. 28-34.

Green, P. (1836). Tubercular meningitis. *Lancet*, Vol. 2, pp. 232–5.

Guler, N.; Ones, U.; Somer, A.; Salman, N. & Yalcin, I. (1998). The effect of prior BCG vaccination on the clinical and radiographic presentation of tuberculosis meningitis in children in Istanbul, Turkey. *Int J Tuberc Lung Dis*, Vol. 11, pp. 885-90.

Hanekom, M.; van der Spuy, GD.; Streicher, E.; Ndabambi, SL.; McEvoy, CR.; Kidd, M.; Beyers, N.; Victor, T.C.; van Helden, PD. & Warren, RM. (2007). A recently evolved sublineage of the *Mycobacterium tuberculosis* Beijing strain family is associated with an increased ability to spread and cause disease. *J Clin Microbiol*, Vol. 45, No. 5, pp. 1483-90.

Hashemi, M.; Sharifi-Mood, B.; Nezamdoost, M.; Moazeni-Roodi, A.; Naderi, M.; Kouhpayeh, H.; Taheri, M. & Ghavami, S. (2011). Functional polymorphism of interferon-gamma (IFN-gamma) gene +874T/A polymorphism is associated with pulmonary tuberculosis in Zahedan, Southeast Iran. *Prague Med Rep*, Vol. 112, No. 1, pp. 38-43.

Hawn, TR.; Dunstan, SJ.; Thwaites, GE.; Simmons, CP.; Thuong,; NT, Lan, NT.; Quy, HT.; Chau, TT.; Hieu, NT.; Rodrigues, S.; Janer, M.; Zhao, LP.; Hien, TT.; Farrar, JJ. & Aderem, A. (2006). A polymorphism in Toll-interleukin 1 receptor domain containing adaptor protein is associated with susceptibility to meningeal tuberculosis. J Infect Dis, Vol. 194, No. 8, pp. 1127-34.

Henze, K. & Martin, W.; (2003). Evolutionary biology: essence of mitochondria. *Nature*, Vol. 426, No. 6963, pp. 127–8.

Hosoglu, S.; Ayaz, C.; Geyik, MF.; Kokoglu, OF. & Ceviz, A. (1998).Tuberculous meningitis in adults: an eleven-year review. *Int J Tuberc Lung Dis*, Vol. 2, No. 7, pp. 553-7.

Hosoglu, S.; Geyik, MF.; Balik, I.; Aygen, B.; Erol, S.; Aygencel, SG.: Mert, A.; Saltoglu, N.; Dokmetas, I.; Felek, S.; Sunbul, M.; Irmak, H.; Aydin, K.; Kokoglu, OF.; Ucmak, H.; Altindis, M. & Loeb, M. (2002). Predictors of outcome in patients with tuberculous meningitis. *Int J Tuberc Lung Dis*, Vol. 6, No. 1, pp. 64-70.

Hosoglu, S.; Geyik, MF.; Balik, I.; Aygen, B.; Erol, S.; Aygencel, SG.; Mert, A.; Saltoglu, N.; Dokmetas, I.; Felek, S.; Sunbul, M.; Irmak, H.; Aydin, K.; Ayaz, C.; Kokoglu, OF.; Ucmak, H. & Satilmis, S. (2003). Tuberculous meningitis in adults in Turkey: epidemiology, diagnosis, clinic and laboratory [corrected]. *Eur J Epidemiol*, Vol. 18, No. 4, pp. 337-43.

Huempener, HR.; Kingsolver, WR. & Deuschle, KW. (1966).Tuberculous meningitis caused by both *Mycobacterium tuberculosis* and atypical mycobacteria. *Am Rev Respir Dis*, Vol. 94, No. 4, pp. 612-4.

Hughes, AL.; Friedman, R. & Murray, M. (2002). Genomewide pattern of synonymous nucleotide substitution in two complete genomes of *Mycobacterium tuberculosis*. *Emerg Infect Dis*, Vol. 8, pp. 1342–1346.

Humphries, M. (1992). The management of tuberculous meningitis. *Thorax*. Vol. 47, No. 8, pp. 577-81.

Kumar, R.; Singh Jain, SK.; Paul-Satyaseela, M.; Lamichhane, G.; Kim, KS. & Bishai, W. (2006). *Mycobacterium tuberculosis* invasion and transversal across an in vivo human blood-brain barrier as a pathogenic mechanism for central nervous system tuberculosis. *JID*, Vol. 193, pp. 1287-95.

Iwamoto, T.; Fujiyama, R.; Yoshida, S.; Wada, T.; Shirai, C. & Kawakami, Y. (2009). Population structure dynamics of *Mycobacterium tuberculosis* Beijing strains during past decades in Japan. *J Clin Microbiol*, Vol. 47, No. 10, pp. 3340-3.

Iwamoto, T.; Yoshida, S.; Suzuki ,K & Wada, T. (2008). Population structure analysis of the *Mycobacterium tuberculosis* Beijing family indicates an association between certain sublineages and multidrug resistance. *Antimicrobial Agent Chem,* Vol. 52, pp. 3805-9.

Jacobs, WR.; Barletta, RG. & Udani R. (1993). Rapid assessment of drug susceptibilities of MTB by means of luciferase reporter phages. Science, Vol. 260, pp. 819–22.

Jeren, T & Beus, I. (1982). Characteristics of cerebrospinal fluid in tuberculous meningitis. Acta Cytol, Vol. 26, pp. 678–80.

Joint Tuberculosis Committee of the British Thoracic Society. (1998). Chemotherapy and management of tuberculosis in the United Kingdom: recommendations 1998. *Thorax*, 53, 7, pp 536-48.

Kalita, J. & Misra, UK. (1999). Outcome of tuberculous meningitis at 6 and 12 months: a multiple regression analysis. *Int J Tuberc Lung Dis*, Vol. 3, No. 3, pp. 261-5.

Kapur, V.; Whittam, TS. & Musser, JM. (1994). Is *Mycobacterium tuberculosis* 15,000 years old? *J. Infect. Dis*, Vol. 170, pp. 1348–1349.

Karstaedt, AS.; Valtchanova, S.; Barriere, R. & Crewe-Brown, HH. (1998). Tuberculous meningitis in South African urban adults. *Qjm*, Vol. 91, No. 11, pp. 743-7.

Kashyap, RS.; Agarwal, NP.; Chandak, NH.; Taori, GM.; Biswas, SK.; Purohit, HJ & Daginawala, HF. (2002). The application of the Mancini technique as a diagnostic test in the CSF of tuberculous meningitis patients. *Med Sci Monit, Vol.* 8, No. 6, pp. MT95-98.

Katrak, SM.; Shembalkar, PK.; Bijwe, SR. & Bhandarkar, LD. (2000). The clinical, radiological and pathological profile of tuberculous meningitis in patients with and without human immunodeficiency virus infection. *J Neurol Sci*, Vol. 181, No. 1-2, pp. 118-26.

Kaneko, H.; Yamada, H.; Mizuno, S.; Udagawa, T.; Kazumi, Y.; Sekikawa, K. & Sugawara, I. (1999). Role of tumor necrosis factor-alpha in Mycobacterium-induced granuloma formation in tumor necrosis factor-alpha-deficient mice. *Lab Invest*, Voo. 79, No. 4, pp. 379-86.

Kent, SJ.; Crowe, SM.; Yung, A.; Lucas, CR. & Mijch, AM. (1993). Tuberculous meningitis: a 30-year review. *Clin Infect Dis*, Vol. 17, pp. 987–94.

Kim, SH.; Chu, K.; Choi, SJ.; Song, KH.; Kim, HB.; Kim, NJ.; Park, SH.; Yoon, BW.; Oh, MD. & Choe, KW. (2008). Diagnosis of central nervous system tuberculosis by T-cell-based assays on peripheral blood and cerebrospinal fluid mononuclear cells. Clin Vaccine Immunol, Vol. 15, No. 9, pp. 1356-62.

Koch, R. (1882). Die aetiologie der Tuberculosos. *Ber Klin Wochenschr*, Vol. 19, ISSN 2211.

Kohli, SN. (1999). A diagnostic rule for tuberculous meningitis. *Arch Dis Child*, Vol. 81, No. 3, pp. 221-4.

Kong, Y.; Cave, MD.; Zhang, L.; Foxman, B.; Marrs, CF.; Bates, JH. &Yang, ZH. (2007). Association between *Mycobacterium tuberculosis* Beijing/W lineage strain infection and extrathoracic tuberculosis: Insights from epidemiologic and clinical characterization of the three principal genetic groups of *M. tuberculosis* clinical isolates. *J Clin Microbiol*, Vol. 45, No. 2, pp. 409-14.

Kruijshaar, ME. & Abubakar I. (2009). Increase in extrapulmonary tuberculosis in England and Wales 1999-2006. *Thorax*, Vol. **64**, pp. 1090-5.

Kumar, R.; Dwivedi, A.; Kumar, P. & Kohli, N. (2005). Tuberculous meningitis in BCG vaccinated and unvaccinated children. *J Neurol Neurosurg Psychiatry*, Vol. 76, No. 11, pp. 1550-4.

Lee, SH.; Han, SK.; Shim, YS. & Yim, JJ. (2009). Effect of matrix metalloproteinase-9 -1562C/T gene polymorphism on manifestations of pulmonary tuberculosis. Tuberculosis (Edinb). Vol. 89, No. 1, pp. 68-70.

Li, Q.; Whalen, CC.; Albert, JM.; Larkin, R.; Zukowski, L.; Cave, MD.; & Silver, RF. (2002). Differences in rate and variability of intracellular growth of a panel of *Mycobacterium tuberculosis* clinical isolates within a human monocyte model. *Infect Immun*, Vol. 70, No. 11, pp. 6489-93.

Leonard, J. & Des Prez, RM. (1990). Tuberculous meningitis. Infect Dis Clin North Am. Vol. 4, pp. 769–87.

Lopez, B.; Aguilar, D.; Orozco, H.; Burger, M.; Espitia, C.; Ritacco, V.; Barrera, L.; Kremer, K.; Hernandez-Pando, R.; Huygen, K.; van Soolingen, D. (2003). A marked difference in pathogenesis and immune response induced by different *Mycobacterium tuberculosis* genotypes. *Clin Exp Immunol*, Vol. 133, No. 1, pp. 30-7.

Lan, NT.; Lien, HT.; Tung le, B.; Borgdorff, MW.; Kremer, K. & van Soolingen, D. (2003). *Mycobacterium tuberculosis* Beijing genotype and risk for treatment failure and relapse, *Vietnam Emerg Infect Dis*, Vol. 9, No. 12, pp. 1633-5.

Mahasirimongkol, S.; Yanai, H.; Nishida, N.; Ridruechai, C.; Matsushita, I.; Ohashi, J.; Summanapan, S.; Yamada, N.; Moolphate, S.; Chuchotaworn, C.; Chaiprasert, A.; Manosuthi, W.; Kantipong, P.; Kanitwittaya, S.; Sura, T.; Khusmith, S.; Tokunaga, K.; Sawanpanyalert, P. & Keicho, N. (2009). Genome-wide SNP-based linkage analysis of tuberculosis in Thais. Genes Immun, Vol. 10 No. 1, pp. 77-83.

Manca, CTL.; Bergtold, A.; Freeman, S.; Tovey, M.; Musser, JM.; Barry, C. E., 3rd; Freedman, V. H. & Kaplan, G. (2001). Virulence of a *Mycobacterium tuberculosis* clinical isolate in mice is determined by failure to induce Th1 type immunity and is associated with induction of IFN-alpha /beta. *Proc Natl Acad Sci USA*, Vol. 98, pp. 5752-7.

Manwaring, WH. (1912). The Effects of Subdural Injections of Leucocytes on the Development and Course of Experimental Tuberculous Meningitis. *J Exp Med*, Vol. 15, No. 1, pp. 1-13.

Maree, F.; Hesseling, AC.; Schaaf, HS.; Marais, BJ.; Beyers, N.; van Helden, P.; Warren, RM. & Schoeman, JF. (2007). Absence of an association between *Mycobacterium tuberculosis* genotype and clinical features in children with tuberculous meningitis. *Pediatr Infect Dis J*, Vol. 26, No. 1, pp. 13-8. pp.

Mastroianni, CM.; Paoletti, F.; Lichtner, M.; D'Agostino, C.; Vullo, V. & Delia, S. (1997). Cerebrospinal fluid cytokines in patients with tuberculous meningitis. *Clin Immunol Immunopathol*, Vol. 84, No. 2, pp. 171-6.

Matsubara, T. (1956). Experimental formation of tuberculous meningitis in rabbit. II. Experiment with bovine type Tbc. bacillus. *Kekkaku*, Vol. 31, No. 7, pp. 411-7.

Mathai, A.; Radhakrishnan, VV.; George, SM. & Sarada C. (2001). A newer approach for the laboratory diagnosis of tuberculous meningitis. Diagn Microbiol Infect Dis, Vol. 39, No.4, pp. 225-8.

Mittal, SK.; Aggarwal, V.; Rastogi, A. & Saini, N. (1996). Does B.C.G. vaccination prevent or postpone the occurrence of tuberculous meningitis? *Indian J Pediatr*, Vol. 63, No. 5, pp. 659-64.

Mokrousov, I.; Jiao, WW.; Valcheva, V.; Vyazovaya, A.; Otten, T.; Ly, HM. & Ly, H. M.; Lan, NN.; Limeschenko, E.; Markova, N.; Vyshnevskiy, B.; Shen, AD.& Narvskaya, O. (2006). Rapid detection of the *Mycobacterium tuberculosis* Beijing genotype and its ancient and modern sublineages by IS*6110*-based inverse PCR. *J Clin Microbiol,* Vol. 44, pp. 2851-56.

Mori, MA.; Leonardson, G. & Welty, TK. (1992). The benefits of isoniazid chemoprophylaxis and risk factors for tuberculosis among Oglala Sioux Indians,,Arch Intern Med, Vol. No. 3, pp. 547–50.

Murphree, R.; Warkentin, JV.; Dunn, JR.; Schaffner, W. & Jones, TF. (2009). Elephant-to-human transmission of tuberculosis. *Emerg Infect Dis,* Vol. 17, pp. 366-371.

Nagarathna, S.; Rafi, W.; Veenakumari, HB.; Mani, R.; Satishchandra, P. & Chandramuki, A. (2008). Drug susceptibility profiling of tuberculous meningitis. *Int J Tuberc Lung Dis,* Vol. 12, No. 1, pp. 105-7.

Nau, R.; Prange, HW.; Menck, S.; Kolenda, H.; Visser, K. & Seydel, JK. (1992). Penetration of rifampicin into the cerebrospinal fluid of adults with uninflamed meninges. *J Antimicrob Chemother,* Vol. 29, No. 6, pp. 719-24.

Pablos-Mendez, A.; Blustein, J. & Knirsch, CA. (1997). The role of diabetes mellitus in the higher prevalence of tuberculosis among Hispanics. *Am J Public Health.* Vol. 87, No. 4, pp. 574-9.

Padayatchi, N.; Bamber, S.; Dawood, H. & Bobat, R. (2006). Multidrug-resistant tuberculous meningitis in children in Durban, South Africa. *Pediatr Infect Dis J,* Vol. 25, No. 2, pp. 147-50.

Prammananan, T.; Arjratanakool, W.; Chaiprasert, A.; Leechawengwong, M.; Asawapokee, N.; Leelarasamee, A. & Dhiraputra C. (2005). Second-line drug susceptibilities of Thai multidrug-resistant Mycobacterium tuberculosis isolates. Int J Tuberc Lung Dis, Vol. 9, No. 2, pp. 216-9.

Prammananan, T.; Chaiprasert, A. & Leechawengwongs, M. (2011) 8-years experience of fluoroquinolone susceptibility testing of multidrug-resistant *Mycobacterium tuberculosis* isolates from Siriraj Hospital, Thailand. Intern J Antimicrob Agent, Vol. 37, No. 84-5.

Prammananan, T.; Chaiprasert, A. & Leechawengwongs, M. (2009). *In vitro* activity of linezolid against multidrug-resistant tuberculosis (MDR-TB) and extensively drug-resistant (XDR-TB) isolates. Intern J Antimicrobial Agents, Vol. 33, pp. 190-1.

Prammananan, T.; Cheunoy, W.; Taechamahapun, D.; Yorsangsukkamol, J.; Phunpruch, S.; Phdarat, P.; Leechawengwong, M. & Chaiprasert, A. (2006). Distribution of *rpoB* mutations among MDRTB strains from Thailand and development of a rapid method for detection mutation. Clin Microbiol Infec Dis, Vol. 14, pp. 446-53.

Patel, VB.; Padayatchi, N.; Bhigjee, AI.; Allen, J.; Bhagwan, B.; Moodley, AA. & Mthiyane, T. (2004). Multidrug-resistant tuberculous meningitis in KwaZulu-Natal, South Africa. *Clin Infect Dis,* Vol. 38, No. 6, pp. 851-6.

Pethe, K.; Alonso, S.; Biet, F.; Delogu, G.; Brennan, MJ.; Locht, C. & Menozzi, F. D. (2001). The heparin-binding haemagglutinin *of M. tuberculosis* is required for extrapulmonary dissemination. *Nature,* Vol. 412, No. 6843, pp. 190-4.

Patrick, J.& Keeling (2004). Diversity and evolutionary history of plastids and their hosts. *American Journal of Botany, Vol.* 91, pp. 1481–1493. doi:10.3732/ajb.91.10.1481

Puvacic, S.; Dizdarevic, J.; Santic, Z. & Mulaomerovic, M. (2004). Protective effect of neonatal BCG vaccines against tuberculous meningitis. *Bosn J Basic Med Sci,* Vol. 4, No. 1, pp. 46-9.

Radhakrishnan, VV., Mathai, A. & Mohan PK. (1994). Diagnosis of tuberculous meningitis by enzyme-linked immuno-sorbent assay (ELISA), using an affinity chromatography purified mycobacterial antigen. J Assoc Physicians India 1994, Vol. 42, No. 9, pp. 684-7.

Reed, MB.; Domenech, P.; Manca, C.; Su, H.; Barczak, AK.; Kreiswirth, BN.; Kaplan, G. & Barry, CE., 3rd (2004). A glycolipid of hypervirulent tuberculosis strains that inhibits the innate immune response. *Nature*, Vol. 431, No. 7004, pp. 84-7.

Rich, AR. (1933). The pathogenesis of tuberculous meningitis. *Bulletin of John Hopkins Hospital*. Vol. 52. pp. 5–37.

Rienthong, D.; Ajawatanawong, P.; Rienthong, S.; Smithtikarn, S.; Akarasewi, P.; Chaiprasert, A. & Palittapongarnpim, P. (2005). Restriction fragment length polymorphism study of nationwide samples of *Mycobacterium tuberculosis* in Thailand, 1997-1998. *Int J Tuberc Lung Dis*, Vol. 9, No. 5, pp. 576-81.

Robertson, GH. & Bersohn, I. (1950). The laboratory diagnosis of tuberculous meningitis. S Afr Med J. Vol. 24, No. 22, pp. 411-4.

Roca, B.; Tornador, N. & Tornador, E. (2008). Presentation and outcome of tuberculous meningitis in adults in the province of Castellon, Spain: a retrospective study. *Epidemiol Infect*, Vol. 136, No. 11, pp. 1455-62.

Sanchez-Castanon, M.; Baquero, IC.; Sanchez-Velasco, P.; Farinas, MC.; Ausin, F.; Leyva-Cobian, F.; & Ocejo-Vinyals, J G.. (2009). Polymorphisms in CCL5 promoter are associated with pulmonary tuberculosis in northern Spain. *Int J Tuberc Lung Dis*, Vol. 13, No. 4, pp. 480-5.

Selwyn, PA.; Lewis, VA.; Schoenbaum, EE.; Vermund, SH.; Klein, RS.; Walker, AT. & Friedland, GH. (1989). A prospective study of the risk of tuberculosis among intravenous drug users with human immunodeficiency virus infection, N Engl J Med, Vol. 320, No.9, pp. 345–50.

Seth, R. & Sharma, U. (2002). Diagnostic criteria for Tuberculous Meningitis. *Indian J Pediatr*, Vol. 69, No. 4, pp. 299-303.

Sidel'Nikova, EF. & Rozina, RI. (1956). Bromide metabolism in rabbits with experimental tuberculous meningitis. *Vopr Med Khim*, Vol. 2, No. 6, pp. 417-23.

Smith, NH.; Hewinson, RG.; Kremer, K.; Brosch, R. & Gordon, SV. (2009). Myths and misconceptions: the origin and evolution of *Mycobacterium tuberculosis*. *Nat Rev Microbiol*, Vol. 7, No. 7, pp. 537-44.

Srisaimanee, N.; Chaiprasert, A.; Gengvinij, A.; Kunakorn, M. & Prayoonwiwat N. (2002). Evaluation of in-house optimized semi-nested PCR and EIA for direct detection of mycobacterial DNA in CSF. Asian Pac J Aller Immunol, Vol. 20, No. 4, pp. 267-77.

Stead, WW.; Senner, JW.; Reddick, WT. & Lofgren, JP.(1990). Racial differences in susceptibility to infection by *Mycobacterium tuberculosis*. N Engl J Med. Vol. 322, No. 7, pp. 422-7.

Sumi, MG.; Annamma, M.; Sarada, C. & Radhakrishnan, VV. (2000). Rapid diagnosis of tuberculous meningitis by a dot-immunobinding assay. Acta Neurol Scand 2000, Vol. 101, No.1, pp. 61-4.

Sumi, MG., Mathai, A., Reuben, S., Sarada, C & Radhakrishnan, VV. (2002). Immunocytochemical method for early laboratory diagnosis of tuberculous meningitis. *Clin Diagn Lab Immunol. Vol.* 9, No. 2, pp. 344-7.

Sutlas, PN.; Unal, A.; Forta, H.; Senol, S. & Kirbas, D. Tuberculous meningitis in adults: review of 61 cases. *Infection*, Vol. 31, No. 6, pp. 387-91.

Takahashi, S.; Takahashi, T.; Kuragano, T.; Nagura, Y.; Fujita, T.; Nakayama, T. & Matsumoto, K. (2005). A case of chronic renal failure complicated with tuberculous meningitis successfully diagnosed by nested polymerase chain reaction (PCR). *Nippon Jinzo Gakkai Shi*, Vol. 47, No. 2, pp. 113-20.

Tang, NL.; Fan, HP.; Chang, KC.; Ching, JK.; Kong, KP.; Yew, WW.; & Kam, KM.; Leung, CC.; Tam, CM.; Blackwell, J. & Chan, CY. (2009). Genetic association between a chemokine gene CXCL-10 (IP-10, interferon gamma inducible protein 10) and susceptibility to tuberculosis. *Clin Chim Acta*, Vol. 406, No. 1-2, pp. 98-102.

Tardieu, M.; Truffot-Pernot, C.; Carriere, JP.; Dupic, Y. & Landrieu, P. (1988). Tuberculous meningitis due to BCG in two previously healthy children. *Lancet*, Vol. 1, No. 8583, pp. 440-1.

Teasdale, G & Jennett, B. (1974). Assessment of coma and impaired consciousness: a practical scale. Lancet, Vol. 2, pp. 81–4.

Theus, S.; Eisenach, K.; Fomukong, N.; Silver, RF. & Cave, MD. (2007). Beijing family *Mycobacterium tuberculosis* strains differ in their intracellular growth in THP-1 macrophages. *Int J Tuberc Lung Dis*, Vol. 11, No. 10, pp. 1087-93.

Thilothammal, N.; Krishnamurthy, PV.; Runyan, DK. & Banu, K. (1996). Does BCG vaccine prevent tuberculous meningitis? *Arch Dis Child*, Vol. 74, No. 2, pp. 144-7.

Thuong, NT.; Dunstan, SJ.; Chau, TT.; Thorsson, V.; Simmons, CP.; Quyen, NT.; Thwaites, GE.; Thi Ngoc Lan, N.; Hibberd, M.; Teo, YY.; Seielstad, M.; Aderem, A.; Farrar, JJ. & Hawn, TR. (2008). Identification of tuberculosis susceptibility genes with human macrophage gene expression profiles. *PLoS Pathog*, Vol. 4, No. 12, ISSN 1000229.

Thuong, NT.; Hawn, TR.; Thwaites, GE.; Chau, TT.; Lan, NT.; Quy, HT.; Hieu, NT.; Aderem, A.; Hien, TT.; Farrar, JJ.; Dunstan, SJ. (2007). A polymorphism in human TLR2 is associated with increased susceptibility to tuberculous meningitis. *Genes Immun*, Vol. 8, No. 5, pp. 422-8.

Thwaites, GE.; Fisher, M.; Hemingway, C.; Scott, G.; Solomon, T & Innes J. (2009). British Infection Society guidelines for the diagnosis and treatment of tuberculosis of the central nervous system in adults and children. *J Infect*, Vol. 59, No. 3, pp.167-87.

Thwaites, GE. & Schoeman, JF. (2009) Update on tuberculosis of the central nervous system: pathogenesis, diagnosis, and treatment. *Clin Chest Med*, Vol. 30, No. 4, pp. 745-54, ix.

Thwaites, G.; Caws, M.; Chau, TT.; D'Sa, A.; Lan, NT.; Huyen, MN.; Gagneux, S.; Anh, PT.; Tho, DQ.; Torok, E.; Nhu, NT.; Duyen, NT.; Duy, PM.; Richenberg, J.; Simmons, C.; Hien, TT. & Farrar, J. (2008). Relationship between *Mycobacterium tuberculosis* genotype and the clinical phenotype of pulmonary and meningeal tuberculosis. *J Clin Microbiol*, Vol. 46, No. 4, pp. 1363-8.

Thwaites, GE.; Duc Bang, N.; Huy Dung, N.; Thi Quy, H.; Thi Tuong Oanh, D.; Thi Cam Thoa, N.; Quang Hien, N.; Tri Thuc, N.; Ngoc Hai, N.; Thi Ngoc Lan, N.; Ngoc Lan, N.; Hong Duc, N.; Ngoc Tuan, V.; Huu Hiep, C.; Thi Hong Chau, T.; Phuong Mai, P.; Thi Dung, N.; Stepniewska, K.; Simmons, CP.; White, NJ.; Tinh Hien, T. & Farrar, JJ. (2005). The influence of HIV infection on clinical presentation, response to treatment, and outcome in adults with Tuberculous meningitis. *J Infect Dis*, Vol. 192, No. 12, pp. 2134-41.

Thwaites, GE.; Lan, NT.; Dung, NH.; Quy, HT.; Oanh, DT.; Thoa, NT.; & Hien, NQ.; Thuc, NT.; Hai, NN.; Bang, ND.; Lan, NN.; Duc, NH.; Tuan, VN.; Hiep, CH.; Chau, TT.; Mai, PP.; Dung, NT.; Stepniewska, K.; White, NJ.; Hien, TT. & Farrar, JJ. (2005).

Effect of antituberculosis drug resistance on response to treatment and outcome in adults with tuberculous meningitis. J Infect Dis, Vol. 192, No. 1, pp. 79-88.
Thwaites, GE. & Tran, TH. (2005). Tuberculous meningitis: many questions, too few answers. *Lancet Neurol*, Vo. 4, No. 3, pp. 160-70.
Thwaites, GE.; Nguyen, DB.; Nguyen, HD.; Hoang, TQ.; Do, TT.; Nguyen, TC.; Nguyen, QH.; Nguyen, TT.; Nguyen, NH.; Nguyen, TN.; Nguyen, NL.; Nguyen, HD.;Vu, NT.; Cao, HH.; Tran, T H.; Pham, PM. ;Nguyen, TD.; Stepniewska, K.; White, NJ.; Tran, TH. & Farrar, JJ. (2004). Dexamethasone for the treatment of tuberculous meningitis in adolescents and adults. *N Engl J Med*, Vol. 351, No. 17, pp.1741-51.
Thwaites, GE.; Chau, TT.; Caws, M.; Phu, NH.; Chuong, LV.; Sinh, DX.; Drobniewski, F.; White, NJ.; Parry, CM.; Farrar, JJ. (2002). Isoniazid resistance, mycobacterial genotype and outcome in Vietnamese adults with tuberculous meningitis. *Int J Tuberc Lung Dis*, Vol. 6, No. 10, pp. 865-71.
Tsenova, L.; Ellison, E.; Harbacheuski, R.; Moreira, AL.; Kurepina, N.; Reed, MB.; Mathema, B.; Barry, CE., 3rd & Kaplan, G. (2005). Virulence of selected *Mycobacterium tuberculosis* clinical isolates in the rabbit model of meningitis is dependent on phenolic glycolipid produced by the bacilli. *J Infect Dis*, Vol. 192, No 1, pp. 98-106.
Trunz, BB.; Fine, P. & Dye, C. (2006). Effect of BCG vaccination on childhood tuberculous meningitis and miliary tuberculosis worldwide: a meta-analysis and assessment of cost-effectiveness. *Lancet*, Vol. 367, No. 9517, pp. 1173-80.
Tsenova, L.; Bergtold, A.; Freedman, VH.; Young, RA. & Kaplan, G. (1999). Tumor necrosis factor alpha is a determinant of pathogenesis and disease progression in mycobacterial infection in the central nervous system. *Proc Natl Acad Sci U S A*, Vol. 96, No. 10, pp. 5657-62.
Tsenova, L.; Ellison, E.; Harbacheuski, R.; Moreira, AL.; Kurepina, N.; Reed, MB.; Mathema, B.; Barry, CE., 3rd & Kaplan, G. (2005). Virulence of selected *Mycobacterium tuberculosis* clinical isolates in the rabbit model of meningitis is dependent on phenolic glycolipid produced by the bacilli. J Infect Dis, Vol. 192, No. 1, pp. 98-106.
Tsenova, L.; Harbacheuski, R.; Sung, N.; Ellison, E.; Fallows, D. & Kaplan, G. (2007). BCG vaccination confers poor protection against *M. tuberculosis* HN878-induced central nervous system disease. *Vaccine*, Vol. 25, No. 28, pp. 5126-32.
Van der Weert, EM.; Hartgers, NM.; Schaaf, HS.; Eley, BS.; Pitcher, RD.; Wieselthaler, NA.; Laubscher, R.; Donald, PR. & Schoeman, JF. (2006). Comparison of diagnostic criteria of tuberculous meningitis in human immunodeficiency virus-infected and uninfected children. *Pediatr Infect Dis J*, Vol. 25, No. 1, pp. 65-9.
Van Loenhout-Rooyackers, JH.; Keyser, A.; Laheij, RJ.; Verbeek, AL. & van der Meer, JW. (2001). Tuberculous meningitis: is a 6-month treatment regimen sufficient? *Int J Tuberc Lung Dis*, Vol. 5, No. 11, pp. 1028-35.
Van Soolingen, D.; Qian, L.; de Haas, PE.; Douglas, JT.; Traore, H.; Portaels, F.; Qing, HZ.; Enkhsaikan, D.; Nymadawa, P. & van Embden, JD. (1995). Predominance of a single genotype of *Mycobacterium tuberculosis* in countries of east Asia. *J Clin Microbiol*, Vol. 33, No. 12, pp. 3234-8.
Van Well, GT.; Wieland, CW.; Florquin, S.; Roord, JJ.; van der Poll, T. & van Furth, AM. (2007). A new murine model to study the pathogenesis of tuberculous meningitis. *J Infect Dis*, Vol. 195, No. 5, pp. 694-7.
Verdon, R.; Chevret, S.; Laissy, JP. & Wolff. (1996). M. Tuberculous meningitis in adults: review of 48 cases. *Clin Infect Dis*, Vol. 22, No. 6, pp. 982-8.

Wada, T.; Fujihara, S.; Shimouchi, A.; Harada, M.; Ogura, H.; Matsumoto, S.; & Hase, A. (2009). High transmissibility of the modern Beijing *Mycobacterium tuberculosis* in homeless patients of Japan. *Tuberculosis (Edinb)*, Vol. 89, No. 4, pp. 252-5.

Walsh, GP.; Tan, EV.; dela Cruz, EC.; Abalos, RM.; Villahermosa, LG.; Young, LJ.; Cellona, RV.; Nazareno, JB. & Horwitz, MA. (1996). The Philippine cynomolgus monkey (Macaca fasicularis) provides a new nonhuman primate model of tuberculosis that resembles human disease. *Nat Med*, Vol. 2, No. 4, pp. 430-6.

Wirth, T.; Hildebrand, F.; Allix-Beguec, C.; Wolbeling, F.; Kubica, T.; Kremer, K.; van Soolingen, D.; Rusch-Gerdes, S.; Locht, C.; Brisse, S.; Meyer, A.; Supply, P. & Niemann, S. (2008). Origin, spread and demography of the *Mycobacterium tuberculosis* complex. *PLoS Pathog*, Vol. 4, ISSN e1000160.

World Health Organization. (2009).Global tuberculosis control report 2009. Epidemiology, strategy, financing. Accessed 2011, Available from http://whqlibdoc.who.int/publications/2009/9789241563802_eng.pdf.

World Health Organization. (2008). Ani-tuberculous drug resisatnce in the world; Fourth Global Report, Accessed 2011, Available from http://wwwwhoint/mediacentre/news/releases/2008/pr05/en/indexhtml

World Health Organization. (2003) Tuberculosis: Advocacy Report. World Health Organization, Accessed 2003, Available from http://www.who.int/tb/publications/advocacy_report_2003/en/index.html

World Health Organization. (1997) Global Tuberculosis Control Reports 1997. Accessed 2011, Available from http://whqlibdoc.who.int/hq/1997/WHO_TB_97.225_(part1).pdf

Wunsch Filho, V.; de Castilho, EA.; Rodrigues, LC. & Huttly, SR. (1990). Effectiveness of BCG vaccination against tuberculous meningitis: a case-control study in Sao Paulo, Brazil. *Bull World Health Organ*, Vol. 68, No. 1, pp. 69-74.

Xiao, J.; Sun, L.; Yan, H.; Jiao, W.; Miao, Q.; Feng, W.; Wu, X.; Gu, Y.; Jiao, A.; Guo, Y.; Peng, X. & Shen, A. (2010). Metaanalysis of P2X7 gene polymorphisms and tuberculosis susceptibility. *FEMS Immunol Med Microbiol*, Vol. 60, No. 2, pp. 165-70.

Xiong, CH.; Liang, XF. & Wang, HQ. (2009). A systematic review on the protective efficacy of BCG against children tuberculosis meningitis and millet tuberculosis. *Zhongguo Yi Miao He Mian Yi*, Vol. 15, No. 4, pp. 358-62.

Yorsangsukkamol, J.; Chaiprasert, A.; Prammananan, T.; Palittapongarnpim, P.; Limsoontarakul, S. & Prayoonwiwat, N. (2009). Molecular analysis of *Mycobacterium tuberculosis* from tuberculous meningitis patients in Thailand. *Tuberculosis (Edinb)*, Vol. 89, No. 4, pp. 304-9.

Yorsangsukkamol, J.; Chaiprasert, A.; Palaga, T.; Prammananan, T.; Faksri, K.; Palittapongarnpim, P. & Prayoonwiwat, N. (2011). Apoptosis, production of MMP9, VEGF, TNF-α and intracellular growth of *M. tuberculosis* different genotypes and different *pks*15/1 genes. APJAI, Vol. 29, No. 3, pp. 240-51.

9

Aseptic Meningitis Caused by Enteroviruses

Takeshi Hayashi, Takamasa Shirayoshi and Masahiro Ebitani
Department of Neurology,
Fuji Heavy Industries Health Insurance Corporation,
Ota General Hospital,
Japan

1. Introduction

A broad range of microorganisms cause meningitis; viruses, bacteria, mycobacteria, mycoplasma, spirochetes, fungi, and protozoa have all been identified as causative agents. Some pathogens almost exclusively affect immunocompromised hosts, and some are confined only to endemic areas, but viruses are the most common pathogen worldwide. It is estimated that about 75,000 people in the United States suffer from viral meningitis annually. The annual incidence of bacterial meningitis in the United States is approximately 3 per 100,000 (Tunkel & Sheld, 1993), therefore, viral meningitis is far more common. Although the exact number of cases varies among countries, viral meningitis is the most common meningitis in almost all countries throughout the world.

Although many patients with viral meningitis are not admitted to a hospital because of an uneventful clinical course, 25,000-50,000 are hospitalized every year in the United States (Khetsuriani et al., 2003; Wang et al., 2002). The estimated mean charge for viral meningitis-associated hospitalization from 1993-1997 was between USD 6,562 and 8,313, resulting in annual estimated hospitalization costs between USD 234 and 310 million (Khetsuriani et al., 2003,; Parasuraman et al., 2001). Viral meningitis is, in most cases, a benign disease with a self-limiting clinical course, but the economic impact it imposes is large. Furthermore, the disease may appear as a small to large outbreak. If large outbreak occurs, they are likely to be enormous economic losses. To better characterize the features of viral meningitis and the causative agents are therefore of importance.

Many viruses can cause meningitis, and the frequency at which each virus is identified differs geographically and yearly. In addition, a causative virus is not identified in many cases of aseptic meningitis. In spite of extensive investigation, no causative agents are identified in about one-third of the cases of aseptic meningitis. When identified, however, enteroviruses are the most frequent agent in every investigated series (CDC, 2003; Kao et al., 2003; Meyer et al., 1960; Tyler & Martin, 1993; Wang et al., 2002), being detected in from 30 to 83% of the cases. Some studies have revealed that enteroviruses are also the most common cause of meningitis in infants; more than 90% of patients younger than 1 year old who develop aseptic meningitis are identified to have an enterovirus infection, although this virus is responsible for only about 50% of adult cases of aseptic meningitis (Berlin et al., 1993; Marier et al., 1975). In this chapter, we review the features of enteroviruses and meningitis caused by this pathogen, with reference to an outbreak we recently experienced (Hayashi et al., 2009).

2. Virology

Enteroviruses are single-stranded RNA viruses, and belong to the Picornaviridae family. Other viruses which belong to this family include rhinovirus, which is the major cause of the common cold. Enteroviruses are divided into 5 subgenera, which are polioviruses, coxsackieviruses (group A and B), and echoviruses. Each subgenus comprises many serotypes, making the total number of serotypes more than 60. Some serotypes have a strong association with meningitis, while others seldom cause it. A list of serotypes associated with aseptic meningitis is summarized in Table 1. Enteroviruses also cause other neurological disorders and the association of serotypes with specific neurological disorders is described in Table 2. Although rare, opsoclonus-myoclonus syndrome and infantile hemipleia have been attributed to enteroviruses in some cases (Kuban et al., 1983; Rodden et al., 1975).

	Frequently associated	Occasionally associated
Polivirus		1-3
Group A coxsackievirus	2, 4, 5, 7, 9, 10, 16	1, 3, 6, 8, 11, 14, 17, 18, 22, 24
Group B coxsackievirus	1-5	6
Echovirus	4, 6, 9, 11, 16, 30, 33	1-3, 5, 7, 8, 12-15, 17-25, 31, 32
Enterovirus	70, 71	

Table 1. The association of enterovirus serotypes with viral meningitis

Enteroviruses lack the envelope, and are stable even in an acidic environment, which allows this virus to transit through the stomach (Rosenthal, 1994). The capsid protein is made of four virion polypeptides (VP1-4), among which VP1 serves as a structure to bind its receptor. The virus is internalized by receptor-mediated endocytosis, and then the genome is released into the cytoplasm. Cytolysis ensues in many cases, depending on the virus and the types of infected cells.

Because the gene encoding this protein undergoes a high rate of mutation during replication, this virus is able to avoid immune detection, and sometimes causes large outbreaks. In the coxsackievirus B3-associated meningitis outbreak in Hong Kong in 2008, for example, an amino acid change of this virus was documented (Wong et al., 2011). There was also a large outbreak of aseptic meningitis caused by echovirus 30 in Korea in 2008. A gene analysis of the sequence of VP1 revealed that the causative strain was of a distinct lineage (Choi et al., 2010). There have also been other reports which demonstrated that changes in the immunogenic portion of the viral protein was related to a large outbreak of meningitis (Cui et al., 2010; Mao et al., 2010).

Encephalitis	Poliovirus	1-3
	Group A coxsackievirus	2, 4, 5-9, 10, 16
	Group B coxsackievirus	1-6
	Echovirus	2-4, 6, 7, 9, 11, 14, 17-19, 22, 25, 30, 33
	Enterovirus	70, 71
Paralysis	Poliovirus	1-3
	Group A coxsackievirus	2-11, 14, 16, 21, 24
	Group B coxsackievirus	1-6
	Echovirus	1, 2, 4, 6, 7, 9, 11, 14, 16-19, 30
	Enterovirus	70, 71
Cerebellar ataxia	Poliovirus	1, 3
	Group A coxsackievirus	2, 4, 7, 9
	Group B coxsackievirus	1-6
	Echovirus	6, 9
	Enterovirus	71
Polyneuropathy	Group A coxsackievirus	2, 5, 9
	Group B coxsackievirus	14
	Echovirus	5, 6, 22

Table 2. The association of enterovirus serotypes with neurological disorders

After initial replication in the oropharynx, the enterovirus transits the stomach and reaches the intestinal loop. In the submucosal lymphatic tissue, the viruses actively replicate and cause viremia, which then targets many organs. The best temperature for enterovirus to replicate is 37°C, and conditions with lower temperatures are unsuitable for the development of this viremia. This is one of the reasons why enterovirus meningitis is most prevalent in hot seasons. A large study showed that enterovirus meningitis is more than 5 times more common in summer than in winter, although mumps or arenavirus meningitis is more common in the winter and spring (Meyer et al., 1960). Exercise, which raises the body temperature, may also promote viral replication. In a mouse model of poliomyelitis, the degree of exercise correlated with the severity of paresis (Rosenbaum & Harford, 1953). Clinical data also shows that hard physical exercise has often preceded the establishment of paresis in this disease (Horstmann, 1950). Cardiac muscle damage caused by the coxsackievirus is also augmented by exercise (Gatmaitan et al., 1970). It is thus believed that severe exercise makes the disease more severe in cases of enteroviruses infection (Modlin, 2008).

We recently experienced an outbreak of aseptic meningitis caused by echovirus 30 in a high school baseball club (Hayashi et al., 2009). Among the 43 members of the baseball club related to our case, 12 were admitted to our hospital, 5 to other hospitals, and all of the other members developed a fever and headache even though they were not admitted to hospitals. This attack rate was extraordinarily high; that in previous reports ranged from 3 to 13% (Akiyoshi et al., 2007; Dumaidi et al., 2006; Mohle-Boetani et al., 1999; Vieth et al., 1999). This extraordinarily high attack rate could be explained by the physically severe training the club members undertook before or just after virus infection.

The route of central nervous system invasion of this virus has not been fully elucidated, but blood-mediated spread is most plausible. The simultaneous occurrence of neurological and other symptoms supports this route. Experimental data show that viremia precedes central nervous system invasion (Nathanson & Bodian, 1962), which also supports this route. Alternatively, the direct spread from intestinal peripheral nerves is also suspected (Sabin, 1956). In the case of poliomyelitis, virus may spread through the muscle and access the innervating nerves, and then travel to the brain (Rosenthal, 1994).

3. Clinical features

More than 90% of enterovirus-infected people remain asymptomatic (Kogon et al., 1969). Even if the infection becomes symptomatic, most of the patients develop only mild febrile illness; less than 5% of febrile patients develop meningitis (Rotbart, 1995, 2000). It is estimated that about 1 in 3,000 cases of enterovirus infection causes meningitis. Females are more prone to evolve meningitis (the male:female ratio is 1.3-1.5:1), although the exact reason for this is unknown. There are no specific findings for the febrile illness caused by enterovirus. It is known that the fever may last for one week or longer (Kogon et al., 1969; Rotbart et al., 1998). Headache, throat pain, emesis, and diarrhea are also common findings in cases of enterovirus infection, all of which are also common in mild febrile illnesses caused by other pathogens.

Organs other than the nervous system are also the targets of this virus, and therefore, various disorders are caused by this infection. Acute hemorrhagic conjunctivitis, exanthems, hand-foot-and-mouth disease, herpangina, myositis, and pericarditis are well-known disorders caused by this virus. As seen for the neurological symptoms (Table 1 and 2), these disorders are also associated with specific enterovirus serotypes. Acute hemorrhagic conjunctivitis, for example, has a strong association with enterovirus 70 and coxsackievirus A24. Herpangina is mainly caused by coxsackievirus A or E71.

As described above, most cases of aseptic meningitis follow an uneventful course. However, a few people show complications such as seizure, coma, and movement disorders. There were no such cases in the outbreak we experienced (Hayashi et al., 2009), but 5 to 10% of infant cases show severe complications (Rorabaugh et al., 1993). Infant cases may suffer from neurological sequela such as altered language development, which suggests a higher vulnerability of infants to this virus. On the other hand, other studies have suggested that older people are more vulnerable to poliovirus infections (Nathanson & Martin, 1979; Weinstein 1957). There is also data suggesting that adults show a more prolonged course of enterovirus infection (Rotbart et al., 1998). The reason why younger people suffer from enterovirus infections more frequently may be related to the absence of specific immunity. The reason older people tend to have a prolonged clinical course, on the other hand, remains unknown.

Although most cases of enterovirus meningitis take a quite benign course, electroencepharograms may show slowing of the waves (Lepow et al., 1962). We investigated the electroencepharograms in several cases of enterovirus meningitis (Hayashi et al., 2009), but no cases revealed abnormal findings. The results of electroencephalograms may be different based on the causative serotype, but this issue has not been fully elucidated. Eleven to twenty-two percent of the cases of viral encephalitis are caused by enteroviruses (Modlin, 2008), which indicates that some serotypes are highly neurotropic and take an aggressive form. Echoviruses 9 and 71 are notorious for their frank brain damage (Fowlkes et al., 2008). However, even in the same serotype-caused outbreak, the clinical picture may be different for those affected by the viruses (Akiyoshi et al., 2007; Faustini et al., 2006; Hayashi et al., 2009; Helfand et al., 1994; Mohle-Boetani et al., 1999; Vieth et al., 1999). Mutations in VP1 change the virulence, as may other mutations.

The classic clinical presentation of bacterial meningitis is the triad of fever, neck stiffness and an altered mental state. Viral meningitis, on the other hand, usually lacks mental state alteration. In our experience, all patients with enterovirus meningitis suffered from headache and fever, but the mental state was unaltered in all of the cases (Hayashi et al., 2009). However, there were other symptoms in these patients (summarized in Table 3). Most previous reports show similar results: headache and fever in all patients, vomiting in 60 to 90%, diarrhea in 11%, and rash in 3 to 9% (Bernit et al., 2004; Gosbell et al., 2000; Ihekwaba et al., 2008; Kao et al., 2003). Why a rash was not observed in our case series remains uncertain. Some serotypes, such as enterovirus 71, tend to be more aggressive, but to speculate the causative serotype based on the clinical presentation alone is impossible. In cases of aseptic meningitis caused by other viruses, some symptoms are informative about the causative agent; concomitant parotitis or genital lesions, for example, indicates a mumps infection or herpes simplex 2 infection, respectively. However, even in mumps-related meningitis, only half of all patients show parotitis. In addition, only 3 of 23 herpes simplex virus 2-related aseptic meningitis cases had shown prior genital lesions (Landry et al., 2009). Whether the meningitis is caused by an enterovirus or another viruses cannot be inferred clinically.

Meningeal irritation signs are important for diagnosing meningitis. Unless meningeal irritation signs are confirmed, the clinician does not generally investigate the cerebrospinal fluid (Attia et al., 2009). In our case series, however, neck stiffness was confirmed in only 60% of cases (Hayashi et al., 2009). Previous reports also showed that this sign was confirmed in only 70% of cases. The absence of this sign does not exclude meningitis. Kernig signs, a common symptom of meningeal irritation, is less sensitive than neck stiffness; as shown in Table 3, only 23.5% of cases showed this sign. Among the three meningeal irritation signs we investigated, the Jolt accentuation signs showed the highest sensitivity (Table 3), which was compatible to that shown in previous report (Uchihara et al., 1991). The Brudzinski sign has high sensitivity in cases of bacterial and tuberculous meningitis (Brody & Wilkins, 1969), but how often this sign is observed in enterovirus-associated meninigitis remains uncertain. Although we did not carry out an exact analysis, this sign was only rarely observed in our case series of echovirus 30-associated meningitis. When a patient with a possible diagnosis of meningitis is encountered, then the Jolt accentuation test is considered to be of great importance.

As the disease usually takes benign clinical course, no specific treatment is required in most cases. Analgesics or anti-emetics are used for relief of symptoms. Pleconaril may reduce the duration of headache or fever, but is not approved for use in the United States.

When immunocompromised patients develop enterovirus meningitis, the outcome is often poor. It tends to become a chronic infection. Even with intravenous administration of immunoglobulin, the disease often has a fatal outcome (Modlin, 2008).

Symptoms	Headache	100%
	Fever	100%
	Emesis	90.5%
	Throat pain	23.8%
	Diarrhea	9.5%
	Rash	0%
Signs	Jolt accentuation	87.5%
	Neck stiffness	60.0%
	Kerni sign	23.5%

Table 3. The signs and symptoms of patients hospitalized with enterovirus meningitis

4. Laboratory data

Pleocytosis in the cerebrospical fluid, with predominance of mononuclear cells, is one of the most important findings for diagnosing viral meningitis. However, many previous studies of enterovirus meningitis have reported results that contradict this rule (Bernit et al., 2004; Carrol et al., 2006; Kao et al., 2003; Lee & Davies, 2007). Our case series also revealed that 59.7±28.9% of the cells in the cerebrospinal fluid were of polymorphonuclear origin (Table 4). Therefore, polymorphonuclear cell predominance in the cerebrospinal fluid is not unusual in enterovirus meningitis. In herpesvirus infection of the central nervous system, polymorphonuclear cell predominance is also common. Although it is sometimes insisted that an inflammatory response in the cerebrospinal fluid tends to be more prominent in herpesvirus infection than in enterovirus infection, to differentiate them by the cerebrospinal fluid findings is impossible. Our case series showed that the cells in the cerebrospinal fluid ranged from 0 to 370/μl, and a study of herpesvirus infection showed 4 to 755/μl (Olson et al., 1967). The results are therefore highly variable among cases, and are not sufficiently informative to speculate on the causative agent.

In cases of bacterial meningitis, some parameters such as a low glucose level in the cerebrospinal fluid, predict a poor outcome of disease. In cases of aseptic meningitis caused by enteroviruses, however, the cerebrospinal fluid profile does not predict the clinical course. Furthermore, the pleocytosis or an increased protein level in the cerebrospinal fluid was not related to the severity of headache or emesis. This may be, at least in part, because the time when the cerebrospinal fluid was obtained varied among the cases; the inflammatory response in the cerebrospinal fluid may be mild when a lumbar puncture is performed early in the course of infection (Jiménez Caballero et al., 2011).

As shown in Table 4, white blood cells and/or C-reactive protein elevation in the blood are generally mild in cases of aseptic meningitis. This profile is similar to that of other viral infections. These findings are useful when viral meningitis needs to be differentiated from bacterial meningitis.

Isolation of the virus in cell culture was the traditional method used to identify the causative agent of viral meningitis, but it usually has low sensitivity, ranging from 60 to 75% (Trabelsi et al., 1995). Serological examinations and RT-PCR have, therefore, now become commonplace, and RT-PCR has recently become preferred because of its high sensitivity and shorter time required for the test. The sensitivity and specificity of RT-PCR are 100 and 97%, respectively (Halonen et al., 1995; Rotbart et al., 1994). We have examined the cerebrospinal fluid and pharyngeal swabs to identify causative agents, and found that both serological and RT-PCR studies have high sensitivity (Hayashi et al., 2009). The amount of sample and the time it was obtained may influence the results.

Cerebrospinal fluid	Initial pressure	216.4±43.6 mmH2O
	Cells	108.9±114.0 /μl
	Polymorphonuclear cells	59.7±28.9 %
	Protein	33.8±16.2 mg/dl
	Glucose (% of blood glucose)	55.5±7.8 %
Blood	White blood cells	10205±2157 /μl
	C-reactive protein	1.65±1.72 mg/dl

Table 4. The laboratory findings of patients hospitalized with enterovirus meningitis

5. Mode of transmission and outbreak prevention

Enteroviruses begin to be excreted when the infection is still asymptomatic. It is thus possible for a person to transmit the virus even when he/she is not aware of being infected. The time from enterovirus exposure to symptom onset differs between disorders; it is 12 to 24 hours for conjunctivitis, 2 to 3 days for gastroenteritis, and 3 to 10 days for aseptic meningitis (Modlin, 2008; Tyler & Martin, 1993). Even during this period, the virus may be propagated.

Viral particles are shed in the upper respiratory tract secretions and feces, the former for about 1 to 3 weeks and the latter for 5 to 6 weeks. There are some exceptions, such as enterovirus 70 in tears, which cause acute hemorrhagic conjunctivitis (Onorato et al., 1985). For the transmission and outbreak of enterovirus meningitis, the fecal-oral route plays the pivotal role. Respiratory secretions could theoretically be involved, but whether this route actually plays a role in meningitis transmission is uncertain. When one became infected by an enterovirus, a member in the same family becomes infected in 43 to 76% of cases (Kogon et al., 1969). Living in crowded conditions increases the probability of transmission. Poor hygiene also facilitates the spread of infection. Consequently, enterovirus infection is more prevalent in people of lower socioeconomic status.

In order to prevent transmission and outbreaks, hand washing is important. Sharing cups or bottles should be forbidden. The outbreak we recently experienced was, at least in part, caused by sharing drink bottles (Hayashi 2009). When the patient is an infant who still needs diapers, caregivers should take special precautions to decrease the spread of infection. Indeed, child-care centers sometimes become the center of outbreaks (Akiyoshi et al., 2007; Dumaidi et al., 2006; Mohle-Boetani et al., 1999; Vieth et al., 1999). To use gloves is warranted.

Not only the above-mentioned limited-community outbreaks, but also larger outbreaks, which involve a city to a country, sometimes occur (Choi et al., 2010; Cui et al., 2010; Gobbi et al., 2010; Kao et al., 2003; Mao et al., 2010; Perevoscikovs et al., 2010). In most of such cases, a mutation of the immunogenic viral protein is involved. In such outbreaks, the attack rate for each person is quite low. Careful hand washing and maintaining quality standards are important. Virus-containing water occasionally pours into a pond, lake, or sea. Relatively small open-community outbreaks can take place under such circumstances (Begier et al., 2008; Hauri et al., 2005). Although exposure to the virus is inevitable when one swims in such pond, the rate of symptomatic infection is variable. What determines whether the infection is symptomatic or asymptomatic is not clear, but the time spent swimming correlated with the occurrence of clinically apparent meningitis (Begier et al., 2008; Hauri et al., 2005). Therefore, it is best to limit the time spent swimming in a pond for a long time, when meningitis is prevalent.

Serum IgG against enteroviruses persists for life, and IgA (secretory immunoglobulin) continues to circulate for approximately 15 years. Infants and young people are less likely to possess serotype-specific antibodies against enteroviruses. Special attention should be paid in order not to expose young people to prevailing virus. In the outbreak we experienced, we notified all schools, kindergartens, and nurseries that an enterovirus infection had been detected. We asked public health centers to teach the school staff in the city how to prevent transmission. Owing to these activities, we successfully contained the echovirus 30-associated meningitis outbreak within a limited-community.

6. References

Akiyoshi, K.; Nakagawa, N. & Suga, T. (2007). An outbreak of aseptic meningitis in a nursery school caused by echovirus type 30 in Kobe, Japan. *Jpn J Infect Dis*. Vol.60, pp. 66-68.

Attia, J.; Hatala, R.; Cook, D.J. & Wong, J.G. (2009). Does this patient have acute meningitis?. In: *The rational clinical examination*. Simel, D.L. & Rennie, D. (Ed.). 395-406, Mc Graw Hill Medical, New York.

Begier, E.M.; Oberste, M.S.; Landry, M.L.; Brennan, T.; Mlynarski, D.; Mshar, P.A.; Frenette, K.; Rabatsky-Her, T.; Purviance, K.; Nepaul, A.; Nix, W.A.; Pallansch, M.A.; Ferguson, D.; Cartter, M.L. & Hadler, J.L. (2008). An outbreak of concurrent echovirus 30 and coxsackievirus A1 infections associated with sea swimming among a group of travelers to Mexico. *Clin Infect Dis*. Vol.47, pp. 616-623.

Berlin, L.E.; Rorabauch, M.L.; Heldrich, L.; Roberts, K.; Doran, T. & Modlin, J.F. (1993). Aseptic meningitis in infants <2 years of age: diagnosis and etiology. *J Infect Dis.* Vol.168, pp. 888-892.

Bernit, E.; de Lamballerie, X.; Zandotti, C.; Berger, P.; Veit, V.; Schleinitz, N.; de Micco, P.; Harlé, J.R. & Charrel, R.N. (2004). Prospective investigation of a large outbreak of meningitis due to echovirus 30 during summer 2000 in marseilles, france. *Medicine (Baltimore).* Vol.83, pp. 245-253.

Brody, I.A. & Wilkins, R.H. (1969). The signs of Kernig and Brudzinski. *Arch Neurol.* Vol.21, pp. 215-218.

Carrol, E.D.; Beadsworth, M.B.; Jenkins, N.; Ratcliffe, L.; Ashton, I.; Crowley B.; Nye, F.J. & Beeching, N.J. (2006). Clinical and diagnostic findings of an echovirus meningitis outbreak in the north west of England. *Postgrad Med J.* Vol.82, pp. 60-64.

CDC. (2003). Outbreaks of aseptic meningitis associated with enteroviruses 9 and 30 and preliminary surveillance reports on enterovirus activity - United States, 2003. *MMWR* Vol.52, pp. 761-764.

Choi, Y.J.; Park, K.S.; Baek, K.A.; Jung, E.H.; Nam, H.S.; Kim, Y.B.& Park, J.S. (2010). Molecular characterization of echovirus 30-associated outbreak of aseptic meningitis in Korea in 2008. *J Microbiol Biotechnol.* Vol.20, pp. 643-649.

Cui, A.; Yu, D.; Zhu, Z.; Meng, L.; Li, H.; Liu, J.; Liu, G.; Mao, N. & Xu, W. (2010). An outbreak of aseptic meningitis caused by coxsackievirus A9 in Gansu, the People's Republic of China. *Virol J.* Vol. 7, pp. 72.

Dumaidi, K.; Frantzidou, F.; Papa, A.; Diza, E. & Antoniadis, A. (2005). Enterovirus meningitis in Greece from 2003-2005: diagnosis, CSF laboratory findings, and clinical manifestations. *J Clin Lab Anal.* Vol.20, pp. 177-183.

Faustini, A.; Fano, V.; Muscillo, M.; Zaniratti, S.; La Rosa, G.; Tribuzi, L. & Perucci, C.A. (2006). An outbreak of aseptic meningitis due to echovirus 30 associated with attending school and swimming in pools. *Int J Infect Dis.* Vol.10, pp. 291-297.

Fowlkes, A.L.; Honarmand, S.; Glaser, C.; Yagi, S.; Schnurr, D.; Oberste, M.S.; Anderson, L.; Pallansch, M.A. & Khetsuriani, N. (2008). Enterovirus-associated encephalitis in the California encephalitis project, 1998-2005. *J Infect Dis.* Vol.198, pp. 1685-1691.

Gatmaitan, B.G.; Chason, J.L. & Lerner, A.M. (1970). Augmentation of the virulence of murine coxsackie-virus B-3 myocardiopathy by exercise. *J Exp Med.* Vol.131, pp. 1121-1136.

Gobbi, F.; Calleri, G.; Spezia, C.; Lipani, F.; Balbiano, R.; De Agostini, M.; Milia, M.G. & Caramello P. (2010). Echovirus-4 meningitis outbreak imported from India. *J Travel Med.* Vol.17, pp. 66-68.

Gosbell, I.; Robinson, D.; Chant, K. & Crone, S. (2000). Outbreak of echovirus 30 meningitis in Wingecarribee Shire, New South Wales. *Commun Dis Intell.* Vol.24, pp. 121-124.

Halonen, P.; Rocha, E.; Hierholzer, J.; Holloway, B.; Hyypiä, T.; Hurskainen, P. & Pallansch, M. (1995). Detection of enteroviruses and rhinoviruses in clinical specimens by PCR and liquid-phase hybridization. *J Clin Microbiol.* Vol.33, pp. 648-653.

Hauri, A.M.; Schimmelpfennig, M.; Walter-Domes, M.; Letz, A.; Diedrich, S.; Lopez-Pila, J. & Schreier, E. (2005). An outbreak of viral meningitis associated with a public swimming pond. *Epidemiol Infect.* Vol.133, pp. 291-298.

Hayashi, T.; Shirayoshi, T.; Nagano, T.; Yaoita, H.; Kogure, S.; Nariai, H.; Natsumeda, T.; Taniuchi, M.; Sandoh, M. & Sato, Y. (2009). An outbreak of aseptic meningitis due to echovirus 30 in a high school baseball club - possible role of severe exercise for a high attack rate. *Inter Med.* Vol.48, pp. 1767-1771.

Helfand, R.F.; Khan, A.S.; Pallansch, M.A.; Alexander, J.P.; Meyers, H.B.; DeSantis, R.A.; Schonberger, L.B. & Anderson, L.J. (1994). Echovirus 30 infection and aseptic meningitis in parents of children attending a child care center. *J Infect Dis.* Vol.169, pp. 1133-1137.

Horstmann, D.M. (1950). Acute poliomyelitis relation of physical activity at the time of onset to the course of the disease. *J Am Med Ass.* Vol.142, pp. 236-241.

Ihekwaba, U.K.; Kudesia, G. & McKendrick, M.W. (2008). Clinical features of viral meningitis in adults: significant differences in cerebrospinal fluid findings among herpes simplex virus, varicella zoster virus, and enterovirus infections. *Clin Infect Dis.* Vol.47, pp. 783-789.

Jiménez Caballero, P.E.; Muñoz Escudero, F.; Murcia Carretero, S. & Verdú Pérez, A. (2011). Descriptive analysis of viral meningitis in a general hospital: differences in the characteristics between children and adults. *Neurologia.* Epub ahead of print..

Kao, C.H.; Lee, S.S.; Liu, Y.C.; Yen, M.Y.; Chen, Y.S.; Wan, S.R.; Lin, H.H.; Lin, W.R.; Huang, C.K. & Chin, C. (2003). Outbreak of aseptic meningitis among adults in southern Taiwan. *J Microbiol Immunol Infect.* Vol.36, pp. 192-196.

Khetsuriani, N.; Quiroz, E.S.; Holman, R.C. & Anderson, L.J. (2003). Viral meningitis-associated hospitalizations in the United States, 1988-1999. *Neuroepidemiology.* Vol.22, pp. 345-52.

Kogon, A.; Spigland, I.; Frothingham, T.E.; Elveback, L.; Williams, C.; Hall, C.E. & Fox, J.P. (1969). The virus watch program: a continuing surveillance of viral infections in metropolitan New York families. VII. Observations on viral excretion, seroimmunity, intrafamilial spread and illness association in coxsackie and echovirus infections. *Am J Epidemiol.* Vol.89, pp. 51-61.

Kuban, K.C.; Ephros, M.A.; Freeman, R.L.; Laffel, L.B. & Bresnan, M.J. (1983). Syndrome of opsoclonus-myoclonus caused by coxsackie B3 infection. *Ann Neurol.* Vol.13, pp. 69-71.

Landry, M.L.; Greenwold, J. & Vikram, H.R. (2009). Herpes simplex type-2 meningitis: presentation and lack of standardized therapy. *Am J Med.* Vol.122, pp. 688-691.

Lee, B.E. & Davies, H.E. (2007). Aseptic meningitis. *Curr Opin Infect Dis.* Vol.20, pp. 272-277.

Lepow, M.L.; Coyne, N.; Thompson, L.B.; Carver, D.H. & Robbins, F.C. (1962). A clinical, epidemiological, and laboratory investigation of aseptic meningitis during the four-year period 1955-1958. II. The clinical disease and its sequalae. *N Engl J Med.* Vol. 266, pp. 1188-1193.

Mao, N.; Zhao, L.; Zhu, Z.; Chen, X.; Zhou, S.; Zhang, Y.; Cui, A.; Ji, Y.; Xu, S. & Xu, W. (2010). An aseptic meningitis outbreak caused by echovirus 6 in Anhui province, China. *J Med Virol.* Vol.82, pp. 441-445.

Marier, R.; Rodriguez, W.; Chloupek, R.J.; Brandt, C.D.; Kim, H.W.; Baltimore, R.S.; Parker, C.L. & Artenstein, M.S. (1975). Coxsackievirus B5 infection and aseptic meningitis in neonates and children. *Am J Dis Child.* Vol.129, pp. 321-325.

Meyer, H.M.; Johnson, R.T.; Crawford, I.P., Dascomb, H.E. & Rogers, N.G. (1960). Central nervous system syndromes of viral etiology. A study of 713 cases. *Am J Med.* Vol.29, pp. 334-347.

Modlin, J.F. (2008). Enterovirus infections. In: *Cecil Medicine. 23rd ed.* Goldman, L. & Ausiello, D. (Ed.). 2514-2519, Elsevier, Philadelphia.

Mohle-Boetani, J.C.; Matkin, C.; Pallansch, M.; Helfand, R.; Fenstersheib, M.; Blanding, J.A. & Solomon, S.L. (1999). Viral meningitis in child care center staff and parents: an outbreak of echovirus 30 infections. *Public Health Rep.* Vol.114, pp. 249-256.

Nathanson, N. & Bodian, D. (1962). Experimental poliomyelitis following intramuscular virus injection. III. The effect of passive antibody. *Bull Johns Hopkins Hosp.* Vol.111. pp. 198-220.

Nathanson, N. & Martin, J.R. (1979). The epidemiology of poliomyelitis: enigmas surrounding its appearance, epidemicity, and disappearance. *Am J Epidemiol.* Vol.110, pp. 672-692.

Olson, L.C.; Buescher, E.L.; Artenstein, M.S. & Parkman, P.D. (1967). Herpesvirus infections of the human central nervous system. *N Engl J Med.* Vol.277, pp. 1271-1277.

Onorato, I.M.; Morens, D.M.; Schonberger, L.B.; Hatch, M.H.; Kaminski, R.M. & Turner, J.P. (1985). Acute hemorrhagic conjunctivitis caused by enterovirus type 70: an epidemic in American Samoa. *Am J Trop Med Hyg.* Vol.34, pp. 984-991.

Parasuraman ,T.V.; Frenia, K. & Romero, J. (2001). Enteroviral meningitis. Cost of illness and considerations for the economic evaluation of potential therapies. *Pharmacoeconomics.* Vol.19, pp.3-12.

Perevoscikovs, J.; Brila, A.; Firstova, L.; Komarova, T.; Lucenko, I.; Osmjana, J.; Savrasova, L.; Singarjova, I.; Storozenko, J.; Voloscuka, N. & Zamjatina, N. (2010). Ongoing outbreak of aseptic meningitis in South-Eastern Latvia, June - August 2010. *Euro Surveill.* Vol. 15, pii. 19639.

Rodden, V.J.; Cantor, H.E.; O'Coner, D.M.; Schmidt, R.R. & Cherry, J.D. (1975). Acute hemiplegia of childhood associated with coxsackie A9 viral infection. *J Pediatr.* Vol.86, pp. 56-58.

Rorabaugh, M.L.; Berlin, L.E.; Heldrich, F.; Roberts, K.; Rosenberg, L.A.; Doran, T. & Modlin, J.F. (1993). Aseptic meningitis in infants younger than 2 years of age: acute illness and neurologic complications. *Pediatrics.* Vol.92, pp. 206-211.

Rosenbaum, H.E. & Harford, C.G. (1953). Effect of fatigue on susceptibility of mice to poliomyelitis. *Proc Soc Exp Biol Med.* Vol.83, pp. 678-681.

Rosenthal, K.S. (1994). Picornaviruses, In: *Medical Microbiology.* Murray, F.R.; Kobayashi, G.S.; Pfaller, M.A. & Rosenthal, K.S. (Ed.), 607-619, Mosby, St. Louis.

Rotbart, H.A.; Sawyer, M.H.; Fast, S.; Lewinski, C.; Murphy, N.; Keyser, E.F.; Spadoro, J.; Kao, S.Y. & Loeffelholz, M. (1994). Diagnosis of enteroviral meningitis by using PCR with a colorimetric microwell detection assay. *J Clin Microbiol.* Vol.32, pp. 2590-2592.

Rotbart, H.A. (1995). Enteroviral infections of the central nervous system. *Clin Infect Dis.* Vol.20, pp. 971-981.

Rotbart, H.A.; Brennan, P.J.; Fife, K.H.; Romero, J.R.; Griffin, J.A.; McKinlay, M.A. & Hayden, F.G. (1998). Enterovirus meningitis in adults. *Clin Infect Dis.* Vol.27, pp. 896-898.

Rotbart, H.A. (2000). Viral meningitis. *Semin Neurol.* Vol.20, pp. 277-292.

Sabin, A.B. (1956). Pathogenesis of poliomyelitis. Reappraisal in the light of new data. *Science.* Vol.123, pp. 1151-1157.

Trabelsi, A.; Grattard, F.; Nejmeddine, M.; Aouni, M.; Bourlet, T. & Pozzetto, B. (1995). Evaluation of an enterovirus group-specific anti-VP1 monoclonal antibody, 5-D8/1, in comparison with neutralization and PCR for rapid identification of enteroviruses in cell culture. *J Clin Microbiol*. Vol.33, pp. 2454-2457.

Tunkel, A.R. & Scheld, W.M. (1993). Pathogenesis and pathophysiology of bacterial meningitis. *Clin Microbiol Rev*. Vol.6, pp. 18-136.

Tyler, K.L. & Martin, J.B. (1993). *Infectious Diseases of the Central Nervous System*. F.A. Davis Company, Philadelphia.

Uchihara, T. & Tsukagoshi, H. (1991). Jolt accentuation of headache: the most sensitive sign of CSF pleocytosis. *Headache*. Vol.31, pp. 167-171.

Vieth, U.C.; Kunzelmann, M.; Diedrich, S.; Timm, H.; Ammon, A.; Lyytikäinen, O. & Petersen LR. (1999). An echovirus 30 outbreak with a high meningitis attack rate among children and household members at four day-care centers. *Eur J Epidemiol*. Vol.15, pp. 655-658.

Wang, J.R.; Tsai, H.P.; Huang, S.W.; Kuo, P.H.; Kiang, D.; & Liu, C.C. (2002) Laboratory diagnosis and genetic analysis of an echovirus 30-associated outbreak of aseptic meningitis in Taiwan in 2001. *J Clin Microbiol*. Vol.40, pp. 4439-4444.

Weinstein, L. (1957). Influence of age and sex on susceptibility and clinical manifestations in poliomyelitis. *N Engl J Med*. Vol.257, pp. 47-52.

Wong, A.H.; Lau, C.S.; Cheng, P.K.; Ng. A.Y. & Lim, W.W. (2011). Coxsackivirus B3-associated aseptic meningitis: an emerging infection in Hong Kong. *J Med Virol*. Vol.83, pp. 483-489.

10

An Overview on Cryptococcal Meningitis

Marcia S. C. Melhem and Mara Cristina S. M Pappalardo
Adolfo Lutz Institute, Laboratory Reference Center and Emilio Ribas, Research Institute of the Secretary of Health of São Paulo State, Brazil

1. Introduction

Cryptococcosis is a systemic disease caused by the yeast *Cryptococcus* spp. *Cryptococcus neoformans* and *C. gattii* are the etiological agents of fungal meningoencephalitis. Chronic meningitis is the most common clinical presentation of cryptococcosis. In contrast with the acute meningitis, patients with chronic meningitis develop an indolent course of symptoms for at least four weeks like headache, nausea, decreased memory and comprehension. Cerebral cryptococcomas can also cause significant neurological morbidity, and these mass lesions require relief of increased intracranial pressure and prolonged antifungal therapy. Although cryptococcosis is considered one opportunistic infection of the central nervous system and lungs, extra neural and non-pulmonary forms may be found. The disease is almost always associated with impaired immunity, and occurs in patients with lymph proliferative disorders, steroid therapy and organ transplantation. Before the acquired immune deficiency syndrome (AIDS) the cases with cryptococcosis were sporadic. Despite of the highly active antiretroviral therapy-HAART, acute mortality due to HIV-associated cryptococcal meningitis remains unacceptably high (Lortholary et al., 2006), and consequently, this disease remains a leading cause of death in Africa, Asia, and Brazil (French et al., 2002; Vidal et al., 2008; Pappalardo et al., 2009).

Cryptococcosis has been documented in few (~3%) of solid-organ transplant recipients with 68% of the cases occurring one year after transplantation., and almost half cases have pulmonary cryptococcal infection. The disease is limited to the lungs only in 6% to 33% of cases, although cryptococcal meningitis and disseminated infections have been documented in up to 60% of patients (Husain et al., 2001; Vilchez et al., 2002; Singh et al., 2007; Shaariah et al., 1992). Data on non-transplant patients or presumably immunocompetent hosts presenting cryptococcal meningitis are scarse, because the majority of patients prior to the HIV epidemic were significantly immunosuppressed, receiving steroids or having cancer or other degenerative diseases (Perfect et al., 2010).

2. Cryptococcosis and AIDS

Cryptococcus neoformans is yeast with a tropism for the central nervous system, and 70-90% of infections caused by this species manifested as meningitis, after spores inhalation and hematologic dissemination. Meningitis is frequently associated to the pulmonary form. In immunosuppressed patients with pulmonary cryptococcosis, meningitis should be always ruled out by lumbar puncture (Mitchell & Perfect, 1995). Cryptococcal meningitis is a common and often fatal opportunistic infection in HIV-infected patients, especially in developing countries and in patients with CD4 cells < 100/µL. Incidence of cryptococcosis decreased in the era HAART, but the incidence and mortality of the disease are still high in some areas of the world. Recent review suggests that there are ~1 million new cases and at least 500.000 annual deaths world-wide due to HIV-associated cryptococcosis (Park et al., 2009).

Computed tomography or magnetic resonance imaging head scans should be done in all patients prior to any diagnostic or therapeutic lumbar puncture, with focal neurological signs or impaired mental functions. Patients with HIV disease generally do not have hydrocephalus or cryptococcal mass lesions and these exams commonly are normal or show cerebral atrophy without obstruction or other abnormality (Graybill et al., 2000).

The most common signs and symptoms are headaches, fever, nausea, vomiting, lethargy, coma, memory loss over 2 to 4 weeks; however, sometimes patients only refer general bodily discomfort. Patients can also present with pulmonary or cutaneous manifestations with or without apparent neurologic disease (Perfect et al., 2010).

The diagnosis of the meningeal cryptococcosis through mycological procedures is easy and based on the visualization of encapsulated yeast cells in the cerebral spinal fluid specimen, and immunological assays. If cryptococal meningitis is confirmed, extra neural sites should be discharged by means of screening of cutaneous lesions, procedures for blood cultures, examination of urine, pleural fluid, sputum, prostatic fluid, and others clinical specimens for detect the etiological agent..

Antifungal drugs more commonly used for treat cryptococcal meningitis are amphotericin B deoxycholate, amphotericin B lipid complex or liposomal formulation, flucytosine, and fluconazole (Perfect et al., 2010). Ideally, antifungal therapy should rapidly sterilize the central nervous system and this should be the primary focus of any induction strategy (Bicanic et al., 2007). The antifungal therapy in cryptococcal meningitis in AIDS patients is divided into 3 phases: induction (for at least 2 weeks), consolidation (for a minimum of eight weeks) and maintenance or suppression phase.

The induction phase aims the achievement of sterilization of cerebral spinal fluid, or reduction of fungal burden. The consolidation phase warrants maintenance of negative cultures and normalization of clinical parameters. Some experts and guidelines suggest a routine lumbar puncture at the second week, with prolongation of the induction phase if the cerebrospinal fluid culture is not yet sterile. The drug of choice for induction is amphotericin B (0,7-1,0 mg/kg per day intravenously), and fluconazole is the choice for consolidation [400 mg (6 mg/kg) per day orally]. Fluconazole should be introduced for consolidation regimen whenever the mental status recovered, fever, headache and meningeal symptoms disappear, and/or yeast culture results are negative at the second week. Despite the theoretic antagonism between amphotericin B and fluconazole, most animal model data suggests that both drugs together are a very effective combination against *C. neoformans* (Menichetti et al., 1996; Larsen et al., 2004; Larsen et al., 2005; Pappas et al., 2009; Perfect et al., 2010).

Maintenance therapy should be initiated after completion of primary therapy with an induction and consolidation regimen, and continued until there is evidence of persistent immune reconstitution with successful HAART. Since a cure doesn't exist in AIDS patients, maintenance should be done for at least one year with 200 mg/daily of fluconazole (standard for consolidation and maintenance), with CD4 cell count > 100 cells/µL and undetectable or very low HIV RNA level sustained for ≥3 months (minimum of 12 months of antifungal therapy). Itraconazole is an alternative, albeit less effective, choice for maintenance therapy. Oral itraconazole if patient is intolerant of fluconazole, may be administered (200 mg per day or a higher dosage 200 mg twice per day orally) (Denning et al, 1989).

The management of cryptococcosis is difficult, particularly in some developing countries where flucytosine is no more commercialized and liposomal or lipid complex amphotericin B formulations are not affordable. The nephrotoxicity of amphotericin B deoxycholate represents a big challenge for the physicians in such regions (Sharkey et al., 1996). Furthermore the treatment of increased intracranial pressure represents another serious issue since approximately one-half of HIV-infected patients have elevated baseline opening intracranial pressures requiring drainage of cerebral spinal fluid daily (Bicanic et al., 2009). Medications other than antifungal drugs are not useful in the management of increased intracranial pressure in cryptococcal meningoencephalitis (Perfect et al. 2010)

The rapid clearance of infection by sterilization of cerebrospinal fluid associated with clinical improvement on day 14 of treatment is predictive of a good evaluation in the 10th week (Robinson et al., 1999). The rate of clearance of cryptococcal colony-forming units is a clinically meaningful endpoint. Maybe deaths within two weeks are nearly all related to cryptococcal infection, whereas, after this time, deaths are increasingly related to other complications of late-stage HIV infections or extended hospitalization (Bicanic et al., 2009). The good control of elevated CSF pressure and symptoms are very important, and they are some of the most critical determinants in the outcome of cryptococcal meningitis (Perfect et al., 2010). This elevated CSF pressure level is generally linked to a high burden of yeast in the cerebrospinal fluid (Bicanic et al., 2009). Factors that indicate a bad outcome in cryptococcal meningitis include abnormal mental status, poor host inflammatory response (cerebrospinal fluid white cells <20/mL), raised CSF opening pressure (> 25 cm H_2O), high organism burden, extra neural sites and the lack of effective antifungal treatment. Some studies confirm the greater fungicidal activity of amphotericin B plus flucytosine to improve prognosis (Brouwer et al., 2004).

Potential complications in management of cryptococcal infection, includes increased intracranial pressure, immune reconstitution inflammatory syndrome, drug resistance, and cryptococcomas. Opportunistic infections such bacteremia, toxoplasmosis, histoplasmosis, or oropharingeal candidosis, tumors, drug-related complications may occur in heavily immunocompromised patients. Moreover, the long-time of hospitalization, never less than two weeks, increased the risk for hospital infections Development of classic hydrocephalus later during treatment and follow-up can occur. Furthermore, impaired vision, mental deficit and cranial nerve palsies are described sequels of cryptocccosis.

After discontinuation of maintenance therapy, relapses with positive culture result may occur and so careful follow-up of patients is necessary. Patients will need follow-up lumbar punctures and intracranial pressure should be measured. Reinstitution of fluconazole maintenance therapy should be considered if the CD4 cell count decreases to <100 cells/mL and/or the serum cryptococcal antigen titer increases [Zolopa et al., 2009)

2.1 Cryptococcosis and IRIS

Immune reconstitution inflammatory syndrome (IRIS) consists of clinical manifestations compatible with enormous tissue inflammation in patients with rapid improvement in cellular immunity and worsening in central nervous system signs and/ or symptoms of the disease. About 30% of patients with cryptococcal meningitis will develop IRIS when HAART is initiated (Bicanic et al., 2006; Antinori et al., 2009). Perfect et al. (2010) suggest a wide range of two to ten weeks after initiation of cryptococcosis therapy to introduce HAART. The exact moment to start HAART in patients with cryptococcal meningitis to avoid immune reconstitution inflammatory syndrome, is still uncertain.

3. Etiologic agents

Cryptococcus neoformans and *Cryptococcus gattii* cause nearly all human and animal cryptococcal infections. In addition to these common species, there are nearby 15 other members of this genus which have appeared as human clinical isolates, such as *C. laurentii, C. luteolus* (80% of non-*neoformans* and non-*gattii* cases), *C. albidus, C. diffluens,* and *C. uniguttulatus* (Heitman et al. 2011). *Cryptococcus gattii* can be discerned from *C. neoformans* using a wide range of microbiological and molecular techniques. A simple and classical method is the use of canavanine-glycine-bromothymol blue (CGB) medium, which allows *C. gattii* but not *C. neoformans* to grow changing the color medium from green-yellowish to blue. Molecular approaches yield determine distinct genotypes among the species. Polymerase chain reaction (PCR) fingerprinting, restriction fragment length polymorphism (RFLP), analysis of specific loci, and amplified fragment length polymorphism (AFLP) fingerprint analysis, and multi-locus sequence typing scheme (Meyer et al., 2009) are molecular tools (Meyer et al., 2009). Furthermore, interspecies hybrid forms have been isolated from clinical samples, and they seem to present a higher virulence potential than regular *C. gattii* or *C. neoformans* isolates (Boekhout et al., 2001).

The species differs in many aspects and improved surveillance should enable better assessment of the local incidence of these two species and also clinical manifestation and course associated to each species. Whereas *C. neoformans* primarily affects persons infected with human immunodeficiency virus worldwide, *C. gattii* primarily affects HIV-uninfected persons in tropical and subtropical regions (Pappalardo and Melhem, 2003; Chaturvedi et al, 2005; Martins et al., 2007; Heitman et al. 2011).

It noteworthy the emergence of *C. gattii* in temperate climate regions that suggests the pathogen might have adapted to a new climatic niche or that climatic warming might have created an environment for spore survival and propagation of this species. *Cryptococcus gattii* is more likely to cause cryptococcomas, and seems to be less responsive to antifungal drugs (Gomez-Lopes et al., 2008).

The profile of antifungal susceptibility can be assessed through *in vitro* antifungal susceptibility testing. Performance of these tests may help not only to monitor the development of resistance in *Cryptococcus* isolates, but could also determine the best antifungal therapy, predicting possible failures due to a resistant strain. Antifungal susceptibility testing is indeed a recognized useful tool to aid the treatment of *Candida* infections. References broth microdilution methods for this genus are described in document M27-A3 of the Clinical and Laboratory Standards Institute - CLSI, and in the doc.

E.Def 7.1 of the European Committee on Antimicrobial Susceptibility Testing (EUCAST) (CLSI, 2008, Subcommittee on Antifungal Susceptibility Testing of the ESCMID, 2008). Although the reference methodologies of CLSI and EUCAST are different, the results are very similar and results are comparable.

Determination of resistance in isolates of *Cryptococcus,* quite distinct yeast in which fermentation is absent, the micro dilution methods present some technical problems. The most relevant one is the low growth of *Cryptococcus* strains due to the oxygen limited environment found in the microdilution plates. So, the standard methods developed for *Candida* are not still completely reliable for test *Cryptococcus* isolates and efforts have been made toward standardization of antifungal susceptibility testing of *Cryptococcus* and other non-fermentative yeasts (Zaragoza et al., 2011).

The minimum inhibition concentration (MIC) of antifungal drugs against clinical and environmental *Cryptococcus* strains has been extensively studied. *Cryptococcus neoformans* has been more frequently assessed for its *in vitro* susceptibility to a wide variety of antifungal compounds, including the new triazoles posaconazole, voriconazole, ravuconazole, and isavuconazole. Otherwise, few studies using relatively small sets of *C. gattii* isolates have been performed to investigate their *in vitro* susceptibilities to these drugs. Since fluconazole may last for a very long period of time, development of resistance to this agent has been reported both *in vivo* and *in vitro.* Many studies pointed out a significant emergence of clinical isolates of *C. neoformans* which present high fluconazole-MICs (MIC >4 mg/L) in different geographical regions (Aller et al., 2000; Dias et al., 2006; Pfaller et al, 2004). Resistance to fluconazole or to other azole compounds is not a cause of concern in the continent of America, where 3% to 10% of strains present high MIC. On opposite, the data from African, Cambodian and Spanish *C. neoformans* isolates showed high fluconazole-MICs (Bicanic et al., 2006; Perkins at al., 2005; Pfaller et al, 2004; Sar et al., 2004). It should be also pointed out that some authors did not find any correlation with clinical failure and the *in vitro* MIC data (Dannaoui et al., 2006). Therefore, the interpretation of the data is quite difficult since there are not interpretative clinical breakpoints for distinguish between resistant or susceptible *Cryptococcus* isolates that could predict failure or clinical success. However, breakpoints have not been defined yet, it is worth performing antifungal susceptibility testing against sequential isolates obtained from patients under antifungal therapy. An increased in MICs values during the monitoring could predict development of resistance of the original strain resulting in therapeutic concerning. Moreover, heteroresistance to fluconazole in *C. neoformans* or *C. gattii* is a phenomen that could play a role in clinical failure (Mondon et al., 1999; Varma, and Kwon-Chung, 2010).

The identification of amphotericin B resistant organisms seems to be more difficult however, as reference methods fail to detect it and trustworthy comparisons have not been done. Consistent detection of AMB resistance *in vitro* in *Cryptococcus neoformans* has proven difficult, and few studies demonstrated that majority of the initials isolates are susceptible to the polyene (Lozano-Chiu et al., 1998; Rodero et al., 2000a). Time-kill curves, a methodology to measure the fungicidal activity of amphotericin B, have been evaluated to identify resistance or tolerance to this antifungal agent in *Cryptococcus* isolates (Rodero et al., 2000b). Yeast isolates with amphotericin B MICs 2 mg/L are extremely uncommon, and therefore any strain with a MIC > 2 mg/L should be considered as potentially resistant to this polyene (CLSI, 2008).

4. Laboratory identification of *cryptococcus* in a routine clinical laboratory

The distinguishing feature of *Cryptococcus* genus is a polysaccharide capsule, and techniques that detect this cryptococcal structure and its components are the most useful tools as diagnostic tests. Evaluation of spinal fluid is essential in diagnosing central nervous system disease. The yeast cells of *Cryptococcus* are spherical in shape and approximately 5 to 7 µm in diameter while the capsules vary enormously in their thickness and are of a few micrometers of average. A rapid, simple and inexpensive procedure employs India ink staining to detect the encapsulated cells of *Cryptococcus* in pellets from centrifuged cerebrospinal fluid and other specimens. The lower limit of detection of India ink is ~10^3 to 10^4 yeast cell/ml. Disadvantages include the poor sensitivity of the technique in diagnosing cryptococcal meningitis in non-HIV-infected patients (30 to 72%) compared with culture. The sensitivity of India ink in high (~80%) for patients with overwhelming infection such HIV-infected patients (Kwon-Chung and Bennett, 1992; Heitman et al. 2011).

False-positive results can occur if inexperienced readers interpret lymphocytes or fat droplets as fungal cells. The capsular polysaccharide antigen that can be detect using commercial systems and represents the most valuable rapid test for the laboratory diagnosis of cryptococcosis. During infection, the capsular antigen is solubilized in cerebrospinal fluid, serum, urine and fluid recovered from the lungs. Almost all high fungal burden patients will have a positive serum and cerebrospinal fluid. Commercial kits typically demonstrate 90 to 100% sensitivity and 97 to 100% specificity for cerebrospinal fluid compared with culture and clinical diagnosis. However, in patients without AIDS the sensitivity of serum cryptococcal antigen in diagnosing cryptococcal meningitis is ~60%. The level of detection of most kits is at least 10 ng of antigen/ml. The most common testing format to detect antigen is latex agglutination assay. Moreover, antigen detection can be quantitative as the greatest dilution of the fluid that gives a positive result. Uncommon false-positive results can be encountered, particularly in serum contaminated with syneresis fluid, in presence of rheumatoid factor. In addition, false-positive results can occurs in patients with collagen vascular disease, chronic meningitis, malignancy (<0.3%), or even presenting a yeast infection caused by *Trichosporon.* Many kits include an enzymatic or heat pre-treatment in order to minimize the false-positive results, and incorporate a control reagent. In cases in which physicians doubt a positive results, they may ask the laboratory personal to treat the specimen with 2,β-mercaptoethanol, as it eliminates non-specific reactions. False-negative results were described in low organism burden infections and for capsule-deficient *Cryptococcus.* The latex assay also yields false-negative reactions due to a prozone effect that can be improved by specimen serial dilutions. An enzyme immunoassay is also available to detect glucuronoxylomannan, the principal polysaccharide component. The enzymatic assay it is slightly more sensitive than latex assay; similar to latex test, false-positive and false-negative results can occur (Kwon-Chun et al, 1981).

Measuring capsular antigen titers in serial clinical specimens for monitoring cerebrospinal fluid or serum cryptococcal antigen levels is useful in the management of cryptococcosis in non-AIDS patients. Decrease in antigen titers has limited value in the management of meningitis in such cases. Although it is expected that the titers should change after a few weeks of therapy, there is no evidence that titers predict or correlate with clinical and mycological outcomes (Kwon-Chung and Bennett, 1992).

The commercial (1,3) β-D-glucan assay detects a polysaccharide component of the cell wall of several pathogenic fungi, but given the limited experience to date with this test in cryptococcosis cases, there is no recommendation of using this test in the diagnosis of cryptococcosis.

Histological stains for tissue sections for revel *Cryptococcus* cells includes Gomori methenamine silver and calcofluor white, that are broad-spectrum fungal histochemical stains for fungi regardless of type. The best histological procedure uses mucicarmine, alcian blue, and periodic acid-Schiff that stain the capsule and Fontana-Masson stain, which interacts with the cell wall.

Culture techniques will remain the mainstay of the diagnosis of this infection. Culturing for *Cryptococcus* may be appropriate, even when the CSF profile is unremarkable. Blood, CSF, urine, and other clinical specimens should be cultured for fungi. Yeasts cells growth in 2 to 7 days in classical Sabouraud dextrose agar, typically as brilliant, mucous, pale colored colonies. Besides de capsular cell, one of the defining characteristics of *Cryptococcus neoformans* and *C. gattii* is its ability to synthesize a dark cell wall-associated pigment (melanin) when grow in media containing phenolic compounds, such Birdseed agar. Identification based on conventional biochemical and physiological assays, which are routinely used in a clinical laboratory for yeasts, can be difficult or even impossible for conclusive identification of *Cryptococcus* species. Laboratories should recognize that *C. gattii* cannot be differentiated from *C. neoformans* by conventional laboratory methods. *C. gattii* can only be differentiated from *C. neoformans* by specific biochemical or molecular testing. Laboratories should seek for definitive identification at an appropriate reference laboratory.

5. Conclusion

In conclusion, cryptococcosis remains a challenging management issue around the world and all patients presenting symptomatic increased intracranial pressure should be tested for HIC-infection, and screened for cryptococcal meningitis for receive early antifungal therapy. Relapses of symptoms and signs can occur during or after treatment and patients should be monitored for IRIS, drug resistance or compliance issues.

6. References

Aller AI, Martin-Mazuelos E, Lozano F; et al.. Correlation of fluconazole MICs with clinical outcome in cryptococcal infection. Antimicrob Agents Chemother. 2000; 44(6) : 1544-1548

Antinori S, Ridolfo A, Fasan M et al. AIDS-associated cryptococcosis:a comparison of epidemiology,clinical features and outcome in the pre-and-post-HAART eras. Experience of a single centre in Italy. HIV Med 2009;10:6-11

Bicanic T, Harrison TS, Niepieklo A, Dyakopu N, Mentjes G. Symptomatic relapse of HIV-associated cryptococcal meningitis after initial fluconazole monotherapy: the role of fluconazole resistance and immune reconstitution. *Clin Infect Dis* 2006; 43: 1069-1073.

Bicanic T,Meintjes G, Wood R et al. Fungal burden,early fungicidal activity,and outcome in cryptococcal meningitis in antiretroviral-naive or antiretroviral-experienced patients with amphotericin B or fluconazole.Clin Infect Dis 2007 ;45 :76-80

Bicanic T, Brouwer AE, Meintjes G et al. Relationship of cerebrospinal fluid pressure,fungal burden and outcome in patients with cryptococcal meningitis undergoing serial lumbar punctures. AIDS 2009; 23:701-706

Bicanic T, Muzoora C, Brouwer AE, Meintjes G, Longley N et al. Independent association between rate of clearance of infection and clinical outcome of HIV-associated cryptococcal meningitis:analysis of a combined cohort of 262 patients. Clin Infect Dis 2009; 49:702-9

Byrnes, E. J., III, W. Li, Y. Lewit, H. Ma, K. Voelz, P. Ren, D. A. Carter, V. Chaturvedi, R. J. Bildfell, R. C. May, and J. Heitman. Emergence and pathogenicity of highly virulent Cryptococcus gattii genotypes in the northwest United States. PLoS.Pathog. 2010; 6:e1000850.

Boekhout, T., B. Theelen, M. Diaz, J. W. Fell, W. C. Hop, E. C. Abeln, F. Dromer, and W. Meyer. Hybrid genotypes in the pathogenic yeast *Cryptococcus neoformans*. Microbiol. 2001; 147:891–907.

Brouwer AE, Rajanuwong A, Chierakul W et al. Combination antifungal therapies for HIV-associated cryptococcal meningitis: a randomized trial. Lancet 2004; 363:1764-7

Chaturvedi, S., M. Dyavaiah, R. A. Larsen, and V. Chaturvedi. *Cryptococcus gattii* in AIDS patients, southern California. Emerg. Infect. Dis. 2005; 11:1686 –1692.

Chuck MN, Sande MA. Infections with Cryptococcus neoformans in the acquired immunodeficiency syndrome. N Eng J Med 1989;321:794-799

Clinical and Laboratory Standards Institute. Reference Method for broth dilution antifungal susceptibility testing of yeast, Approved standard. Third Edition.M27-A3 2008; 28:1-25.

Dannaoui E, Abdul M, Arpin M, *et al*. Results obtained with various antifungal susceptibility testing methods do not predict early clinical outcome in patients with cryptococcosis. *Antimicrob Agents Chemother* 2006;50: 2464-2470

Denning DW, Tucker RM, Hanson LH, et al. Itraconazole therapy for cryptococcal meningitis and cryptococcosis. Arch Intern Med 1989; 149: 2301–2308.

Dias ALT, Matsumoto F, Melhem MSC, Silva GS, Auler ME, Siqueira AM, Paula CR. Comparative analysis of Etest and broth microdilution method (AFST-EUCAST) for trends on antifungal drug susceptibility testing of Brazilian *Cryptococcus neoformans* Isolates. *J Med Microbiol* 2006; 55: 1693- 1699

French N,Gray K,Watrea C et al. Cryptococcal infection in a cohort of HIV-1-infected Ugandan adults. AIDS 2002;16:1031-8

Graybill JR, Sobel J, Saag M et al. Diagnosis and management of increased intracranial pressure in patients with AIDS and cryptococcal meningitis. The NIAID Mycoses Study Group and AIDS Cooperative Treatment Groups. Clin Infect Dis 2000;30: 47-54

Gomez-Lopez A, Zaragoza O, Anjos Martins MA, Melhem MC, Rodriguez-Tudela JL, Cuenca-Estrella M. *In vitro* susceptibility of *Cryptococcus gattii* clinical isolates. *Clin Microbiol Infect* 2008; 14: 727-730

Heitman J, Kozel TR, Kwon-Chung KJ, Perfect JR, and Casadevall A. *Cryptococcus*: From Human Pathogen to Model Yeast. Washington, D.C., ASM Press, 2011.620pp

Husain S, Wagener MM, Singh N. Cryptococcus neoformans infection in organ transplant recipients: variables influencing clinical characteristics and outcome. Emerg Infect Dis 2001; 7:375–381.

Kwon-Chung KJ, Bennett JE. Medical Mycology. Philadelphia, Lea & Febiger, 1992. 866p

Kwon-Chung KJ, Hill WB,Bennett J. New, special stain for histopathological diagnosis of Cryptococcosis. J.Clin.Microbio. 1981; 13; 383-387

Larsen RA, Bauer M, Thomas AM, Graybill JR. Amphotericin B and fluconazole,a potent combination therapy for cryptococcal meningitis. Antimicrob Agents Chemother 2004;48:985-91

Larsen RA, Bauer M,Thomas AM et al. Correspondence of *in vitro* and *in vivo* fluconazole dose-response curves for *Cryptococcus neoformans*. Antimicrob Agents Chemother 2005; 49: 3297-301

Lortholary O,Poizat G,Zeller V et al. Long-term outcome of AIDS-associated cryptococcosis in the era of combination antiretroviral therapy.AIDS 2006;20:1764-7

Lozano-Chiu M, Paetznick VL; Ghannoum MA, Rex JH Detection of resistance to amphotericine B among *Cryptococcus neoformans* clinical isolates: performances of three different media assessed by using E-test and National Committee for Clinical Laboratory Standards M27-A methodologies. J Clin Microbiol. 1998; 36:2817-2822

Martins MA, Pappalardo MCSM, Melhem MSC, Pereira-Chioccola VL. Molecular diversity of serial Cryptococcus neoformans isolates from AIDS patients in the city of São Paulo, Brazil. Mem Inst Oswaldo Cruz 2007; 102:777–783.

Menichetti F,Fiorio M,Tosti A et al. High-dose fluconazole therapy for cryptococcal meningitis in patients with AIDS. Clin Infect Dis 1996;22:838-40

Meyer, W., A. Castaneda, S. Jackson, M. Huynh, E. Castaneda, and the IberoAmerican Cryptococcal Study Group. Molecular typing of IberoAmerican *Cryptococcus neoformans* isolates. Emerg. Infect. Dis. 2003; 9:189 –195.

Meyer, W., D. M. Aanensen, T. Boekhout, M. Cogliati, M. R. Diaz, M. C. Esposto, M. Fisher, F. Gilgado, F. Hagen, S. Kaocharoen, A. P. Litvintseva, T. G. Mitchell, S. P. Simwami, L. Trilles, M. A. Viviani, and J. Kwon-Chung. Consensus multi-locus sequence typing scheme for *Cryptococcus neoformans* and *Cryptococcus gattii*. Med. Mycol. 2009; 47: 561–570.

Mitchell TG,Perfect JR. Cryptococcosis in the era of AIDS-100 years after the discovery of *Cryptococcus neoformans*. Clin Microbiol Rev 1995; 8:515-548

Mondon P, Petter R, Amalfitano G et al. Heteroresistance to fluconazole and voriconazole in *Cryptococcus neoformans*. Antimicrob Agents Chemother. 1999; 43: 1856–1861

National Committee for Clinical Laboratory Standards (NCCLS) (2008) Reference method for broth dilution antifungal susceptibility testing of yeasts; approved standard - 3nd ed., M27-A3. Wayne, PA: NCCLS.

Pappalardo MCSM, Melhem MSC. Cryptococcosis: a review of the Brazilian experience for the disease. Rev Inst Med Trop Sao Paulo 2003; 45: 299–305

Pappalardo MCSM,Szeszs MW, Martins MA,Baceti LB, Bonfietti LX et al. Susceptibility of clinical isolates of *Cryptococcus neoformans* to amphotericin B using time-kill methodology. Diag Microbiol and Infect Dis 2009; 64: 146-151

Pappas PG, Chetchotisakd P, Larsen RA, Manosuthi W,Morris MI et al. A phase II randomized trial of amphotericin B alone or combined with fluconazole in the treatment of HIV-associated cryptococcal meningitis. Clin Infect Dis 2009; 48:1175-83

Park BJ, Wannemuehler KA, Marston BJ, Govender N,Pappas PG et al. Estimation of the global burden of cryptococcal meningitis among people living with HIV/AIDS. AIDS 2009;23:525-30

Perfect JR, Casadevall A. Cryptococcosis. Infect Dis Clin N Am 2002; 16:837-874

Perfect JR, Dismukes WE, Dromer F, Goldman DL,Graybill JR et al. Clinical practice guidelines for the management of cryptococcal disease:2010 update by the Infectious Diseases Society of America. Clin Infect Dis 2010;50:291-322

Perkins A, Gomez-Lopez A, Mellado E, Rodriguez-Tudela JL, Cuenca-Estrella M. Rates of antifungal resistance among Spanish clinical isolates of *Cryptococcus neoformans* var. *neoformans*. *J Antimicrobial Chemother* 2005; 56: 1144-1147.

Pfaller MA, Messer SA, Boyken L, Hollis RJ, Rice C, *et al.* *In vitro* activities of voriconazole, posaconazole and fluconazole against 4,169 clinical isolates of *Candida* spp and

Cryptococcus neoformans collected during 2001 and 2002 in the ARTEMIS global antifungal surveillance program. *Diag Microbiol Infect Dis* 2004; 48: 201-205.

Robinson PA, Bauer M,Leal ME et al.Early mycological treatment failure in AIDS-associated cryptococcal meningitis. Clin Infect Dis 1999;28:82-92

Rodero L, Cordoba S, Cahn P, Hochenfellner F, Davel G, Canteros C, *et al. In vitro* susceptibility studies of *Cryptococcus neoformans* isolated from patients with no clinical response to amphotericin B therapy. *J Antimicrobiol Chemother* 2000-a; 45: 239- 242.

Rodero L, Córdoba S, Cahn P, Soria M, Lucarini M, Davel G, *et al.* Timed-kill curves for *Cryptococcus neoformans* isolated from patients with AIDS. *Med Mycology* 2000-b;38: 201-207

Rodriguez-Tudela JL, Barchiesi F, Bille J, Chryssanthou E, Cuenca-Estrella M, Denning D *et al.* Method for the determination of minimum inhibitory concentration (MIC) by broth dilution of fermentative yeasts. *Clin. Microbiol. Infect.* 2007; 9(8), 1-7

Rodriguez-Tudela JL, Arendrup MC, Barchiesi F, Bille J, Chryssanthou E, Cuenca-Estrella M *et al.* EUCAST Definitive Document EDef 7.1: method for the determination of broth dilution MICs of antifungal agents for fermentative yeasts. *Clin. Microbiol. Infect.* 2008; 14(4), 398-405

Sar B, Monchy D, Vann M, Keo C, Sarthou JL, *et al.* Increasing in vitro resistance to fluconazole of *Cryptococcus neoformans* Cambodian isolates: April 2000 to March 2002. *J Antimicrob Chemother* 2004; 54: 563-565

Shaariah W, Morad Z, Suleiman AB. Cryptococcosis in renal transplant recipients. Transplant Proc 1992; 24:1898–1899.

Singh N, Alexander BD, Lortholary O, et al. *Cryptococcus neoformans* in organ transplant recipients: impact of calcineurin-inhibitor agents on mortality. J Infect Dis 2007; 195:756–764. 72.

Subcommittee on Antifungal Susceptibility Testing (AFST) of the ESCMID European Committee for Antimicrobial Susceptibility Testing. EUCAST definitive document EDef 7.1: method for the determination of broth dilution MICs of antifungal agents for fermentative yeasts. Clin MicrobiolInfect 14:398-405.

Sharkey PK, Graybill JR,Johnson ES et al. Amphotericin B lipid complex compared with amphotericin B in the treatment of cryptococcal meningitis in patients with AIDS. Clin Infect Dis 1996 ;22 :315-321

Varma, A., and K. J. Kwon-Chung. Heteroresistance of *Cryptococcus gattii* to fluconazole. Antimicrob. Agents Chemother. 2010; 54:2303–2311.

Vilchez RA, Fung J, Kusne S. Cryptococcosis in organ transplant recipients: an overview. Am J Transplant 2002; 2:575–580.

Vidal JE, Penalva de Oliveira AC, Fink MC,Pannuti CS, Trujillo JR. Aids related progressive multifocal leukoencephalopathy :a retrospective study in a referral center in São Paulo,Brazil. Rev Inst Med Trop Sao Paulo 2008;50:209-12

Zaragoza O, Mesa-Arango AC, Gómez-López A, Bernal-Martínez L, Rodríguez-Tudela JL, Cuenca-Estrella M. A process analysis of variables for standardization of antifungal susceptibility testing of non-fermentative yeasts. Antimicrob. Agents Chemother. 20101 doi:10.1128/AAC.01631-10

Zolopa A, Andersen J, Powderly W, et al. Early antiretroviral therapy reduces AIDS progression/death in individuals with acute opportunistic infections: a multicenter randomized strategy trial. PLoS ONE 2009; 4:e5575.

11

Cryptococcal Meningitis

Claudia Fabrizio, Sergio Carbonara and Gioacchino Angarano
Clinic of Infectious Diseases, University of Bari, Italy

1. Introduction

Cryptococcus neoformans is an encapsulated yeast first described in 1894, whose infection can induce a wide spectrum of clinical manifestations that range from a harmless colonization of the airways and asymptomatic infection to meningitis or disseminated disease.

Virulence probably plays a relatively small role in the outcome of this infection: the crucial factor is the immune status of the host. The most serious infections usually develop, in fact, in patients with defective cell-mediated immunity, for example those with AIDS, organ transplantation, reticuloendothelial malignancy, corticosteroid treatment and sarcoidosis, but not in subjects with neutropenia or immunoglobulin deficiency. Cryptococcosis has shown an increasing incidence over the last decades, mainly because of the AIDS pandemic, and still represents a major life-threatening fungal infection in these patients.

2. Mycology

Of the more than 50 species that comprise the genus Cryptococcus, human disease is primarily associated with *C. neoformans* and *C. gattii*. These two species, once considered as two varieties of *C. neoformans*, include five serotypes based on antigenic specificity of the capsular polysaccharide; serotypes A, D, and AD (*C. neoformans*), and serotypes B and C (*C. gattii*). Genome analyses demonstrate that serotypes A and D are actually distinct strains, respectively called *C. neoformans* var. *grubii* and *C. neoformans* var. *neoformans*

C. neoformans forms round, yeast like cells, 3-6 µm in diameter, which are surrounded by a polysaccharide capsule when the yeast is present in the host and in certain culture media; colonies are smooth, convex and they grow in solid media at 20-37°C.

The characteristics that allow identification of *C. neoformans* include microscopical appearance, biochemical features (such as the use of creatinine as a nitrogen source, the production of melanine, etc.) and the ability to grow at 37°C; in fact, most of nonpathogenetic Cryptococcus strains are not able to grow at this temperature.

3. Epidemiology

C. neoformans occurs mainly in immune-impaired subjects, can be recovered in high concentrations in pigeon faeces and bird nests, and is distributed worldwide, with different epidemiological features according to the different strains. Most cases of cryptococcosis involve serotype A (*C. neoformans* var. *grubii),* which is reported especially in patients living in low-income countries, whereas, in Western areas, it represents a clinical problem mainly in late presentation HIV-infected patients and is a marker of poor access to health care. On the other hand, serotype D *(C. neoformans* var. *neoformans)* is predominantly found in Western Europe and its infection is uncommon in the rest of the world.

C. gattii (serotypes B and C) causes 70-80% of Cryptococcal infections among immunocompetent hosts and can be isolated from certain species of eucalyptus trees and from the air beneath them. Infection by these strains is mainly common in tropical and subtropical areas, where the clinical disease occurs sporadically. However, a recent outbreak (1999-2003), involving patients with apparently normal immune system, was reported in some areas of Canada and Northwest US.

The incidence of Cryptococcal infection does not significantly differ in relation to age, race or occupation.

Since the mid 1980s, most Cryptococcal disease has occurred in patients with AIDS. The overall incidence (5-10% of patients with AIDS in Europe and US) decreased after the availability of highly active antiretroviral therapy (HAART). However, cryptococcosis still causes death in 15-44% of all patients with AIDS in sub-Saharan Africa and remains one of the most common AIDS-defining illnesses in some other areas, such as India, Brazil and Thailand.

4. Pathophysiology

Cryptococcal infection develops both in animals and humans, but neither animal-to-animal, animal-to-human transmission nor person-to-person direct respiratory transmission has been documented. The organism is primarily transmitted via the respiratory route. Humans can get Cryptococcal infection by inhalation of airborne fungi which are spread from the sources mentioned above. Following inhalation, the yeast spores are deposited into the pulmonary alveoli, where they are phagocytized by alveolar macrophages. Encapsulated yeasts, however, are often resistant to phagocytosis, because of the antiphagocytic and immunosuppressive properties of the polysaccharidic capsule, which is able to inhibit the recognition of the yeast by phagocytes and the leukocyte migration into the area of fungal replication.

The host response to Cryptococcal infection involves both cellular and humoral components, including natural killer cells, T-lymphocytes, macrophages and anti-Cryptococcal antibodies, which enhance the cell-mediated immune response to the organism.

C. neoformans infection is usually characterized by little or absent necrosis or organ dysfunction until late in the disease; the typical lesion consists of a cystic cluster of yeasts with no well-defined inflammatory response and well-formed granulomas are generally absent.

The initial pulmonary Cryptococcal infection is usually asymptomatic; in immunocompetent hosts the infection can be cleared, contained as latent infection or cause a disease limited to the lungs, inducing development of a pneumonia with poorly defined interstitial nodules. In contrast, in immunosuppressed patients, especially those with defects in the function of T cells, the infection can progress to a meningitis and/or a disseminated disease, which usually is the resultiof a reactivation of a chronic latent pulmonary infection; in fact, from the lungs of these patients, cryptococci disseminate widely and may infect any organ, most frequently the central nervous system (CNS), but also bones, prostate, eyes and skin.

5. Clinical

The CNS is the main site of Cryptococcal disease in both immunocompetent and immunocompromised hosts. The infection usually involves both the meninges and the brain, causing a diffuse, usually subacute or chronic disease.

Immunocompetent hosts may present with either meningitis or, more frequently than immunocompromised hosts, with cryptococcomas, which often manifest with focal neurologic defects.

The clinical presentation and the course of Cryptococcal meningitis vary according to the underlying medical conditions and immune status of the host: the most common symptoms are headache, altered mental status (personality changes, memory loss, reduced level of consciousness, confusion, lethargy, up to coma), nausea and vomiting (often associated with increased intracranial pressure) and cranial nerves paralysis. Other findings, less frequently observed, may include ataxia, aphasia, hearing defects and choreoathetoid movements.

Ocular symptoms such as blurred vision, photophobia or diplopia may result from arachnoiditis, papilledema, optic nerve neuritis or chorioretinitis.

Physical findings, such as fever and stiff neck, are less common because of the limited inflammatory response induced by the encapsulated yeasts. . Some HIV positive patients may have minimal or nonspecific symptoms at presentation and may often be afebrile; this lack or aspecifity of symptoms contribute to delayed diagnosis.

Dementia is a potential sequela and may indicate the presence of hydrocephalus as a late complication.

In the case of CNS disease, Cryptococcal lesions should be carefully searched in other body sites, considering that, especially in AIDS patients, virtually any organ can be involved. In particular, a pneumonia without peculiar features (interstitial patterns or basal unilateral infiltrates are frequently observed) and skin lesions mimicking molluscum contagiosum are frequently observed.

6. Diagnosis

6.1 Laboratory studies

Even with widespread disease, the routine laboratory tests (e.g. leukocyte count, haematocrit, erythrocyte sedimentation rate) may yield normal results.

Evaluation of cerebral spinal fluid (CSF) is essential in diagnosing CNS disease, usually showing depressed CSF glucose concentrations, mild elevated protein concentrations and leukocyte counts of 20/μL or higher, with a lymphocyte predominance. The CSF can be normal at times, such as in AIDS patients with inadequate inflammatory response or in persons with early infection.

It is also important to evaluate the CSF opening pressure, because elevated values (more than 250 mmH_2O) are found in more than half of patients and are associated with a poor prognosis, requiring drainage of CSF to reduce the pressure to 200 mmH_2O or lower. Prior to removal of CSF, CT scanning or MRI should be performed to exclude intracranial masses that could result in cerebral herniation, especially in patients with focal neurological signs.

6.2 Microbiological investigations

Etiological diagnosis of Cryptococcal meningitis is obtained by microbiological investigations performed on the CSF.

An India ink preparation is commonly used with CSF to identify the organism by direct microscopy and to support a presumptive diagnosis; if performed correctly, 25-50% of patients with Cryptococcal meningitis show cryptococci.

In patients with a negative India ink test result, Cryptococcal meningitis can be diagnosed with the highly sensitive and specific Cryptococcal antigen testing in CSF, which it is almost invariably detected at high titre in this disease. The test is performed by an immunoenzimatic procedure. If a lumbar puncture cannot be performed, testing for serum antigen can be useful; this test may also be considered as an initial screening tool to detect Cryptococcal infection in HIV positive patients.

CSF and blood should always be cultured for fungi; CSF culture should be performed from three or more centrifuged specimens in Sabouraud dextrose agar. Blood culture results prove positive in up to 75% of HIV infected patients; this indicates an extensive infection, in which the organism may be observed within peripheral leukocytes or bone marrow macrophages.

A high Cryptococcal burden at the baseline (as detected by quantitative CSF culture or high CSF antigen titre) and an altered mental status are the most important predictors of death.

6.3 Imaging studies

Obtaining a CT or MRI of the brain prior to performing a lumbar puncture is important in patients who present with focal neurologic deficits or a history suggesting slowly progressive meningitis, in order to detect mass lesion that may increase the risk of cerebral herniation following a lumbar puncture.

CT can reveal small, ring-enhancing lesions or non-enhancing 'pseudocystis'. Both CT scanning and MRI can also reveal the presence of hydrocephalus caused by basilar meningitis.

7. Therapeutical management

Cryptococcal meningitis and disseminated disease represent severe clinical conditions which were invariably fatal prior to the use of amphoterycin B, flucytosine and azoles; in fact, without a specific antifungal treatment, mortality rates of 100% have been reported within two weeks after clinical presentation in certain HIV-infected populations. The availability of such antifungal therapy regimens has lead to a dramatic decrease in the mortality. However, the three month mortality rate during a correct management of acute Cryptococcal meningoencephalitis still approximates 20%, even in areas where HAART and advanced medical care are widely available.

Treatment regimens are based on a sequence of induction, consolidation and maintenance regimens, both in AIDS and non-AIDS patients **(Table 1)**. The first and second phase of the treatment aim to obtain a rapid clearance of cryptococcus by the CNS, whereas maintenance therapy is targeted to maintain a stable suppression (latency) of the chronic infection in the human organism.

Clinical Setting	Induction Therapy	Duration	Consolidation/Maintenance therapy	Duration
HIV-infected patients	c-AMB (0,7-1 mg/kg/daily) + flucytosine (100 mg/kg/daily) *or:*	≥2 weeks	Consolidation: fluconazole (400 mg/daily) Maintenance: fluconazole (200 mg/daily)	≥ 8 weeks
	L-AMB (3-4 mg/kg/daily) or ABLC (5mg/kg/daily) (if there are renal concerns) + flucytosine (100 mg/kg/daily) *or:*	≥2 weeks	Consolidation and maintenance: Itraconazole (400 mg daily)[a] *or:* c-AMB (1 mg/kg per week)[a]	≥1 year[b]
	c-AMB or L-AMB or ABLC (for flucytosine-intolerant patients; doses as above)	4-6 weeks		≥1 year[b]
Organ transplant recipients	L-AMB (3-4 mg/kg daily) or ABLC (5 mg/kg daily) + flucytosine (100 mg/kg daily) *or:*	≥2 weeks	Consolidation: fluconazole (400-800 mg daily)	8 weeks
	c-AMB (0.7 mg/kg daily) or L-AMB (6 mg/kg daily) or ABLC (5 mg/kg daily)	≥4-6 weeks	Maintenance: fluconazole (200-400 mg daily)	6-12 months
Non-HIV, non-transplant patients	c-AMB (0.7-1 mg/kg daily) + flucytosine (100 mg/kg daily) *or:*	≥4 weeks	Consolidation: fluconazole (400-800 mg daily)	8 weeks
	L-AMB (3-4 mg/kg daily) or ABLC (5 mg/kg daily) + flucytosine (100 mg/kg daily) *or:*	≥4 weeks	Maintenance: fluconazole (200 mg daily)	6-12 months
	c-AMB or L-AMB or ABLC (for flucytosine-intolerant patients; doses as above)	≥6 weeks		

ABLC, amphotericin B lipid complex; **c-AMB**, amphotericin B deoxycholate; **L-AMB**, liposomal amphotericin B. **a**: Inferior to fluconazole. **b**: Consider discontinuing antifungal therapy after a minimum of one year, if following a successful HAART, CD4+ count ≥100 cells/µL and undetectable viral load are detected for ≥3 months.
Adapted from [Perfect JR, Clin Inf Dis 1010;50:291-322]

Table 1. Antifungal treatment for Cryptococcal meningoencephalitis

7.1 Management of adverse events

Antifungal drugs used for Cryptococcal meningitis may induce adverse reaction and toxicity. Therefore, patients receiving such regimens must be strictly monitored for dose-dependent nephrotoxicity and electrolyte alterations, if treated with amphotericin B; for bone marrow suppression and gastrointestinal disturbance, if receiving flucytosine; for hepatotoxicity, if fluconazole is administrated.

7.2 HIV-infected patients

Induction therapy is based on amphotericin B deoxycholate (c-AMB) plus flucytosine (see **Table 1** for dosage) for at least two weeks; flucytosine can be administered orally or intravenously in severe cases or if oral intake is not possible. This regimen should be followed by a consolidation therapy with fluconazole orally for eight weeks.

In patients with renal function impairment, lipid formulations of amphotericin B, mainly represented by amphotericin B lipid complex (ABLC) and liposomal amphotericin B (L-AMB), appear to be less nephrotoxic and can substitute c-AMB. Lipid formulations of amphotericin B can also be used as monotherapy for four to six weeks or in association with fluconazole in flucytosine-intolerant patients.

Alternative consolidation regimens include flucytosine plus fluconazole for six weeks, fluconazole alone for 10 to 12 weeks or itraconazole for 10 to 12 weeks, although the results of several trials with these therapies are variable and often disappointing.

Maintenance therapy in HIV-infected patients should be started when CSF Cryptococcal culture becomes negative and a substantial clinical improvement is observed; oral fluconazole is the most effective therapy, with a very low relapse rate, if compared with regimens based on oral itraconazole or intravenous c-AMB. It is considered reasonable to discontinue maintenance therapy, if patients have successfully completed a course of initial therapy and, following HAART, their CD4+ cell count increase to ≥200/µl for at least three to six months.

Primary prophylaxis for Cryptococcal disease is not routinely recommended for several reasons: its relative infrequency in areas where HAART is available, potential for drug toxicity or interactions with concurrent medications, risk of antifungal drug resistance and costs. However, according to some studies, a screening strategy (Cryptococcal antigen testing) and a prophylaxis may be useful in areas where the availability of HAART is limited and cryptococcosis incidence is high.

7.3 Organ transplant recipient

Cryptococcosis is the third most common fungal infection among solid organ transplant recipients, usually occurring more than one year post-transplant and generally representing a reactivation of latent infection; CNS involvement and/or disseminated disease are documented in most of these patients. Acquisition of the organism usually occurs via inhalation, but the risk of transmission through donor organs or other tissues has also been recently described, even if in a few cases.

Primary induction therapy is based on either L-AMB or ABLC plus flucytosine (see **Table 1** for doses) for at least two weeks, followed by fluconazole for eight weeks as consolidation regimen and for additional six to 12 months, at lower dosage, as maintenance therapy. The use of c-AMB should be avoided because of the risk of nephrotoxicity, especially with the concurrent use of calcineurine inhibitors which are often administrated to these patients as immunosuppressive therapy.

If induction therapy does not include flucytosine, L-AMB should be administrated for at least four to six weeks. Moreover, a positive CSF culture result after two weeks of induction treatment may indicate a poor outcome and suggests a prolonged induction period with L-AMB in these patients.

During cryptococcosis, a careful reduction of the immunosuppressant therapy (slow dose decrease over time and/or stepwise elimination of immunosuppressants) should be adopted following the initiation of antifungal therapy. Furthermore, reduction of corticosteroids should precede that of calcineurin inhibitors, since the latter drugs have a direct anti-Cryptococcal activity.

7.4 Non-HIV infected, non transplant recipients patients

This represents a heterogeneous category of patients that may include 'presumably immunocompetent hosts', but also people with different immune defects (such as malignancy, connective tissue diseases, severe liver disease and so on).

Antifungal regimens for these patients are substantially the same as the one mentioned above **(see Table 1)**, but there are different opinions about the length of induction therapy: according to some authors, in fact, duration of induction phase should be two weeks, while others suggest to administrate it for four to six weeks. The great variability of features in patients forming this category makes it necessary to adapt the therapeutical management to each case.

8. Indications for the management of complications

8.1 Persistence and relapses

Persistent infection is defined by positive results of CSF cultures after four weeks of effective antifungal therapy; relapse is defined by the recovery of cryptococci from a previously checked sterile body site and/or the recrudescence of signs/symptoms at the previous site of disease after an initial normalization. Most cases of relapse are due to an inadequate primary therapy (dose and/or duration) or to the lack of the patient adherence to the consolidation or maintenance treatment.

Restarting induction regimen for a longer course and with a higher dosage may be the first approach in these situations, using amphotericin B deoxycholate plus fluconazole in flucytosine intolerant patients and high doses of fluconazole plus flucytosine in polyene intolerant patients.

The possibility of development of antifungal drug resistance should also be checked in terms of changes in the MIC from the original isolate: a ≥3-dilution difference, in fact, suggests development of direct drug resistance.

Finally, the use of Voriconazole or Posaconazole as salvage therapy should be considered in cases resistant to the first-line antifungal agents. However, the frequent interactions of these agents with several antiretroviral drugs should be carefully considered in HIV-infected patients. In this regard, the use of therapeutic drug monitoring of the plasma concentrations of these agents may represent a useful tool in clinical practice.

8.2 Elevated CSF pressure

Control of CSF pressure is one of the most important determinants in the outcome of Cryptococcal meningitis because elevated values are associated with a high burden of yeasts in the CNS and with increased morbidity and mortality rates. This association is valid for most HIV-infected patients (there is lack of data about this complication in non-HIV patients with Cryptococcal meningitis), so it is very important to measure the initial opening pressure during the first lumbar puncture. If there is persistent pressure elevation (≥25 cm of CSF) and symptoms, lumbar puncture should be repeated daily, until CSF pressure and symptoms have been stabilized for ≥2 days, considering temporary percutaneous lumbar drains or ventriculostomy if repeated daily lumbar punctures are required.

8.3 Cryptococcoma

Large cryptococcomas should be treated with a combination of antifungal therapy and early surgical removal, as response to antifungal drugs only is poor. Multiple lesions require a prolonged induction/eradication therapy. Corticosteroids may be required if there is a substantial surrounding oedema, especially in the presence of neurological deficits. Moreover, a nonresponsive brain mass in severely immunosuppressed patients may also suggest the presence of a second pathogen or a tumour.

8.4 IRIS

Immune reconstitution inflammatory syndrome (IRIS) consists of a paradoxical worsening of the clinical manifestations or the course of the Cryptococcal disease in spite of an appropriate antifungal therapy and an apparent microbiological efficacy of the latter. IRIS is interpreted as an exuberant inflammatory reaction of the host at the sites of Cryptococcal infection, subsequent to a rapid improvement in the cellular immunity; for example, IRIS may occur in AIDS patients following introduction of HAART and the restoration of pathogen-specific CD4+ cells.

Risk factors for developing IRIS include: severe Cryptococcal disease (high fungemia), HIV infection, extremely low baseline CD4+ cell count, no previous antiretroviral therapy, lack of CSF sterilization at week two of therapy, introduction of HAART during the early part of antifungal induction therapy and rapid decrease in the HIV viral load in response to HAART.

If IRIS occurs, it is not recommended to modify antifungal therapy, neither to administrate any specific treatment for minor manifestations, whereas corticosteroids may be required for major complications, such as severe CNS inflammation. In order to reduce the risk of developing IRIS, according to the principal current guidelines, introduction of HAART should be delayed for two to 10 weeks after the starting of antifungal therapy.

9. Suggested treatment in special clinical situations

9.1 Pregnant women

If Cryptococcal meningitis occurs during pregnancy it is often severe because of the immunological alterations associated with this event. c-AMB or L-AMB should be administrated as induction therapy, while the use of flucytosine (pregnancy category C) must be considered in relationship to benefit versus risk. Fluconazole (pregnancy category C) must be preferably started after delivery and should be avoided in the first trimester. During the last two trimesters the possible benefits following fluconazole use should be carefully weighed against the risks associated to the long-lasting exposure to this drug during pregnancy.

9.2 Children

Cryptococcosis in children is less frequent than in adults and it is associated with some underlying conditions, such as primary immune defects or certain haematological malignancies, peculiar to childhood, and to common risk factors for both adults and children (e.g. AIDS, transplant recipients).

Induction and consolidation therapy for children is based on the use of c-AmB plus flucytosine for two weeks, followed by fluconazole for eight weeks (10-12 mg/kg daily); for AmB-intolerant patients it is possible to administrate either L-AmB or ABLC. Maintenance therapy is based on the use of fluconazole (6 mg/kg daily).

The optimal dosing and duration of therapy for children with cryptococcosis, however, have not been precisely determined because of the lack of literature data concerning this matter. For the non–HIV-infected, non-transplant population, treatment dose and length schedules similar to that indicated above for adults is prescribed (except for fluconazole dose, which is modified as explained above).

9.3 Resource - Limited health care environment

In many areas of the world with high incidence of cryptococcosis the most effective antifungal drugs are often not available and adjustments in the management of patients with Cryptococcal disease often become necessary. The recommendations concerning therapeutical approach in these settings include:

- When flucytosine is not available, induction therapy is represented by c-AmB with or without fluconazole for two weeks, followed by fluconazole as consolidation therapy for eight weeks and as maintenance therapy until immune reconstitution.
- When a polyene is not available, induction therapy is based on fluconazole for at least 10 weeks or until CSF culture results are negative, followed by consolidation/maintenance therapy with the same drug, at a lower dosage.
- When a polyene is not available but flucytosine is available, induction therapy is represented by fluconazole plus flucytosine for two to 10 weeks, followed by maintenance therapy with fluconazole.
- With use of primary fluconazole therapy for induction, both primary or secondary drug resistance of the isolate may be an issue, and MIC testing is advised; for azole-resistant strains, administer c-AmB until CSF, blood, and/or other sites are sterile.

9.4 C. *gattii* infection

Induction, consolidation and suppressive treatment are the same as for *C. neoformans*. A delayed response to treatment frequently occurs. A radiology follow-up focused on cryptococcoma and hydrocephalus is needed as these conditions are often observed in patients with *C. gattii* infection, as described above. For very large and multiple cryptococcomas, a combination of cAmB and flucytosine therapy for four to six weeks should be considered, followed by fluconazole for six to 18 months, depending on whether surgery was performed. Neurosurgical intervention must be considered if there is compression of vital structures, failure to reduce the size of cryptococcoma after four weeks of therapy or failure to thrive.

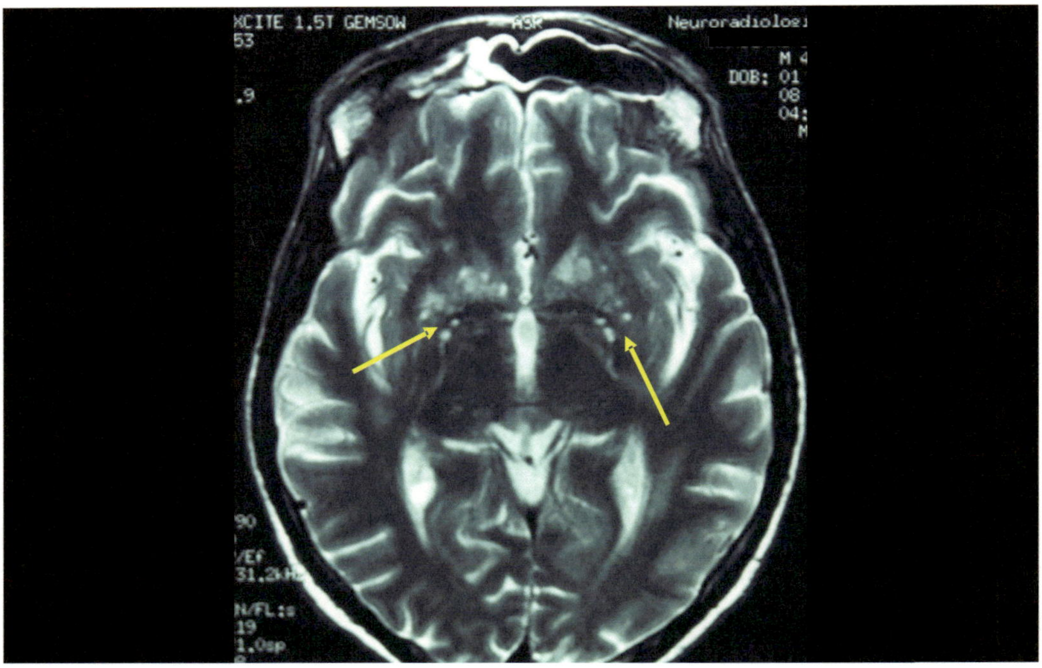

Fig. 1. Brain magnetic resonance of an AIDS patient with Cryptococcal meningitis, highlighting dilatation of the perivascular (Virchow-Robin) spaces

10. References

Centers for Disease Control and Prevention. Guidelines for Prevention and Treatment of Opportunistic Infections in HIV-Infected Adults and Adolescents: recommendations from CDC, the National Institutes of Health, and the HIV Medicine Association/Infectious Diseases Society of America. *MMWR Morb Mortal Wkly Rep* 2009; 58:48-50.

Jarvis JN, Harrison TS. HIV-associated cryptococcal meningitis. *AIDS* 2007, 21:2119–2129

Perfect JR, Dismukes WE, Dromer F, et al. Clinical Practice Guidelines for the Management of Cryptococcal Disease: 2010 Update by the Infectious Diseases Society of America. *Clin Inf Dis* 2010; 50:291–322

Carbonara S, Regazzi M, Ciracì E, et al. Long-term efficacy and safety of TDM-assisted combination of voriconazole plus efavirenz in an AIDS patient with cryptococcosis and liver cirrhosis. *Ann Pharmacother* 2009 May;43(5):978-84.

Sorrell TC, Chen SC-A. Recent advances in management of cryptococcal meningitis: commentary. *F1000 Medicine Reports* 2010, 2:82

Pukkila-Worley R & Mylonakis E. Epidemiology and management of cryptococcal meningitis: developments and challenges. *Expert Opin. Pharmacother* (2008) 9(4):551-560

Baddley JW, Schaine DC et al. Transmission of Cryptococcus neoformans by organ transplantation. *Clin Inf Dis* 2011; 52(4): e94-e98

King JW, DeWitt ML. Cryptococcosis. http://emedicine.medscape.com/article/215354-overview (updated Mar 9, 2011)

12

Human Parechoviruses, New Players in the Pathogenesis of Viral Meningitis

Kimberley Benschop[1], Joanne Wildenbeest[2], Dasja Pajkrt[2] and Katja Wolthers[1]
[1]*Laboratory of Clinical Virology, Dept. of Medical Microbiology,*
[2]*Dept. of Pediatric Hematology, Immunology and Infectious Diseases, Emma Children's Hospital, Academic Medical Center, Amsterdam, The Netherlands*

1. Introduction

Human parechoviruses (HPeVs) belong to the family of *Picornaviridae* and have been recognized as a separate group on the basis of distinct molecular and biological properties since 1999. The identification of HPeV3 in 2004 and its association with neonatal sepsis and meningitis made it particularly clear that HPeVs are related to severe disease in infants. Molecular techniques are increasingly being used for the identification of HPeVs and with the increase in epidemiological and clinical data, HPeVs are now considered to be the second predominant cause of viral meningitis, following enteroviruses (EVs). This review focuses on the role of HPeVs, with particular notice to HPeV3, as a causative agent in viral meningitis as well as neonatal sepsis and encephalitis. Data on epidemiology, clinical manifestations, immunology and molecular and cellular biology, underlying the greater pathogenicity of this novel group of viruses as well as the diagnosis, management and treatment options will be discussed.

2. Classification and biology of HPeV

Human parechoviruses (HPeVs) belong to the large *Picornaviridae* family, comprising small non-enveloped, single-stranded positive-sense RNA viruses infecting both humans and animals. The *Picornaviridae* family currently consists of 12 established genera as of 2011: *Enterovirus, Parechovirus, Hepatovirus, Kobuvirus, Aphthovirus, Erbovirus, Teschovirus, Cardiovirus, Tremovirus, Sapelovirus, Avihepatovirus* and *Senecavirus*. Many new genera such as the *Cosavirus, Klassevirus* and *Aquamovirus* have recently been proposed, and are awaiting genus/type classification (http://www.picornastudygroup.com/).

HPeVs were first discovered in 1956 during a summer diarrhea outbreak in the USA by Wigand & Sabin et al. (1961) and originally classified within the *Enterovirus* genus as echovirus 22 and 23. This was based on their biology in cell culture, exhibiting a similar cytopathogenic effect (CPE) as enteroviruses (EVs), their clinical presentation and non-pathogenicity in both mice and monkeys. Despite these similarities, subtle differences such as a slow progression of CPE of infected cells in cell culture and their more common association with mild gastrointestinal disease, in comparison to the more severe symptoms reported for other enterovirus types, led to their description as atypical enteroviruses. Later, evident differences in genome organization and structure, divergence of encoded proteins and other biological properties (Hyypia et al., 1992; Stanway et al., 2000), prompted their reclassification in 1999 (Stanway et al., 1994; Stanway & Hyypia, 1999) as HPeV types 1 and 2 within the genus *Parechovirus*. Almost half a century after the discovery of HPeV1 and 2, a third HPeV type was discovered in Japan (Ito et al., 2004) and since then the number of HPeV types increased rapidly with the development of more state-of-the-art molecular techniques. Up to date there are 16 HPeV types known (Table, Figure 1). The *Parechovirus* genus also comprises a second group of viruses isolated from rodents; the Ljungan viruses (Niklasson et al., 1999; Stanway et al., 2005).

Type	Strain	Origin	Reference
HPeV1A	Harris	Ohio, USA	Hyypia et al., 1992
HPeV1B	BNI-788 St	Bonn, Germany	Baumgarte et al., 2008
HPeV 2	Williamson	Ohio, USA	Ghazi et al., 1998
HPeV 3	A308/99	Aichi, Japan	Ito et al., 2004
HPeV 4	K251176-02	Amsterdam, the Netherlands	Benschop et al., 2006b
HPeV 5	CT86-6760	Connecticut, USA	Oberste et al., 1998
HPeV 6	NII561-2000	Niigata, Japan	Watanabe et al., 2007
HPeV 7	PAK5045	Badin, Pakistan	Li et al., 2009
HPeV 8	BR/217/2006	Salvador, Brazil	Drexler et al., 2009
HPeV 9	BAN2004-10902	Bangkok, Thailand	Oberste et al., unpub.
HPeV 10	BAN2004-10903	Bangkok, Thailand	Oberste et al., unpub.
HPeV 11	BAN2004-10905	Bangkok, Thailand	Oberste et al., unpub.
HPeV 12	BAN2004-10904	Bangkok, Thailand	Oberste et al., unpub.
HPeV 13	BAN2004-10901	Bangkok, Thailand	Oberste et al., unpub.
HPeV 14	451564	Amsterdam, the Netherlands	Benschop et al., 2008c
HPeV 15	BAN-11614	Bangkok, Thailand	Oberste et al., unpub.
HPeV 16	BAN-11615	Bangkok, Thailand	Oberste et al., unpub.

Table. HPeV prototype strains (http://www.picornastudygroup.com/)

Like other picornaviruses, the HPeV genome is small containing approximately 7300 basepares encoding for a single polyprotein flanked by 5´ and 3´ untranslated regions (UTRs) and a poly A tail at the 3'end (Figure 2) (Stanway & Hyypia, 1999).

Following virus entry, the RNA is directly translated into a long polyprotein, which is subsequently cleaved by the viral protease (3C) into three structural proteins (VP0, VP1 and VP3) forming the capsid structure and seven non-structural proteins (2A–2C and 3A–3D) that are needed for replication. In contrast to other picornaviruses, VP0 is not further cleaved into VP4 and VP2. Additionally, while VP0 is not antigenic in any other genera, the predominant antigenic sites of HPeV have been mapped to the N-terminal region of the VP0 protein (Joki-Korpela et al., 2000). For HPeV1, additional antigenicity eliciting the production of neutralizing antibodies is found to be located at the C-terminal end of the capsid protein VP1, where the receptor binding motif arginine-glycine-aspartic acid (RGD) is located.

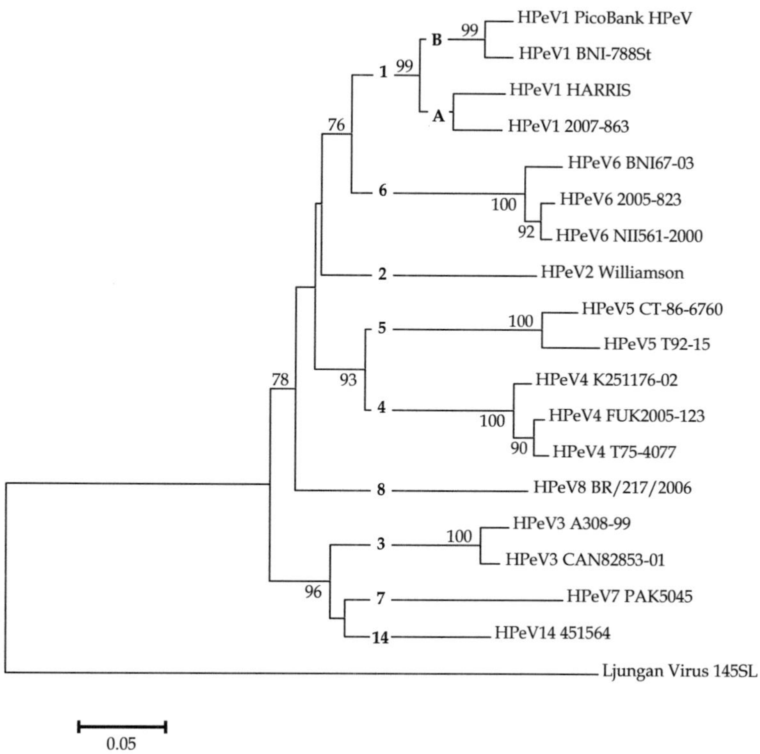

Fig. 1. Neighbour joining tree based on the complete VP1 gene of HPeV types 1-8 and 14 (amino acid p-distance). Complete VP1 sequences for HPeV9-13 and 15-16 were unavailable at the time of publication.

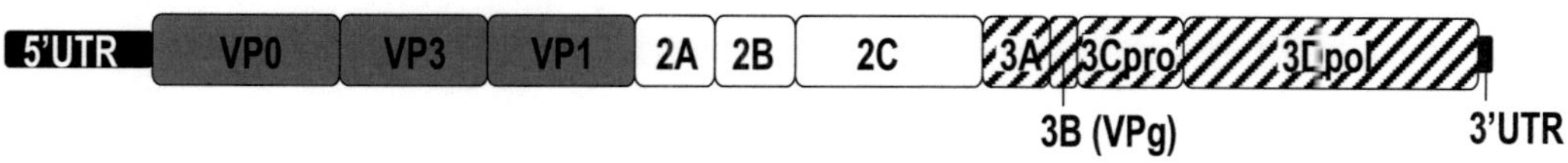

Fig. 2. HPeV genome.

To allow efficient translation, most picornaviruses enable the majority of host cellular mRNA translation to be shut off by the non-structural protein 2A. However, there is little evidence that HPeVs elicit the same shut-off (Stanway et al., 1994).

Replication is driven by the RNA-dependent RNA polymerase (3Dpol) and involves RNA structures present on the 5′UTR (Nateri et al., 2000, 2002) and VP0 (*cis*-acting replication element (CRE)) (Al-Sunaidi et al., 2007) as well as the 2C protein (NTPase activity and RNA binding) (Samuilova et al., 2006). Following binding of the protein VPg (3B) at the 5′end, the positive stranded RNA is copied to produce negative stranded RNA, which in turn can be replicated back to positive stranded RNA needed for assembly and additional translation activity to produce virus particles.

Finally, these particles are released from the cells. In most picornaviruses, virus release is achieved through capsid maturation by the cleavage of VP0 into VP2 and VP4. However, the cleavage of VP0 into VP2 and VP4 does not appear in parechoviruses and the manner of how maturation and virus release is achieved for HPeVs remains largely unknown (Stanway et al., 1994). Nonetheless, the external appearance of HPeV particles has proved consistent with the external appearance of other picornaviruses, most closely resembling Foot and Mouth Disease Virus (FMDV) in the *Aphthovirus* genus as has recently been shown by cryoelectron microscopy and image reconstruction (Seitsonen et al., 2010).

3. HPeV infections, from mild to severe disease

Clinical symptoms of HPeV infections are generally similar to those found in EV infections ranging from mild respiratory and gastrointestinal disease to more severe disease like meningitis and sepsis-like illness. In earlier decades when only HPeV1 and 2 were known, HPeV infections were considered of little clinical importance. Even though occasionally, severe disease was reported for HPeV such as acute flaccid paralysis, myocarditis, meningitis, encephalitis and encephalomyelitis (Benschop et al., 2006a; Figueroa et al., 1989; Koskiniemi et al., 1989; Legay et al., 2002; Maller et al., 1967) the majority of HPeV1 infections caused mild gastrointestinal and/or respiratory symptoms.

This all changed with the discovery of HPeV3 (Ito et al., 2004). By comparing clinical data from children infected with HPeV1 and children infected with HPeV3, we showed the increased clinical relevance of this type. HPeV3 infections were predominantly associated with neonatal sepsis and CNS infections while children infected with HPeV1 had milder symptoms (Benschop et al., 2006a). These findings were later confirmed by others, increasingly detecting this type in the CSF of children with CNS disease, such as meningitis and encephalitis, as well as neonatal sepsis (Harvala et al., 2009; Levorson et al., 2009; van der Sanden et al., 2008; Verboon-Maciolek et al., 2008a; Wolthers et al., 2008).

Children infected with HPeV3 often present with symptoms of fever and irritability as a sign of CNS infection, either meningitis or encephalitis. The majority (54-80%) of the children also show sepsis-like illness, defined as fever or hypothermia with signs of circulatory and/or respiratory dysfunction defined by tachycardia or bradycardia, low blood pressure and/or decreased saturation (Benschop et al., 2006a; Harvala et al., 2009; Selvarangan et al., 2011; Wolthers et al., 2008). Additional clinical symptoms frequently seen in HPeV3 infections are maculopapular rash, gastrointestinal symptoms and respiratory symptoms (Benschop et al., 2006a; Selvarangan et al., 2011; Verboon-Maciolek et al., 2008a; Wolthers et al., 2008).

Severe clinical manifestations are mainly described in relation to HPeV3 infections, although occasionally other HPeV genotypes have been associated with serious illness (Schnurr et al.,

1996; Watanabe et al., 2007). However, similarly to HPeV1 and 2, newer types have mainly been associated with mild gastro-intestinal and respiratory symptoms in children and are often found in children with an underlying illness (Pajkrt et al., 2009).

4. Epidemiology of HPeV in relation to CNS infections

Because HPeVs are reported as being transmitted through the fecal-oral route, epidemiological studies are often performed on stool samples and provide an accurate estimation of the prevalence of the different types. HPeV1 is considered as the predominant strain mainly affecting young children (Baumgarte et al., 2008; Benschop et al., 2006a, 2008c, 2010a; Harvala et al., 2008; Joki-Korpela & Hyypia, 1998; Stanway et al., 2000; Tapia et al., 2008; Watanabe et al., 2007). Epidemiological studies dating back over 30 year ago, showed HPeV1 to be widely spread (Ehrnst & Eriksson, 1993; Grist et al., 1978; Joki-Korpela & Hyypia, 1998; Khetsuriani et al., 2006b). In recent studies, involving the detection of the newer HPeV types, the new HPeV type 3 is identified as the second predominant strain (Benschop et al., 2006a, 2008c, 2010a; Ito et al., 2010; Tapia et al., 2008; Watanabe et al., 2007). HPeV3 comprised 22 to 26% of the HPeV types identified in HPeV positive stool samples collected in the Amsterdam region, while the majority of the HPeV positive stool samples comprised HPeV1 (65-71%)(Benschop et al., 2006a, 2008c, 2010a). Similar data were found in studies on stool samples in other European countries (Baumgarte et al., 2008; Tapia et al., 2008), and Asia (Ito et al., 2010; Pham et al., 2010, 2011a; Watanabe et al., 2007) where HPeV1 was identified as the most prevalent type, followed by HPeV3. HPeV4 is frequently found in stools as well (Benschop et al., 2008c, 2010a; Boros et al., 2010; Pham et al., 2011b; Zhong et al., 2011), while HPeV6 seems to prevail as a secondary respiratory pathogen (Harvala et al., 2008). Infections with HPeV2 and 5 are reported sporadically (Benschop et al., 2010a; Ehrnst & Eriksson, 1996; van der Sanden et al., 2008). Circulation patterns of the newly reported HPeV types 7–16 are yet to be determined (Benschop et al., 2008c, 2010a; van der Sanden et al., 2008).

The distribution of HPeV types is significantly different when only CNS infections are taken into account. Screening of CSF samples show HPeV3 to be the dominant type found in children, in particular neonates (Benschop et al., 2008c; Harvala et al., 2009, 2011; Pineiro et al., 2010; Renaud et al., 2011; Selvarangan et al., 2011; Verboon-Maciolek et al., 2008a, 2008b; Watanabe et al., 2007; Wolthers et al., 2008). These infections account for approximately 3-17% of CNS infections reported as meningitis or encephalitis (Harvala et al., 2009; Pineiro et al., 2010; Watanabe et al., 2007; Wolthers et al., 2008; Yamamoto et al., 2009), far exceeding the percentage of herpes simplex virus infections. In contrast, EV in CSF is still most frequently detected in these samples, with 14-19% positive cases each year in the summer (Harvala et al., 2011; Pineiro et al., 2010; Wolthers et al., 2008). This ranks HPeV as the second dominant pathogen of viral meningitis and encephalitis. HPeV1 infections are rarely described in CSF (Harvala et al., 2011); the other HPeV types have never been described in CSF.

Of interest is that HPeV infections of the CNS circulate intermittently every 2-3 years, and always in the summer months. However, the circulation patterns seem to be geographically distinct. HPeV3 detected in both CSF and stool in Northern Europe is described most commonly every 2 years, in the summer period of the even years (Benschop et al., 2006a, 2008c, 2010a; Ehrnst & Eriksson, 1993; Harvala et al., 2009; van der Sanden et al., 2008;

Wolthers et al., 2008). In contrast, HPeV3 infections in the USA occur most frequently in the uneven years every 2 years (Renaud et al., 2011; Selvarangan et al., 2011). Pineiro et al. (2010) described HPeV3 detection rates in Spain to peak in 2006 and 2009, suggesting a longer cycle of perhaps every 3 years. However more data are needed to confirm this circulation pattern. In Asia, where HPeV3 was first identified, HPeV3 epidemics are more dispersed over the years (Watanabe et al., 2007). This intermittent circulation is also described for EV types, e.g. echovirus 9 and 30 (Antona et al., 2007; Khetsuriani et al., 2006b), and is associated with the emergence of antigenic diverse genetic lineages or novel recombinants for which the community presumably is not immune protected (McWilliam Leitch et al., 2010). However, based upon the lower evolution rate and diversity of circulating HPeV3 strains (Benschop et al., 2010b; Calvert et al., 2010), diversification of HPeV into new lineages that are antigenically distinct is unlikely. The reason for the intermittent circulation of HPeV3 thus remains unclear.

In contrast to HPeV3, HPeV1 circulates every year in high numbers in the fall and winter months in Europe and Asia (Benschop et al., 2006a, 2008c, 2010a; Ehrnst & Eriksson, 1993; Tauriainen et al., 2007; Watanabe et al., 2007). The same is described for HPeV4 and 6 (Benschop et al., 2008c, 2010a; Harvala et al., 2008; Pajkrt et al., 2009). Again, not only in clinical sense, but also from a epidemiological point of view, HPeV3 behaves different from other HPeV types.

5. Risk groups for HPeV infections

While EVs generally affect individuals of all ages, more than 90% of HPeV infections have been described in children younger than 5 years of age, (Abed & Boivin, 2006; Baumgarte et al., 2008; Benschop et al., 2008c, 2010a; Chen et al., 2009; Grist et al., 1978; Khetsuriani et al., 2006a, 2006b; Pham et al., 2010; Tapia et al., 2008). WHO data from 1967-1974 reported that 94% of the HPeV1 infections were found in children < 4 years of age, of which 60% where < 1 year of age. Only 2,6% were isolated from adults (Grist et al., 1978). A survey in Sweden (1966-1990) reported similar findings, where 92% of the 109 patients with an HPeV1 infection were < 2 years old and only 1,8% were adults (Ehrnst & Eriksson, 1993). A more recent survey performed in the USA spanning over the years 1970 and 2005 reported approximately 95% of HPeV1 infection (n=880) to be from children <5 years of age. Children aged < 1 year with an HPeV1 infection were reported in 73% of the 880 infections (Khetsuriani et al., 2006b).

In 2006, we demonstrated in an observational pediatric study that the median age of children infected with HPeV3 was 1.3 months. This was significantly lower than the median age of children infected with HPeV1 (6.6 months) (Benschop et al., 2006a). Since then, the majority of HPeV3 infections have been found in children under the age of 2 months, most frequently in neonates (Benschop et al., 2008a, 2008c; Harvala et al., 2009, 2011; Pineiro et al., 2010; Renaud et al., 2011; Selvarangan et al., 2011; Verboon-Maciolek et al., 2008a; Watanabe et al., 2007; Yamamoto et al., 2009). This age difference in relation to the disease severity between the two HPeV types suggests that neonates in comparison to older children might be less protected against HPeV3 infection. Seroprevalence data showed that 95-99% of neonates had antibodies against HPeV1 which is most likely to be maternal (Joki-Korpela & Hyypia, 1998; Nakao et al., 1970; Stanway et al., 2000; Takao et al., 2001; Tauriainen et al., 2007). The high HPeV1 seroprevalence thus suggests that the majority of infants should be protected from HPeV1 infection early in life via maternal protection. However, this may not always be the case as suggested by Ehrnst et al. (1993). The seroprevalence decreased after 6 months of age, only to rapidly increase among children older than 1-3 year of age to 95%. The low seropositivity from 6 months to 1-3 years is marked by an increase in infection frequencies among children in this age group, (Benschop et al., 2006a; Joki-Korpela & Hyypia, 1998; Stanway et al., 2000; Takao et al., 2001; Tauriainen et al., 2007). Seroprevalence rates among adults remained stable at 97-99% (Joki-Korpela & Hyypia, 1998; Stanway et al., 2000; Tauriainen et al., 2007).

For HPeV3, seroprevalence is approximately 70% among adults (Ito et al., 2004). Data on seroprevalence in neonates are not available, but the seroprevalence rate for children between 7-12 months is 15% which steadily increases to 91% in adolescent adults only to decline again to 56-87% in adults. This is in contrast to what is seen for HPeV1 where over 97% of adults still have antibodies against HPeV1 (Joki-Korpela & Hyypia, 1998; Stanway et al., 2000; Tauriainen et al., 2007). Interestingly, seroprevalence among adults in the child-bearing age (20-39 years) is the lowest (57-74%) (Ito et al., 2004). This may indicate that children are less protected through maternal antibodies specific for HPeV3, explaining the young age and increased disease severity of HPeV3 infected children in comparison to HPeV1 infected children. The reason for the lower seroprevalence of HPeV3 is presumably to be related to its proposed recent emergence in the late eighties, which suggests that HPeV3 circulation is not widespread enough to provide sufficient protection in the neonatal period through maternal antibodies (Calvert et al., 2010; Harvala et al., 2011).

Despite the lower seroprevelance of HPeV3, infection with this type has not been reported in adults or older children (>5 years). HPeV1 infections in adults have been documented but only rarely, and usually in patients with an underlying immune deficiency (Wolthers et al., manuscript in preparation). This confirms that antibodies against HPeV1 protect the adult immune competent population. In this respect, with 20-30% of adults seronegative for HPeV3 antibodies, infection with this type in adults should be described as well. A possible explanation will be discussed in paragraph 7.

6. Laboratory findings and diagnosis of HPeV infection

Diagnosis of viral meningitis typically involves analysis of CSF and the establishment of an etiological agent. CSF analysis of HPeV infected children can show a mildly elevated leukocyte count, but in the majority of the children (especially neonates) pleiocytosis is not detected. Normal values for leukocyte cell count vary with age, and in general a higher value is accepted as normal in younger children. In a recent study normal values for leukocyte counts (under 95th percentile) in children younger than 56 days were redefined as <19/µl for infants aged 0-28 days and <9/µl for infants aged 29-56 days (Kestenbaum et al., 2010). Furthermore, CSF glucose levels in children infected with HPeV are usually normal, while CSF protein levels can be normal or elevated (Pineiro et al., 2010; Selvarangan et al., 2011; Verboon-Maciolek et al., 2008a; Wolthers et al., 2008); thus normal CSF findings therefore do not rule out an HPeV meningitis or encephalitis.

Laboratory evaluation of blood from HPeV infected children typically shows a normal leukocyte blood count, although leukopenia is also reported in 33% of the children (Selvarangan et al., 2011). C-reactive protein remains low or slightly elevated (Pineiro et al.,

2010; Verboon-Maciolek et al., 2008b; own observations). In some cases liver enzymes can be elevated, sometimes leading to hepatitis and liver necrosis (Levorson et al., 2009; Selvarangan et al., 2011; Verboon-Maciolek et al., 2008b).

In children with signs of encephalitis cranial ultrasonography and MRI are useful for the detection of cerebral abnormalities. Cranial ultrasonography showed extensive periventricular echogenicity in one study of neonates with HPeV encephalitis (Verboon-Maciolek et al., 2008a). MRI can demonstrate white matter abnormalities (Gupta et al., 2010; Verboon-Maciolek et al., 2008a). The severity of the imaging abnormalities correlated with neurodevelopmental problems later in age (Verboon-Maciolek et al., 2008a).

Classically, HPeVs, like EVs, can be diagnosed through cell culture isolation, usually involving monkey kidney cells and human fibroblasts (Benschop et al., 2010a; Schnurr et al., 1996). Other cell lines, such as the HT29 cell line (human colon adenocarcinoma cells), A549 (human lung carcinoma cell line), RD (Rhabdomyosarcoma cells) can be used for culturing HPeV isolates as well (Abed & Boivin, 2006; Al-Sunaidi et al., 2007; Benschop et al., 2010a; Watanabe et al., 2007). However, cell culture has its limitations. As shown for culturing EVs, different HPeV types display difference in cell growth in various cell lines, and panels of at least three cell lines may be required to efficiently isolate the subsequent types from clinical material (Abed & Boivin, 2006; Benschop et al., 2010a; Watanabe et al., 2007). The colon carcinoma cell line HT29 was found to efficiently support the growth of HPeV1, 2, and 4-6. However, for the isolation of HPeV3, only a few specific cell lines (e.g. Vero and LLCMK2 monkey kidney cells) were found to support the growth, albeit slow, of this type (Abed & Boivin, 2006; Benschop et al., 2010a; Watanabe et al., 2007). CPE produced by HPeV3 on these cells was scarce as well.

In general, CPE produced by HPeVs is not significantly different from the CPE elicited by EVs and HPeVs can mistakenly be identified as EVs in the event specific serotyping is not routinely performed (Benschop et al., 2006a). This also explains the original classification of HPeVs as EVs (Wigand & Sabin, 1961). The neutralization EV-panel of specific antibodies only includes antisera against HPeV1 and 2 (Kapsenberg, 1988). Other HPeV types cannot be serotyped because antibodies are not available (HPeV3-6), or because they cannot be cultured at all (HPeV7-14).

To isolate viruses from CSF, cell culture is proven to be less sensitive, as the load in patients with meningitis or encephalitis is fairly low ranging from 10 to 1000 TCID50 infectious virus per milliliter CSF (Rotbart, 2000). Therefore, PCR is the preferred method for detection of viruses in this material (Espy et al., 2006; Read et al., 1997; Romero 1999; Rotbart HA & Romero JR, 1995; van Doornum et al., 2007). But while with cell culture, both EVs and HPeVs can be diagnosed, PCR specific for EVs will fail to detect HPeVs because the targeted 5'UTR is too diverse between HPeVs and EVs (Beld et al., 2004; Benschop et al., 2006a; Hyypia, 1989; Hyypia et al., 1989; Oberste et al., 1999). Therefore a separate RT-PCR specifically targeting the 5'UTR of HPeVs is required. Real-time RT-PCRs have been developed and validated for HPeV detection, which are faster, less laborious and with a lower contamination risk than conventional endpoint PCRs (Baumgarte et al., 2008; Benschop et al., 2008b; Corless et al., 2002; Nix et al., 2008; Noordhoek et al., 2008; Tapia et al., 2008). By genotyping methods targeting the variable capsid region VP1, positive CSF samples from infants with CNS associated disease, can be characterized directly from the clinical material (Harvala et al., 2009; Verboon-Maciolek et al., 2008a). Direct genotyping from clinical material avoids secondary cell culture isolation of EV/HPeV from CSF, a material for which virus culture is already an insensitive method of detection (Romero, 1999; Rotbart & Romero, 1995).

Pathogen detection in CSF is the strongest indicator of the pathogen's association to the disease, but it is not uncommon to diagnose an EV or HPeV infection by detection of the virus in other clinical samples while the patient presents neurological symptoms (Benschop et al., 2006a). Several real-time PCRs for HPeV have been validated and tested on stool samples, and/or throat swabs (Baumgarte et al., 2008; Benschop et al., 2008c; Nix et al., 2008; Noordhoek et al., 2008; Tapia et al., 2008). The high viral loads in these samples make them suitable for diagnosis by cell culture as well. However, it should be taken into account that both HPeVs and EVs can be shed in high amount in stool and respiratory material, even after clearance of symptoms (Chung et al., 2001; Harvala et al., 2008).

In summary, HPeV3, which is the most pathogenic HPeV type, and the most prevalent type detected in CNS disease, is difficult to grow in cell culture and is not routinely serotyped by the available antibody pools. Data on prevalence of HPeV types that rely on virus isolation by cell culture alone (Abed & Boivin, 2006; de Vries et al., 2008; van der Sanden et al., 2008; Watanabe et al., 2007) will be biased by the cell panel used for virus culture, the difference in growth characteristics between the HPeV types, and the inability of the newer HPeV types 7-14 to grow in cell culture. Therefore, detection of HPeV for clinical or epidemiological purposes should rely on real-time PCR and subsequent genotyping based on VP1 or VP1/VP3.

7. Pathogenesis

It is not known why HPeV3 is more associated with severe neonatal sepsis and CNS disease in infants in comparison to other HPeV types. But several serological as well as biological and genomic features of HPeV3 in conjunction with preliminary experimental data may provide clues as to why this type has a neurovirulent phenotype and is predominantly identified among neonates.

7.1 Host immune response to HPeV

The defense mechanisme against HPeV meningitis/encephalitis or HPeV infections in general is largely unknown. Most of what we know from picornavirus immunity is distilled from immunological studies with EV infections. An efficient host response against EVs is most likely dependent on a proper humoral immune response with release of neutralizing antibodies. This is underlined by the increased incidence of severe EV infections in patients with primary antibody deficiency (PID), such as X-linked agammaglobulinemia (XLA), in which chronic enteroviral meningoencephalitis (CEMA) is one of the most severe complications (Moin et al., 2004; Plebani et al., 2002; Wildenbeest et al., 2011). In a recent survey in the USA, a mortality rate of 35% was reported in patients with PID due to chronic or disseminated EV infections and 40% of the survivors of the initial illness had long-term neurological symptoms (Halliday et al., 2003). In this large survey echovirus 11 was the most common EV type identified and the CNS was nearly always involved. Interestingly, changes in CSF parameters, such as elevated CSF protein levels did not correlate with changes in neurological signs and symptoms. Successful treatment with therapeutic immunoglobulin therapy (e.g. intravenous immunoglobulins (IVIG)) in PID patients with an EV meningitis/encephalitis provides additional evidence for an important role of neutralizing antibodies for an adequate host immune response in EV meningitis/encephalitis. In neonates, characterized by an impaired humoral immune response, lack of specific maternal EV antibodies is shown to be a risk factor for the development of severe illness (Abzug, 2004).

Knowledge of the host immune response to HPeV is in comparison to EV even more limited. In contrast to the evidence as described in the section above, there are no data available on the protective role of neutralizing antibodies in HPeV infections. The lower seroprevelance of HPeV3 in adults might suggest a lack of maternal protection in the early months of life. To study the protective role of these antibodies against both HPeV1 and 3 infections, our group has set up a case-control study of neonates and children < 1 year that is currently ongoing.

Only recently, toll like receptors (TLR) 7 and 8 were identified as important key players in the innate immune defense against HPeV1 (Triantafilou et al., 2005). TLRs are transmembrane proteins that play an important role in immune responses against microbial pathogens, by inducing inflammatory cytokines in response to bacteria and viruses. Although never published, one can assume that these TLRs are equally important in the defense against HPeV3 infections. Volpe (2008) suggested that HPeV3 infections could result in intracellular binding of TLR8, leading to the release of reactive oxygen and nitrogen and pro-inflammatory cytokines from microglia and as a result neural cell death. Interestingly, TLR8 is specifically distributed in axonal perturbations and only in the developing nervous system which could explain why we specifically observe the severe HPeV3 infections in infants rather than among older children and adults.

7.2 Cell tropism & receptor interactions

The specific detection of HPeV3 in CSF might direct towards a difference in cell tropism between HPeV types. This is already reflected by the slow growth of HPeV3 on a limited number of cell lines and its poor production of CPE (Abed & Boivin, 2006; Benschop et al., 2010a; Watanabe et al., 2007). That HPeV3 infects other cell lines than for example HPeV1, is underlined by recombination studies done in our laboratory. HPeV3 recombination is highly limited, while other HPeV types frequently recombine with each other (Benschop et al., 2008d, 2010b; Calvert et al., 2010). This indicates that HPeV3 rarely gets into contact with other types in the same cell where recombinants are produced during replication of the infected viruses.

The difference in tropism can be explained by a difference in receptor usage. HPeV types 1, 2, and 4-6 contain an RGD motif in the C-terminus of VP1 that is utilized by several other viruses, such as FMDV, Coxsackie A virus 9 and echovirus 9, for their attachment to cell surface integrins. The RGD motif is essential for HPeV1 infection (Boonyakiat et al., 2001; Joki-Korpela et al., 2001; Pulli et al., 1997; Stanway et al., 2000). However, HPeV3 does not contain an RGD motif and thus it is assumed that infection of HPeV3 is established via a different receptor that is RGD independent, but is as yet unknown. Based on receptor studies of different EV types we also know that the cell surface expression of receptors during organ development plays a major role in defining tropism (Harvala et al., 2005; Scassa et al., 2011; Yamayoshi et al., 2009). This shift of specific cell receptor expression during development would support the observation that HPeV3 infections are rarely or never seen in older children and adults and could partly explain why neonates are more prone for HPeV3 infections.

8. Treatment

There is no antiviral treatment against HPeVs currently available (Wildenbeest et al., 2010). Therefore, supportive treatment and administration of IVIG are the only available options. IVIG is sometimes given to neonates to reduce disease burden from EV infection, although its efficacy has not been proven. Neutralizing EV antibody (nAb) titers in IVIG vary between batches and geographic regions (Cao et al., 2010; Galama et al., 1997; Planitzer et al., 2011). For therapeutic purposes, high nAb titers against the specific serotype might be needed (Abzug et al., 1995). The seroprevalence rates of HPeV1 and HPeV3 found in adults would suggest IVIG to contain moderate to high titers of nAbs against these HPeV types. A case-report of a twin with neonatal sepsis and hepatitis infected with HPeV3 showed one child to have recovered after having received IVIG (Al Maamari et al., 2009). However, data on IVIG titers against HPeV3 was not given in this study. We found high HPeV1-specific nAb in two batches of IVIG, but low nAb titers against HPeV3 in these IVIG batches (Westerhuis et al., manuscript in preparation; Wildenbeest et al., 2011). Therefore, IVIG might be beneficial in the treatment of HPeV1 infections and less effective in the treatment of HPeV3, although more data are needed. Moreover, the dispersed circulation of HPeV3 could have effect on the nAb titers in IVIG batches collected in different years and should be taken into account.

Recently, a case report was published on the use of pleconaril in a patient with HPeV-associated enteropathy (van de Ven et al., 2011). Pleconaril inhibits viral replication by integration into the hydrophobic pocket inside the viral capsid. As a result, uncoating and binding of the virus to the host cell are interrupted (Pevear et al., 1999). The hydrophobic pocket is relatively well preserved among EVs and HRVs, resulting in a broad-spectrum anti-enteroviral and -rhinoviral activity of pleconaril. However, the capsid of HPeVs is different (Stanway et al., 2000; Seitsonen et al., 2010), indicating that the hydrophobic pocket differs from that of EVs. Indeed data from our laboratory show that HPeV1 and HPeV3 are resistant against pleconaril *in vitro* (Wildenbeest et al., 2010). In agreement, pleconaril did not have any effect on replication of an unspecified HPeV found in the patient with enteropathy, nor did ribavirin (van de Ven et al., 2011).

In summary, no systematic data are available on HPeV treatment, and clinical experience with severity and treatment of HPeV infections is just beginning to build up. Treatment options for HPeV and the related EV are urgently needed. In the meantime, administration of IVIG is the only option.

9. Concluding remarks: HPeV3 infection of the CNS

Before the turn of the century, HPeVs infections were described as mild infections in children. At that time only two types were known, and severe symptoms were occasionally reported. With the discovery of a third HPeV type (HeV3), the view on HPeVs as relevant pathogens in viral CNS infections such as meningitis and encephalitis has changed drastically. While various EV types are known to be commonly involved in meningitis, (echovirus 9 and 30, EV71 and CBV5), of the 16 HPeV types currently described, HPeV3 is the primary type to cause CNS disease in children.

The introduction of rapid PCR detection for both EVs and HPeVs in CSF demonstrate that both viruses play an important role in the pathogenesis of meningitis/encephalitis. Increased routine screening of HPeVs will lead to an increase in the identification of HPeV infected children and a decrease in the use of antibiotics. Differences in maternal protection and its genetic make up in relation to its biological characteristics should provide clues in the near future on how HPeV3 type specifically infects the CNS of particularly newborns. This will aid in the development of new treatment options that will allow effective care of these children, possibly preventing neurological sequelae in these children.

10. References

Abed, Y. & Boivin, G. (2006). Human parechovirus infections in Canada. *Emerg.Infect.Dis.*, Vol.12, No.4, pp. 969-975.

Abzug, M.J. (2004). Presentation, diagnosis, and management of enterovirus infections in neonates. *Paediatr.Drugs*, Vol.6, No.1, pp. 1-10.

Abzug, M.J., Keyserling, H.L., Lee, M.L., Levin, M.J. & Rotbart, H.A. (1995). Neonatal enterovirus infection: virology, serology, and effects of intravenous immune globulin. *Clin.Infect.Dis.*, Vol.20, No.5, pp. 1201-1206.

Al Maamari, K., Docherty, C. & Aitken, C. (2009). "Twin" viruses. *J.Clin.Virol.*, Vol.44, No.3, pp.vi (Q)/I (A).

Al-Sunaidi, M., Williams, C.H., Hughes, P.J., Schnurr, D.P. & Stanway, G. (2007). Analysis of a new human parechovirus allows the definition of parechovirus types and the identification of RNA structural domains. *J.Virol.*, Vol.81, No.2, pp. 1013-1021.

Antona, D., Leveque, N., Chomel, J.J., Dubrou, S., Levy-Bruhl, D. & Lina, B. (2007). Surveillance of enteroviruses in France, 2000-2004. *Eur.J.Clin.Microbiol.Infect.Dis.*, Vol.26, No.6, pp. 403-412.

Baumgarte, S., de Souza Luna, L.K., Grywna, K., Panning, M., Drexler, J.F., Karsten, C., Huppertz, H.I. & Drosten, C. (2008). Prevalence, types, and RNA concentrations of human parechoviruses, including a sixth parechovirus type, in stool samples from patients with acute enteritis. *J.Clin.Microbiol.*, Vol.46, No.1, pp. 242-248.

Beld, M., Minnaar, R., Weel, J., Sol, C., Damen, M., van der Avoort, H., Wertheim-Van Dillen, P.M., van Breda, A. & Boom, R. (2004). Highly sensitive assay for detection of enterovirus in clinical specimens by reverse transcription-PCR with an armored RNA internal control. *J.Clin.Microbiol.*, Vol.42, No.7, pp. 3059-3064.

Benschop, K., Stanway, G. & Wolthers, K. (2008a). New Human Parechoviruses: six and counting. In: *Emerging Infections,* Scheld W.M, Hammer S.M & Hughes J.M, pp/ 53-74, ASM Press, ISBN 978-1-55581-444-1, Washington, DC.

Benschop, K., Minnaar, R., Koen, G., van Eijk H., Dijkman, K., Westerhuis, B., Molenkamp, R. & Wolthers, K. (2010a). Detection of human enterovirus and human parechovirus (HPeV) genotypes from clinical stool samples: polymerase chain reaction and direct molecular typing, culture characteristics, and serotyping. *Diagn.Microbiol.Infect.Dis.*, Vol.68, No.2, pp. 166-173.

Benschop, K., Molenkamp, R., van der Ham, A., Wolthers, K. & Beld, M. (2008b). Rapid detection of human parechoviruses in clinical samples by real-time PCR. *J.Clin.Virol.*, Vol.41, No.2, pp. 69-74.

Benschop, K., Thomas, X., Serpenti, C., Molenkamp, R. & Wolthers, K. (2008c). High prevalence of human Parechovirus (HPeV) genotypes in the Amsterdam region and identification of specific HPeV variants by direct genotyping of stool samples. *J.Clin.Microbiol.*, Vol.46, No.12, pp. 3965-3970.

Benschop, K.S., de, V.M., Minnaar, R.P., Stanway, G., van der, H.L., Wolthers, K.C. & Simmonds, P. (2010b). Comprehensive full-length sequence analyses of human parechoviruses: diversity and recombination. *J.Gen.Virol.*, Vol.91, No.1, pp. 145-154.

Benschop, K.S., Schinkel, J., Minnaar, R.P., Pajkrt, D., Spanjerberg, L., Kraakman, H.C., Berkhout, B., Zaaijer, H.L., Beld, M.G. & Wolthers, K.C. (2006a). Human parechovirus infections in Dutch children and the association between serotype and disease severity. *Clin.Infect.Dis.*, Vol.42, No.2, pp. 204-210.

Benschop, K.S., Williams, C.H., Wolthers, K.C., Stanway, G. & Simmonds, P. (2008d). Widespread recombination within human parechoviruses: analysis of temporal dynamics and constraints. *J.Gen.Virol.*, Vol.89, No.4, pp. 1030-1035.

Benschop, K.S.M., Schinkel, J., Luken, M.E., van den Broek, P.J.M., Beersma, M.F.C., Menelik, N., van Eijk, H.W.M., Zaaijer, H.L., VandenBroucke-Grauls, C.M.J.E., Beld, M.G.H.M. & Wolthers, K.C. (2006b). Fourth Human Parechovirus Serotype. *Emerg.Infect.Dis.*, Vol.12, No.10, pp. 1572-1575.

Boonyakiat, Y., Hughes, P.J., Ghazi, F. & Stanway, G. (2001). Arginine-glycine-aspartic acid motif is critical for human parechovirus 1 entry. *J.Virol.*, Vol.75, No.20, pp. 10000-10004.

Boros, A., Uj, M., Pankovics, P. & Reuter, G. (2010). Detection and characterization of human parechoviruses in archived cell cultures, in Hungary. *J.Clin.Virol.*, Vol.47, No.4, pp. 379-381.

Calvert, J., Chieochansin, T., Benschop, K., William Leitch, E.C., Drexler, J.F., Grywna, K., da Costa, R.H., Drosten, C., Harvala, H., Poovorawan, Y., Wolthers, K. & Simmonds, P. (2010). The recombination dynamics of human parechoviruses; investigation of type-specific differences in frequency and epidemiological correlates. *J.Gen.Virol.* Vol.91, No.5, pp. 1229-1238.

Cao, R., Han, J., Deng, Y., Yu, M., Qin, E. & Qin, C. (2010). Presence of high-titer neutralizing antibodies against enterovirus 71 in intravenous immunoglobulin manufactured from Chinese donors. *Clin.Infect.Dis.*, Vol.50, No.1, pp. 125-126.

Chen, B.C., Cheng, M.F., Huang, T.S., Liu, Y.C., Tang, C.W., Chen, C.S. & Chen, Y.S. (2009). Detection and identification of human parechoviruses from clinical specimens. *Diagn.Microbiol.Infect.Dis.*, Vol.65, No.3, pp. 254-260.

Chung, P.W., Huang, Y.C., Chang, L.Y., Lin, T.Y. & Ning, H.C. (2001). Duration of enterovirus shedding in stool. *J.Microbiol.Immunol.Infect.*, Vol.34, No.3, pp. 167-170.

Corless, C.E., Guiver, M., Borrow, R., Edwards-Jones, V., Fox, A.J., Kaczmarski, E.B. & Mutton, K.J. (2002). Development and evaluation of a 'real-time' RT-PCR for the detection of enterovirus and parechovirus RNA in CSF and throat swab samples. *J.Med.Virol.*, Vol.67, No.4, pp. 555-562.

de Vries, M., Pyrc, K., Berkhout, R., Vermeulen-Oost, W., Dijkman, R., Jebbink, M.F., Bruisten, S., Berkhout, B. & van der, H.L. (2008). Human parechovirus type 1, 3, 4, 5, and 6 detection in picornavirus cultures. *J.Clin.Microbiol.*, Vol.46, No.2, pp. 759-762.

Ehrnst, A. & Eriksson, M. (1993). Epidemiological features of type 22 echovirus infection. *Scand.J.Infect.Dis.*, Vol.25, No.3, pp. 275-281.

Ehrnst, A. & Eriksson, M. (1996). Echovirus type 23 observed as a nosocomial infection in infants. *Scand.J.Infect.Dis.*, Vol.28, No.2, pp. 205-206.

Espy, M.J., Uhl, J.R., Sloan, L.M., Buckwalter, S.P., Jones, M.F., Vetter, E.A., Yao, J.D., Wengenack, N.L., Rosenblatt, J.E., Cockerill, F.R., III & Smith, T.F. (2006). Real-time PCR in clinical microbiology: applications for routine laboratory testing. *Clin.Microbiol.Rev.*, Vol.19, No.1, pp. 165-256.

Figueroa, J.P., Ashley, D., King, D. & Hull, B. (1989). An outbreak of acute flaccid paralysis in Jamaica associated with echovirus type 22. *J.Med.Virol.*, Vol.29, No.4, pp. 315-319.

Galama, J.M., Vogels, M.T., Jansen, G.H., Gielen, M. & Heessen, F.W. (1997). Antibodies against enteroviruses in intravenous Ig preparations: great variation in titres and poor correlation with the incidence of circulating serotypes. *J.Med.Virol.*, Vol.53, No.2, pp. 273-276.

Grist, N.R., Bell, E.J. & Assaad, F. (1978). Enteroviruses in human disease. *Prog.Med.Virol.*, Vol.24, pp. 114-157.

Gupta, S., Fernandez, D., Siddiqui, A., Tong, W.C., Pohl, K. & Jungbluth, H. (2010). Extensive white matter abnormalities associated with neonatal Parechovirus (HPeV) infection. *Eur.J.Paediatr.Neurol.* Vol. 14, No.6, pp 531-534.

Halliday, E., Winkelstein, J. & Webster, A.D. (2003). Enteroviral infections in primary immunodeficiency (PID): a survey of morbidity and mortality. *J.Infect.*, Vol.46, No.1, pp. 1-8.

Harvala, H., Kalimo, H., Bergelson, J., Stanway, G. & Hyypia, T. (2005). Tissue tropism of recombinant coxsackieviruses in an adult mouse model. *J.Gen.Virol.*, Vol.86, No.7, pp. 1897-1907.

Harvala, H., McLeish, N., Kondracka, J., McIntyre, C.L., McWilliam Leitch, E.C., Templeton, K. & Simmonds, P. (2011). Comparison of human parechovirus and enterovirus detection frequencies in cerebrospinal fluid samples collected over a 5-year period in edinburgh: HPeV type 3 identified as the most common picornavirus type. *J.Med.Virol.*, Vol.83, No.5, pp. 889-896.

Harvala, H., Robertson, I., Chieochansin, T., William Leitch, E.C., Templeton, K. & Simmonds, P. (2009). Specific Association of Human Parechovirus Type 3 with Sepsis and Fever in Young Infants, as Identified by Direct Typing of Cerebrospinal Fluid Samples. *J.Infect.Dis.*, Vol.199, No.12, pp. 1753-1760.

Harvala, H., Robertson, I., William Leitch, E.C., Benschop, K., Wolthers, K.C., Templeton, K. & Simmonds, P. (2008). Epidemiology and clinical associations of human parechovirus respiratory infections. *J.Clin.Microbiol.*, Vol.46, No.10, pp. 3446-3453.

Hyypia, T. (1989). Identification of human picornaviruses by nucleic acid probes. *Mol.Cell Probes*, Vol.3, No.4, pp. 329-343.

Hyypia, T., Auvinen, P. & Maaronen, M. (1989). Polymerase chain reaction for human picornaviruses. *J.Gen.Virol.*, Vol.70 (Pt 12), No.12, pp. 3261-3268.

Hyypia, T., Horsnell, C., Maaronen, M., Khan, M., Kalkkinen, N., Auvinen, P., Kinnunen, L. & Stanway, G. (1992). A distinct picornavirus group identified by sequence analysis. *Proc.Natl.Acad.Sci.U.S.A*, Vol.89, No.18, pp. 8847-8851.

Ito, M., Yamashita, T., Tsuzuki, H., Kabashima, Y., Hasegawa, A., Nagaya, S., Kawaguchi, M., Kobayashi, S., Fujiura, A., Sakae, K. & Minagawa, H. (2010). Detection of human parechoviruses from clinical stool samples in Aichi, Japan. *J.Clin.Microbiol.*, Vol.48, No.8, pp. 2683-2688.

Ito, M., Yamashita, T., Tsuzuki, H., Takeda, N. & Sakae, K. (2004). Isolation and identification of a novel human parechovirus. *J.Gen.Virol.*, Vol.85, No.2, pp. 391-398.

Joki-Korpela, P. & Hyypia, T. (1998). Diagnosis and epidemiology of echovirus 22 infections. *Clin.Infect.Dis.*, Vol.27, No.1, pp. 129-136.

Joki-Korpela, P., Marjomaki, V., Krogerus, C., Heino, J. & Hyypia, T. (2001). Entry of human parechovirus 1. *J.Virol.*, Vol.75, No.4, pp. 1958-1967.

Joki-Korpela, P., Roivainen, M., Lankinen, H., Poyry, T. & Hyypia, T. (2000). Antigenic properties of human parechovirus 1. *J.Gen.Virol.*, Vol.81, No.7, pp. 1709-1718.

Kapsenberg, J.G. (1988). Picornaviridae; the enteroviruses (polioviruses, coxsackieviruses, echoviruses. In: *Laboratory diagnosis of infectious diseases. Principles and Practice,* Balows, A., Hausler, W.J. & Lennette, E, pp. 692-722, Springer-Verlag, ISBN 978-0387967561, NY, USA.

Kestenbaum, L.A., Ebberson, J., Zorc, J.J., Hodinka, R.L. & Shah, S.S. (2010). Defining cerebrospinal fluid white blood cell count reference values in neonates and young infants *Pediatrics,* Vol.125, No.2, pp. 257-264.

Khetsuriani, N., Lamonte, A., Oberste, M.S. & Pallansch, M. (2006a). Neonatal enterovirus infections reported to the national enterovirus surveillance system in the United States, 1983-2003. *Pediatr.Infect.Dis.J.*, Vol.25, No.10, pp. 889-893.

Khetsuriani, N., Lamonte-Fowlkes, A., Oberst, S. & Pallansch, M.A. (2006b). Enterovirus surveillance--United States, 1970-2005. *MMWR Surveill Summ.*, Vol.55, No.8, pp. 1-20.

Koskiniemi, M., Paetau, R. & Linnavuori, K. (1989). Severe encephalitis associated with disseminated echovirus 22 infection. *Scand.J.Infect.Dis.*, Vol.21, No.4, pp. 463-466.

Legay, V., Chomel, J.J., Fernandez, E., Lina, B., Aymard, M. & Khalfan, S. (2002). Encephalomyelitis due to human parechovirus type 1. *J.Clin.Virol.*, Vol.25, No.2, pp. 193-195.

Levorson, R.E., Jantausch, B.A., Wiedermann, B.L., Spiegel, H.M. & Campos, J.M. (2009). Human parechovirus-3 infection: emerging pathogen in neonatal sepsis. *Pediatr.Infect.Dis.J.*, Vol.28, No.6, pp. 545-547.

Maller, H.M., Powars, D.F., Horowitz, R.E. & Portnoy, B. (1967). Fatal myocarditis associated with ECHO virus, type 22, infection in a child with apparent immunological deficiency. *J.Pediatr.*, Vol.71, No.2, pp. 204-210.

McWilliam Leitch, E.C., Cabrerizo, M., Cardosa, J., Harvala, H., Ivanova, O.E., Kroes, A.C., Lukashev, A., Muir, P., Odoom, J., Roivainen, M., Susi, P., Trallero, G., Evans, D.J. & Simmonds, P. (2010). Evolutionary dynamics and temporal/geographical correlates of recombination in the human enterovirus echovirus types 9, 11, and 30. *J.Virol.*, Vol.84, No.18, pp. 9292-9300.

Moin, M., Aghamohammadi, A., Farhoudi, A., Pourpak, Z., Rezaei, N., Movahedi, M., Gharagozlou, M., Ghazi, B.M., Zahed, A., Abolmaali, K., Mahmoudi, M., Emami, L. & Bashashati, M. (2004). X-linked agammaglobulinemia: a survey of 33 Iranian patients. *Immunol.Invest*, Vol.33, No.1, pp. 81-93.

Nakao, T., Miura, R. & Sato, M. (1970). ECHO virus type 22 infection in a premature infant. *Tohoku J.Exp.Med*, Vol.102, No.1, pp. 61-68.

Nateri, A.S., Hughes, P.J. & Stanway, G. (2000). In vivo and in vitro identification of structural and sequence elements of the human parechovirus 5' untranslated region required for internal initiation. *J.Virol.*, Vol.74, No.14, pp. 6269-6277.

Nateri, A.S., Hughes, P.J. & Stanway, G. (2002). Terminal RNA replication elements in human parechovirus 1. *J.Virol.*, Vol.76, No.24, pp. 13116-13122.

Niklasson, B., Kinnunen, L., Hornfeldt, B., Horling, J., Benemar, C., Hedlund, K.O., Matskova, L., Hyypia, T. & Winberg, G. (1999). A new picornavirus isolated from bank voles (Clethrionomys glareolus). *Virology*, Vol.255, No.1, pp. 86-93.

Nix, W.A., Maher, K., Johansson, E.S., Niklasson, B., Lindberg, A.M., Pallansch, M.A. & Oberste, M.S. (2008). Detection of all known parechoviruses by real-time PCR. *J.Clin.Microbiol.*, Vol.46, No.8, pp. 2519-2524.

Noordhoek, G.T., Weel, J.F.L., Poelstra, E., Hooghiemstra, M. & Brandenburg, A.H. (2008). Clinical validation of a new real-time PCR assay for detection of enteroviruses and parechoviruses, and implications for diagnostic procedures. *J.Clin.Virol.*, Vol.41, No.2, pp. 75-80.

Oberste, M.S., Maher, K. & Pallansch, M.A. (1999). Specific detection of echoviruses 22 and 23 in cell culture supernatants by RT-PCR. *J.Med.Virol.*, Vol.58, No.2, pp. 178-181.

Pajkrt, D., Benschop, K.S., Westerhuis, B., Molenkamp, R., Spanjerberg, L. & Wolthers, K.C. (2009). Clinical Characteristics of Human Parechoviruses 4-6 Infections in Young Children. *Pediatr.Infect.Dis.J.* Vol. 28, No.11, pp 1008-1010.

Pevear, D.C., Tull, T.M., Seipel, M.E. & Groarke, J.M. (1999). Activity of pleconaril against enteroviruses. *Antimicrob.Agents Chemother.*, Vol.43, No.9, pp. 2109-2115.

Pham, N.T., Chan-It, W., Khamrin, P., Nishimura, S., Kikuta, H., Sugita, K., Baba, T., Yamamoto, A., Shimizu, H., Okitsu, S., Mizuguchi, M. & Ushijima, H. (2011a). Detection of human parechovirus in stool samples collected from children with acute gastroenteritis in Japan during 2007-2008. *J.Med.Virol.*, Vol.83, No.2, pp. 331-336.

Pham, N.T., Takanashi, S., Tran, D.N., Trinh, Q.D., Abeysekera, C., Abeygunawardene, A., Khamrin, P., Okitsu, S., Shimizu, H., Mizuguchi, M. & Ushijima, H. (2011b). Human parechovirus infection in children hospitalized with acute gastroenteritis in Sri Lanka. *J.Clin.Microbiol.*, Vol.49, No.1, pp. 364-366.

Pham, N.T., Trinh, Q.D., Khamrin, P., Maneekarn, N., Shimizu, H., Okitsu, S., Mizuguchi, M. & Ushijima, H. (2010). Diversity of human parechoviruses isolated from stool samples collected from Thai children with acute gastroenteritis. *J.Clin.Microbiol.*, Vol.48, No.1, pp. 115-119.

Pineiro, L., Vicente, D., Montes, M., Hernandez-Dorronsoro, U. & Cilla, G. (2010). Human parechoviruses in infants with systemic infection. *J.Med.Virol.*, Vol.82, No.10, pp. 1790-1796.

Planitzer, C.B., Farcet, M.R., Schiff, R.I., Ochs, H.D. & Kreil, T.R. (2011). Neutralization of different echovirus serotypes by individual lots of intravenous immunoglobulin. *J.Med.Virol.*, Vol.83, No.2, pp. 305-310.

Plebani, A., Soresina, A., Rondelli, R., Amato, G.M., Azzari, C., Cardinale, F., Cazzola, G., Consolini, R., De, M.D., Dell'Erba, G., Duse, M., Fiorini, M., Martino, S., Martire, B., Masi, M., Monafo, V., Moschese, V., Notarangelo, L.D., Orlandi, P., Panei, P., Pession, A., Pietrogrande, M.C., Pignata, C., Quinti, I., Ragno, V., Rossi, P., Sciotto, A. & Stabile, A. (2002). Clinical, immunological, and molecular analysis in a large cohort of patients with X-linked agammaglobulinemia: an Italian multicenter study. *Clin.Immunol.*, Vol.104, No.3, pp. 221-230.

Pulli, T., Koivunen, E. & Hyypia, T. (1997). Cell-surface interactions of echovirus 22. *J.Biol.Chem.*, Vol.272, No.34, pp. 21176-21180.

Read, S.J., Jeffery, K.J. & Bangham, C.R. (1997). Aseptic meningitis and encephalitis: the role of PCR in the diagnostic laboratory. *J.Clin.Microbiol.*, Vol.35, No.3, pp. 691-696.

Renaud, C., Kuypers, J., Ficken, E., Cent, A., Corey, L. & Englund, J.A. (2011). Introduction of a novel parechovirus RT-PCR clinical test in a regional medical center. *J.Clin.Virol.*, Vol.51, No.1, pp. 50-53.

Romero, J.R. (1999). Reverse-transcription polymerase chain reaction detection of the enteroviruses. *Arch.Pathol.Lab Med.*, Vol.123, No.12, pp. 1161-1169.

Rotbart HA & Romero JR. (1995). Laboratory diagnosis of enteroviral infections. In: *Human Enterovirus Infections,* Rotbart H, pp. 401-418ASM Press, ISBN 978-1-55581-092-4, Washington, DC.

Rotbart, H.A. (2000). Viral meningitis. *Semin.Neurol.*, Vol.20, No.3, pp. 277-292.

Samuilova, O., Krogerus, C., Fabrichniy, I. & Hyypia, T. (2006). ATP hydrolysis and AMP kinase activities of nonstructural protein 2C of human parechovirus 1. *J.Virol.*, Vol.80, No.2, pp. 1053-1058.

Scassa, M.E., de Giusti, C.J., Questa, M., Pretre, G., Richardson, G.A., Bluguermann, C., Romorini, L., Ferrer, M.F., Sevlever, G.E., Miriuka, S.G. & Gomez, R.M. (2011). Human embryonic stem cells and derived contractile embryoid bodies are susceptible to Coxsakievirus B infection and respond to interferon Ibeta treatment. *Stem Cell Res.*, Vol.6, No.1, pp. 13-22.

Schnurr, D., Dondero, M., Holland, D. & Connor, J. (1996). Characterization of echovirus 22 variants. *Arch.Virol.*, Vol.141, No.9, pp. 1749-1758.

Seitsonen, J., Susi, P., Heikkila, O., Sinkovits, R.S., Laurinmaki, P., Hyypia, T & Butcher, S.J. (2010). Interaction of {alpha}V{beta}3 and {alpha}V{beta}6 integrins with Human parechovirus 1. *J.Virol.* Vol. 84, No.17, pp 8509-8519.

Selvarangan, R., Nzabi, M., Selvaraju, S.B., Ketter, P., Carpenter, C. & Harrison, C.J. (2011). Human parechovirus 3 causing sepsis-like illness in children from midwestern United States. *Pediatr.Infect.Dis.J.*, Vol.30, No.3, pp. 238-242.

Stanway, G., Brown, F., Christian, P., Hovi, T., Hyypiä, T., King, A.M.Q., Knowles, N.J., Lemon, S.M., Minor, P.D., Pallansch, M.A., Palmenberg, A.C. & Skern, T. (2005). Picornaviridae. In: *Virus Taxonomy. Classification and Nomenclature of Viruses, Eight Report of the ICTV,* C.M.Fauquet, M.A.Mayo, J.Maniloff, U. Desselberger, L.A. Ball, pp 757-778, Elsevier/Academic Press, ISBN 0122499514, London.

Stanway, G. & Hyypia, T. (1999). Parechoviruses. *J.Virol.*, Vol.73, No.7, pp. 5249-5254.

Stanway, G., Joki-Korpela, P. & Hyypia, T. (2000). Human parechoviruses--biology and clinical significance. *Rev.Med.Virol.*, Vol.10, No.1, pp. 57-69.

Stanway, G., Kalkkinen, N., Roivainen, M., Ghazi, F., Khan, M., Smyth, M., Meurman, O. & Hyypia, T. (1994). Molecular and biological characteristics of echovirus 22, a representative of a new picornavirus group. *J.Virol.*, Vol.68, No.12, pp. 8232-8238.

Takao, S., Shimazu, Y., Fukuda, S., Noda, M. & Miyazaki, K. (2001). Seroepidemiological study of human Parechovirus 1. *Jpn.J.Infect.Dis.*, Vol.54, No.2, pp. 85-87.

Tapia, G., Cinek, O., Witso, E., Kulich, M., Rasmussen, T., Grinde, B. & Ronningen, K.S. (2008). Longitudinal observation of parechovirus in stool samples from Norwegian infants. *J.Med.Virol.*, Vol.80, No.10, pp. 1835-1842.

Tauriainen, S., Martiskainen, M., Oikarinen, S., Lonnrot, M., Viskari, H., Ilonen, J., Simell, O., Knip, M. & Hyoty, H. (2007). Human parechovirus 1 infections in young children--no association with type 1 diabetes. *J.Med.Virol.*, Vol.79, No.4, pp. 457-462.

Triantafilou, K., Vakakis, E., Orthopoulos, G., Ahmed, M.A., Schumann, C., Lepper, P.M. & Triantafilou, M. (2005). TLR8 and TLR7 are involved in the host's immune response to human parechovirus 1. *Eur.J.Immunol.*, Vol.35, No.8, pp. 2416-2423.

van de Ven, A.A., Douma, J.W., Rademaker, C., van Loon, A.M., Wensing, A.M., Boelens, J.J., Sanders, E.A. & van Montfrans, J.M. (2011). Pleconaril-resistant chronic parechovirus-associated enteropathy in agammaglobulinaemia. *Antivir.Ther.*, Vol.16, No.4, pp. 611-614.

van der Sanden, S., de Bruin E., Vennema, H., Swanink, C., Koopmans, M. & van der Avoort, H. (2008). Prevalence of human parechovirus in the Netherlands in 2000 to 2007. *J.Clin.Microbiol.*, Vol.46, No.9, pp. 2884-2889.

van Doornum, G.J., Schutten, M., Voermans, J., Guldemeester, G.J. & Niesters, H.G. (2007). Development and implementation of real-time nucleic acid amplification for the detection of enterovirus infections in comparison to rapid culture of various clinical specimens. *J.Med.Virol.*, Vol.79, No.12, pp. 1868-1876.

Verboon-Maciolek, M.A., Groenendaal, F., Hahn, C.D., Hellmann, J., van Loon, A.M., Boivin, G. & de Vries, L.S. (2008a). Human parechovirus causes encephalitis with white matter injury in neonates. *Ann.Neurol.*, Vol.64, No.3, pp. 266-273.

Verboon-Maciolek, M.A., Krediet, T.G., Gerards, L.J., de Vries, L.S., Groenendaal, F. & van Loon, A.M. (2008b). Severe neonatal parechovirus infection and similarity with enterovirus infection. *Pediatr.Infect.Dis.J.*, Vol.27, No.5, pp. 241-245.

Volpe, J.J. (2008). Neonatal encephalitis and white matter injury: more than just inflammation? *Ann.Neurol.*, Vol.64, No.3, pp. 232-236.

Watanabe, K., Oie, M., Higuchi, M., Nishikawa, M. & Fujii, M. (2007). Isolation and characterization of novel human parechovirus from clinical samples. *Emerg.Infect.Dis.*, Vol.13, No.6, pp. 889-895.

Wigand, R. & Sabin, A.B. (1961). Properties of ECHO types 22, 23 and 24 viruses. *Arch.Gesamte Virusforsch.*, Vol.11, pp. 224-247.

Wildenbeest, J.G., Harvala, H., Pajkrt, D. & Wolthers, K.C. (2010). The need for treatment against human parechoviruses: how, why and when? *Expert.Rev.Anti.Infect.Ther.*, Vol.8, No.12, pp. 1417-1429.

Wildenbeest J.G., van den Broek P.J., Benschop K.S.M., Koen G., Wierenga P.C., Vossen A.C.T.M., Kuijpers T.W. & Wolthers K.C. (2011). Pleconaril revisited: clinical course of chronic enterovirus meningoencephalitis after treatment correlates with in vitro susceptibility. *Antiviral Therapy*. In press.

Wolthers, K.C., Benschop, K.S., Schinkel, J., Molenkamp, R., Bergevoet, R.M., Spijkerman, I.J., Kraakman, H.C. & Pajkrt, D. (2008). Human parechoviruses as an important viral cause of sepsislike illness and meningitis in young children. *Clin.Infect.Dis.*, Vol.47, No.3, pp. 358-363.

Yamamoto, M., Abe, K., Kuniyori, K., Kunii, E., Ito, F., Kasama, Y., Yoshioka, Y. & Noda, M. (2009). Epidemic of human parechovirus type 3 in Hiroshima city, Japan in 2008. *Jpn.J.Infect.Dis.*, Vol.62, No.3, pp. 244-245.

Yamayoshi, S., Yamashita, Y., Li, J., Hanagata, N., Minowa, T., Takemura, T. & Koike, S. (2009). Scavenger receptor B2 is a cellular receptor for enterovirus 71. *Nat.Med.*, Vol.15, No.7, pp. 798-801.

Zhong, H., Lin, Y., Sun, J., Su, L., Cao, L., Yang, Y. & Xu, J. (2011). Prevalence and genotypes of human parechovirus in stool samples from hospitalized children in Shanghai, China, 2008 and 2009. *J.Med.Virol.*, Vol.83, No.8, pp. 1428-1434.

13

Strategies for the Prevention of Meningitis

J.J. Stoddard[1], L.M. DeTora[1], M.M. Yeh[4], M. Bröker[2] and E.D.G. McIntosh[3]
[1]*Novartis Vaccines and Diagnostics, Cambridge MA,*
[2]*Novartis Vaccines and Diagnostics, Marburg,*
[3]*Novartis Vaccines and Diagnostics, Amsterdam,*
[4]*Tapestry Networks, Waltham, Massachusetts,*
[1,4]*USA*
[2]*Germany*
[3]*The Netherlands*

1. Introduction

Meningitis is a clinical condition involving inflammation of the meninges that most commonly affects otherwise healthy people. Generally, the meningitides are of infectious etiology that can be viral, bacterial, fungal, or parasitic in nature, although iatrogenic causes are rarely reported (Table 1). Inflammation of the meninges can pose serious dangers to patients, given that many of the areas affected are encased by bony structures that can exacerbate tissue damage caused by swelling. Collapse of the blood vessels, causing hypoxic damage, is a particularly dangerous effect of inflammation in the brain. In fact, permanent disability and death may result from all forms of meningitis. Further, sepsis bacteremia, or other disease processes can be caused by the same infectious agents that cause meningitis. Epidemics associated with certain pathogens, like the meningococcus, pose a serious public health risk, and therefore require prevention and control strategies. The quest to limit the

	Viruses*	Bacteria	Fungi
Vaccine preventable	Japanese and tick-borne encephalitis Polio Measles Mumps	*Streptococcus pneumoniae* ("Pneumococcus") *Neisseria meningitidis* serogroups A, C, W-135, Y *Haemophilus influenzae* type b Tuberculosis	
Vaccines under clinical investigation		Group B streptococcus *Neisseria meningitidis* serogroup B *Staphylococcus aureus*	
No vaccines available	West Nile Herpes simplex	*Neisseria meningitidis* serogroup X *Escherichia coli* *Listeria monocytogenes* Lyme (*Borrelia burgdorferi*)	*Candida albicans* *Cryptococcus neoformans* Histoplasma

*Most commonly enteroviruses, arboviruses, herpes, measles and mumps
Rarely, meningitis may be caused by parasites or as a side effect of medication.

Table 1. Examples of pathogens associated with meningitides, encephalitis, or sepsis (2-3)

public health impact of meningitis has led to the application of various public health strategies, including vaccine campaigns, over the last century (1-2). This chapter places meningitis vaccine policy in the context of several forces: public perception and media activity, clinical diagnosis and laboratory testing, antibiotic effectiveness and vaccine safety, efficacy and cost-effectiveness. Country and situational examples will be given.

2. Disease factors that impact policy decisions

The global epidemiology of meningitis changed dramatically during the twentieth century as vaccines and antibiotics became available to prevent and treat this deadly disease (4-5). The potential public health impact of meningitis-causing organisms is affected by disease incidence, severity and scope, case fatality ratio, risk of contagion, rate of disease progression and additional acute and chronic disease caused by the pathogen. The Meningitis Research Foundation notes that, with the exception of measles and mumps (6) which have been vaccine-preventable for decades, the relatively mild severity and generally good prognosis associated with the viral meningitides makes for mild concern among policymakers (3). The World Health Organization and the Pan American Health Organization consider bacterial, particularly meningococcal, meningitis to be among the world's most important public health problems (2).

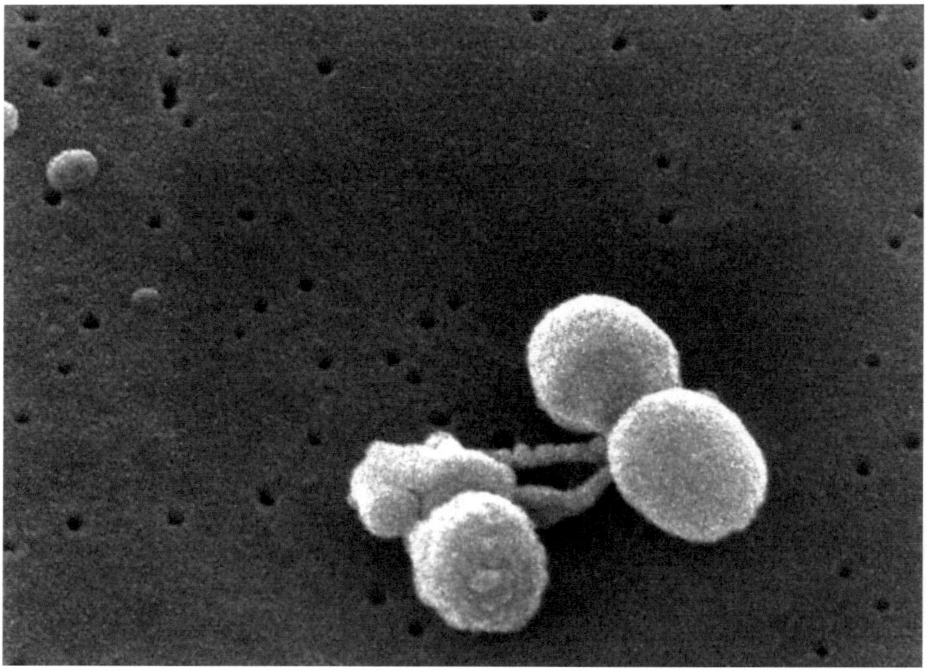

Fig. 1. Scanning electromicrograph of the pneumococcus. photo by Janice Haney Carr. Centers for Disease Control and Prevention Public Health Image Library ID # 265. (15)

The most common causes of bacterial meningitis in the United States, Europe and many other developed countries since the 1980s have been the pneumococcus, *Haemophilus influenzae* type b, the meningococcus, group B streptococcus, and *Listeria monocytogenes* (4-5, 7). In Africa, seasonal outbreaks and epidemics of meningococcal meningitis and septicemia numerically represent the greatest public health impact in this context (1, 8-9). The three polysaccharide-encapsulated bacteria for which licensed vaccines are widely available, the pneumococcus, *Haemophilus influenzae* type b , and the meningococcal serogroups A, C, W-135 and Y, have been the major focus of vaccine development and policy efforts (1-2, 10-11). Following the initial introduction of conjugate polysaccharide vaccines against these pathogens during the 1980s and 1990s the epidemiology of bacterial meningitis has changed dramatically. Further challenges to reducing the global burden of meningitis remain, among them the need for vaccines against Group B streptococcus, which accounts for a large proportion of newborn and very young infant infections, and meningococcal serogroup B (11-12). Indeed, in a recent report, Group B streptococcus was responsible for more than 85% of bacterial meningitis among US infants less than 2 months of age (5). In regions where vaccines against pneumococcus and *Haemophilus influenzae* type b are not available, Group B streptococcus is also an important cause of meningitis in the first 3 months of life (13-14).

The clinical characteristics of various meningitides are discussed in detail in other chapters. Risk factors for bacterial meningitis include age (the very young, the elderly, adolescents), underlying medical conditions (innate or acquired immunosuppression, complement deficiency, shunts, cochlear implants) and lifestyle factors such as poverty, college attendance, or travel. Increasing evidence suggests that genetic factors increase the risk of contracting bacterial meningitis (Table 2).

Genetic condition	Arising infection
Severe congenital neutropenia	Recurrent infections
Immunoglobulin deficiency	Pneumococcal infection
Severe combined immune deficiency	Recurrent infections
Complement deficiency	Meningococcal infection
TLR and NEMO	Pneumococcal infection
Mal/TIRAP gene	*Haemophilus influenzae* type b vaccine failure

TLR: toll-like receptor; NEMO: NF-kappa-B essential modulator; TIRAP: toll-interleukin 1 receptor (TIR) domain containing adaptor protein.
(1, 16-20)

Table 2. Known genetic predispositions to bacterial meningitis

Unique risk factors (Table 3) for meningococcal meningitis have been observed in adolescents and young adults: close social contact (e.g. bars, discotheques, dormitories), kissing, smoking (1, 3, 17-18). For *Haemophilus influenzae* type b, and pneumococcus, low socioeconomic status and ethnic minority group status represent risk factors of special note (5).

Exposure to antibiotics can increase the risk of infection with an antibiotic-resistant organism, as observed for pneumococcal infections, while vaccine policy has exerted a downward pressure on antibiotic resistance (26). For newborn Group B streptococcus infection, maternal colonization alone is a risk factor – accordingly some regions recommend administration of prophylactic antibiotics during labor and delivery for all women known to be colonized (27).

Crowding factors
Moving into a college dormitory, particularly freshmen
Moving into army barracks, particularly new military recruits
Travel
Attendance at the Hajj or Umrah pilgrimages
Travel to areas with hyperendemic or epidemic disease
Social factors
Pub or discotheque attendance
Kissing
Smoking and exposure to second-hand smoke

(1,21-25)

Table 3. Examples of risk factors for developing meningococcal meningitis

Rates of asymptomatic carriage may affect the transmission of encapsulated pathogenic bacteria and thereby lead to colonization, invasion and invasive disease. The ability to adhere to or penetrate the mucosa, or to survive and multiply in blood or infect organs (especially the brain) are commonly-recognized virulence factors that, like epidemiology, may differ among strains, serogroups or types of encapsulated bacteria within a species (1, 5, 24, 28-32). Susceptibility to disease or asymptomatic carriage may coincide or occur in distinct population groups (Table 4).

Carriage in infants, disease in infants
Pneumococcal diseases: bacteremia, meningitis, otitis media, pneumonia
Invasive *Haemophilus influenzae* type b disease: bacteremia, meningitis, epiglotitis
Carriage in adolescents and/or adults, disease in adolescents and/or adults
Invasive meningococcal meningitis and septicemia in travelers
Invasive meningococcal meningitis and septicemia in military recruits
Carriage in adolescents and adults, disease in infants
Invasive meningococcal meningitis in infants in developed countries
Maternal colonization with Group B streptococcus, disease in infants

(1,5, 16, 20, 22-23, 31-32)

Table 4. Examples of carriage versus invasive disease profiles

Ideally, definitive laboratory tests would rapidly confirm or exclude bacterial meningitis, determine the organism and identify its pattern of antibiotic susceptibility. Unfortunately, diagnosis of bacterial meningitis in the absence of a positive culture remains at best imprecise, despite numerous algorithms and putative biomarkers (Table 5). A recent early diagnostic model relies on dichotomized variables of peripheral blood polymorphonuclear cell count >16 × 10^9/l, serum C-reactive protein >100 mg/l and hemorrhagic rash, with a predicted probability of bacterial meningitis or meningococcal septicemia >95% with the presence of any one variable and >99% for two or more (33). Serum procalcitonin distinguished viral from bacterial meningitis more effectively than C-reactive protein or leukocyte counts (34-35). However, methods must approach 100% sensitivity to avoid missed cases. Immediate and urgent administration of antibiotics until the results of microbiological tests become available is therefore recommended, (24, 36-37) although this practice may hinder diagnostic methods and surveillance that rely on culture. More sensitive molecular diagnostic techniques such as polymerase chain reaction (PCR) can enable definitive diagnosis in these cases (1, 38). Administration of preemptive antibiotics to viral meningitis patients can be costly and may indirectly contribute to antibiotic resistance. Suboptimal dosing of preemptive antibiotics may result in penetration into the cerebrospinal fluid or across the blood-brain barrier that is inadequate to eradicate bacterial pathogens (36-37).

Clinical criteria: hemorrhagic nonblanching rash, neck stiffness, altered mental state, shock, hypotension, back rigidity, photophobia, toxic or moribund state, seizures headache, vomiting, fever, etc.
Bacterial antigen testing
Gram staining
Blood markers: C-reactive protein level, white blood cell count
Cerebrospinal fluid markers: protein level, glucose level, white blood cell count, neutrophil count
Cultures of blood or cerebrospinal fluid
Serum procalcitonin
Blood polymorphonuclear cell count >16 × 10^9/l, serum C-reactive protein >100 mg/l and/or hemorrhagic rash

(33-39)

Table 5. Examples of algorithms and biomarkers for bacterial meningitis.

Difficulties in differential diagnosis, combined with the severe consequences of disease, including sepsis, shock, gangrene, deafness, seizures, CNS damage, or limb amputation, taken together support vaccination as the best approach for preventing the most epidemiologically and clinically important forms of bacterial meningitis.

While the brain and meninges are relatively anatomically inaccessible, once breached by a pathogen the blood-brain barrier tends to become more permeable to medicines because of resultant inflammation. *Haemophilus influenzae* type b, the meningococcus and the pneumococcus are generally highly sensitive to antibiotics, although resistance has been increasingly reported with pneumococci and a few meningococcal strains, leading to recommendations for the empiric use of third-generation cephalosporins. Therapies are also available for other forms of meningitis. Corticosteroids may be recommended as adjunctive therapy to reduce some symptoms (36-37).

3. Prevention of meningitis

Strategies and policies to prevent and control meningitis tend to involve narrow, categorical, pathogen-specific programs. Few if any broad policies spanning the gamut of pathogens responsible for causing meningitis exist. This shortcoming reflects the differences in the epidemiology of the etiologic agents, the limited antigenic composition and coverage of the available vaccines, the complexity of primary prevention and secondary prevention modalities, and the cost and complexity of instituting large scale programs.

In epidemic situations, antibiotics may be used to prevent bacterial meningitis in close contacts or communities within a reasonable period (1 week in the case of meningococcal meningitis) from the diagnosis of an index case. Current recommendations often call for third-generation cephalosporins to address possible drug-resistant strains. (22-23, 36-37). In addition, intrapartum antibiotics are routinely administered to mothers colonized with Group B streptococcus to prevent infant disease. Nevertheless, vaccination remains the most effective means of preventing both the most common causes of bacterial meningitis and some viral pathogens, like measles and mumps. Although vaccines have been licensed steadily throughout the late twentieth and early twenty-first centuries for encapsulated bacteria, areas for improvement remain.

Investigation into vaccines that limit meningitis followed work against other deadly diseases such as rabies, yellow fever, and smallpox. The diphtheria and tetanus toxoid vaccines originally designed in the 1920s were later adapted to act as protein carriers in the current polysaccharide-protein conjugate vaccines. Another early twentieth-century vaccine to prevent a range of illnesses, including meningitis, was the Bacille Calmette-Guérin (BCG) vaccine against tuberculosis, which has become the most widely used vaccine in the WHO Expanded Programme for Immunisation. Measles and mumps vaccines were developed during the second half of the twentieth century, and, like diphtheria and tetanus vaccines, remain an essential part of early childhood universal vaccination programs (40).

The first vaccines against encapsulated bacterial meningitis-causing pathogens during the 1960s and 1970s employed the purified outer polysaccharide capsule to provide immune responses in persons over 2 years of age who were able to mount B-cell responses. Such vaccines have been used successfully in situations where individual protection is needed for a limited amount of time. However, these vaccines may have blunted or diminished responses with repeat dosing, possibly due to B-cell depletion and do not offer protection in infants and others who cannot mount B-cell responses. The next generation of conjugated pneumococcal, meningococcal and *Haemophilus influenzae* type b vaccines offer protection to infants and young children and allow for booster responses with repeat dosing. Extensive vaccination of infants and young children with pneumococcal vaccines has led to considerable reductions in disease in non-target age groups by means of herd protection, which was also evident in meningococcal serogroup C vaccine programs that include the primary carriage population (1, 2, 40-41).

Policy makers and health care providers generally consider the full spectrum of clinical disease caused by meningitis-causing pathogens when making decisions about therapy, prevention, or vaccination. For example, meningococci can cause a range of clinical syndromes including septicemia, bacteremia, and localized suppurative infections such as arthritis. Similarly, pneumococci cause otitis media and pneumonia, which create serious public health consequences. Further, *Haemophilus influenzae* type b vaccine policy was strongly affected by the possibility to prevent pneumonia and epiglottitis, which is very difficult to manage. Meningococcal vaccine policy must also address the possibility for unpredictable, severe

VACCINE	PRIMARY DISEASE TARGETED	CURRENT ROUTINE USE EXAMPLES
Early Twentieth Century		
Bacille-Calmette-Guérin (BCG) Vaccine	Tuberculosis	WHO countries
Mid-Twentieth Century		
Measles virus vaccine	Measles	Infants and toddlers
Mumps virus vaccine	Mumps	Infants and toddlers
Late twentieth Century		
Meningococcal polysaccharide vaccines	Meningitis and septicemia	Hajj travel in countries without access to conjugate vaccines
Pneumococcal polysaccharide vaccine	Meningitis and pneumonia	Elderly persons in countries without conjugate vaccines against all significant serotypes
Haemophilus influenzae type b conjugate vaccine	Meningitis and epiglotitis	Infants and toddlers
Pneumococcal conjugate vaccine	Meningitis, pneumonia and otitis media	Infants and toddlers
Meningococcal conjugate vaccines	Meningitis and septicemia	Infants, toddlers, adolescents, travelers, Hajj pilgrims

Note: vaccines against Japanese and tick-borne encephalitis also became available during the twentieth century. (1,2, 5, 40-41)

Table 6. Vaccines against pathogens that cause meningitis

outbreaks and epidemics that may prevent adequate distribution of antibiotics fast enough to treat individuals and to curtail the spread of infection through a community. The possibility of drug resistance can also impact vaccine policy and treatment decisions (2).

3.1 *Haemophilus influenza* type b vaccines

No single intervention has done more to prevent cases of bacterial meningitis than the successful introduction of conjugate *Haemophilus influenzae* type b vaccines, which stands as a major triumph in the history of vaccinology (42-43). The virulence of *Haemophilus influenzae* type b results from its unique polyribosylribitol phosphate (PRP) capsule, which is thought to be particularly effective at enabling the organism to evade complement-mediated lysis and avoid splenic clearance (44-45). Previous to the development of conjugate vaccines, *Haemophilus influenzae* type b was the most common cause of bacterial meningitis, and disease incidence remains high in countries that do not immunize infants (42-43). *Haemophilus influenzae* type b meningitis occurs primarily in older infants and toddlers, during a "window of vulnerability" corresponding to a gap in anti-capsular antibody titers that occurs between a decline in maternal antibody and the second year of life. Conjugated *Haemophilus influenzae* type b PRP (or PRP derivative) vaccines enabled the

Vaccine	Diseases/pathogens covered	Regions used
Haemophilus influenzae type b (Hib) conjugate vaccines		
PRP-T PRP-OMPC PRP-D PRP-CRM197	*Haemophilus influenzae* type b	North America and Europe
Haemophilus influenzae type b and pertussis-containing vaccine combinations		
DTaP-IPV/Hib	Diphtheria, tetanus, pertussis, polio, *Haemophilus influenzae* type b	North America
DTaP-IPV/Hib-HBV	Diphtheria, tetanus, pertussis, polio, *Haemophilus influenzae* type b , hepatitis B	Europe
DTP-Hib	Diphtheria, tetanus, pertussis, *Haemophilus influenzae* type b	Africa, Asia, Latin America
DTP-Hib-HBV	Diphtheria, tetanus, pertussis, *Haemophilus influenzae* type b , hepatitis B	Africa, Asia, Latin America
Haemophilus influenzae type b meningitis combinations		
MenCY-Hib	Meningococcal serogroups C and Y, *Haemophilus influenzae* type b	Not yet in use
MenC-Hib	Meningococcal serogroup C, *Haemophilus influenzae* type b	UK
Other *Haemophilus influenzae* type b combinations		
Hib-HBV	*Haemophilus influenzae* type b and hepatitis B	North America Europe

-aP: acellular pertussis; CRM197: cross-reacting material; D: diphtheria toxoid; HBV: hepatitis B virus; IPV: inactivated poliovirus vaccine; MenC meningococcal serogroup C; MenCY: meningococcal serogroups C and Y; OMPC: outer membrane protein complex; P: whole-cell pertussis; PRP: polyribosylribitol phosphate; T: tetanus toxoid. (40-52)

Table 7. Examples of vaccines against *Haemophilus influenzae* type b

institution of immunization policies shaped by an understanding of epidemiology. Universal use of *Haemophilus influenzae* type b conjugate vaccines in the first year of life provided protection from invasive disease, reductions in carriage, and herd effects, an approach that was tailored to fit existing routine infant immunization schedules. Combining conjugate *Haemophilus influenzae* type b vaccine with other routine infant vaccines has allowed for ease of implementation in increasingly crowded immunization schedules (42-52).

3.1.1 Pneumococcal vaccines

The pneumococcus comprises antigenically distinct types based on the chemistry of the polysaccharide outer capsule. Vaccines have therefore been designed to provide protection against the broadest number of serotypes in a specific population (Table 8).

Pneumococcal Types	23-valent polysaccharide vaccine	7-valent CRM-conjugate vaccine	10-valent protein D-conjugate	13-valent CRM-conjugate vaccine
Target age group	Adults	Infants	Infants	infants
1	X		X	X
2	X			
3	X			X
4	X	X	X	X
5	X		X	X
6A				X
6B	X	X	X	X
7F	X		X	X
8	X			
9N	X			
9V	X	X	X	X
10A	X			
11A	X			
12F	X			
14	X	X	X	X
15B	X			
17F	X			
18C	X	X	X	X
19F	X	X	X	X
19A	X			X
20	X			
22F	X			
23F	X	X	X	X
33F	X			

CRM: cross reacting material 197; protein D is derived from nontypeable *Haemophilus influenzae* (40, 63)

Table 8. Pneumococcal types covered by available polysaccharide vaccines for use in adults and polysaccharide-protein conjugate vaccine for use in infants and young children

The UK has been a leader in implementing universal infant vaccination against bacterial meningitides. Awareness raised by charities such as the Meningitis Research Foundation or the Meningitis Trust and the media helped support the inclusion of pneumococcal vaccines in not only routine infant schedules but also into at-risk programs. At-risk programs may have little impact on disease burden (54), particularly given that immunization of infants and young children provides some protection in older age groups by virtue of herd protection (55). Pneumococcal conjugate vaccine also provided unexpected benefits such as the prevention of secondary bacterial super-infection in influenza (56).

The 7-valent pneumococcal conjugate vaccine has been in use in the US since 2000 with subsequent licensing in the EU and elsewhere. Although the initial European recommendation was for at-risk groups, by 2006 more countries were making universal recommendations and providing funding. Cost-effectiveness data from the US, some European countries and Australia (57) have been reported and indicate that vaccination can be cost-saving, as in Germany, partly as a result of reduction of high-incidence but also lower severity infections such as otitis media. Favorable pharmacoeconomic results tend to drive routine (universal use) policy implementation. Pneumococcal conjugate vaccine is funded in many countries including Turkey, Mexico, and South Africa, and in some GAVI-eligible countries.

The safety, efficacy and effectiveness of the 7-valent pneumococcal conjugate vaccine were established through pivotal trials, long-term surveillance, and monitoring. In a multi-centre study of 1379 pneumococcal meningitis cases in the US from 1998 to 2005 (58), incidence declined from 1.13 to 0.79 cases per 100,000 persons, a 30.1% reduction ($P<0.001$). Reductions were most marked in those less than 2 years and more than 65 years of age, respectively 64.0% and 54.0% ($P<0.001$). Non-vaccine serotypes were noted to cause more disease after the introduction of vaccine. Newer 10- and 13-valent pneumococcal vaccines have been studied in clinical trials and are appearing in some markets. A 15-valent pneumococcal conjugate vaccine is also in clinical trials.

Questions regarding the efficacy of 23-valent pneumococcal polysaccharide vaccine have led the UK to consider eliminating its routine use in the elderly and confining use to specific at-risk groups (59). Licensing of the 13-valent pneumococcal conjugate vaccine for adults should provide an alternative. In France, the 13-valent pneumococcal vaccine, which is already licensed for use in children, may reduce disease where serotypes 7F and 19A have come to predominate (60) while in the African meningitis belt there is potential for the reduction in the burden of disease through coverage of serotype 1 (61).

3.2 Meningococcal vaccines

The epidemiology of meningococcal disease is characterized by dynamic shifts in serogroup incidence over time and across geography. In addition, hypervirulent strains cause unpredictable outbreaks, and epidemics are reported annually in the sub-Saharan meningitis belt. Six meningococcal serogroups, A, B, C, W-135, X, and Y cause the majority of disease worldwide and are considered epidemiologically important by the WHO (1, 5, 9). Currently, conjugate vaccines are available against serogroups A, C, W-135 and Y. Routine immunization with the serogroup C conjugate vaccines dramatically reduced disease incidence and asymptomatic carriage, thus leading to herd protection in many countries including the UK, Ireland, the Netherlands, and Canada. Effective vaccination policy mandated immunization of both infants and adolescents, an important reservoir for meningococcal carriage. These findings have yet to be replicated with additional serogroups (1, 9). Quadrivalent meningococcal vaccines against serogroups A, C, W-135 and Y are routinely recommended in North America for use in adolescents, and a booster dose is recommended in the US. Additional recommendations for meningococcal vaccination include the military, persons travelling to regions with endemic or epidemic disease, and those attending the annual Hajj pilgrimage to Mecca (1, 25, 62). A very significant new advance in this field is the recent implementation of serogroup A conjugate vaccine in the African meningitis belt (8).

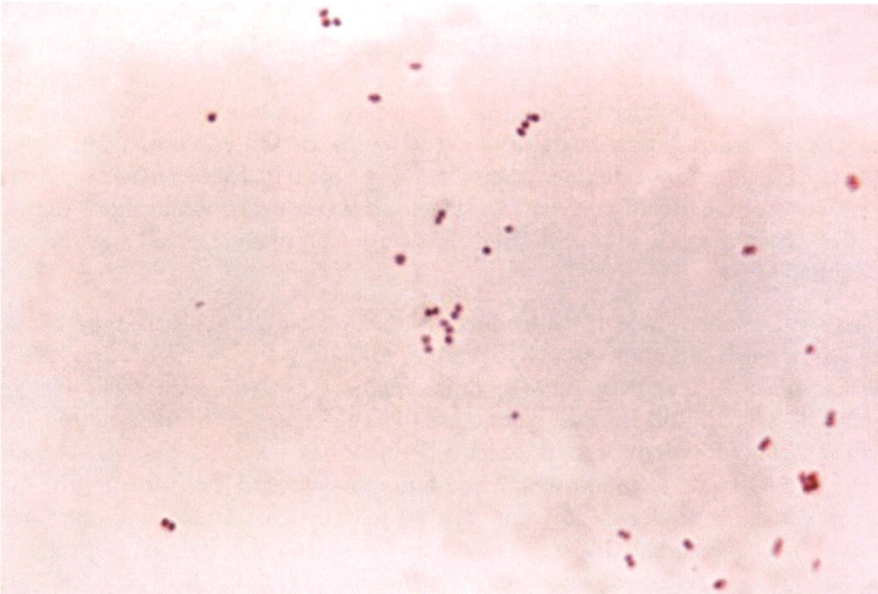

Fig. 2. Micrograph at 1150 X magnification of meningococci. Image by Dr Brodsky c. 1966. Centers for Disease Control and Prevention Public Health Image Library ID #6423 (15).

Serogroup B presents special challenges because its capsular polysaccharide is non-immunogenic, resulting in the need for subcapsular antigenic approaches (1, 11). Serogroup B vaccines using outer membrane vesicles (OMVs) as the primary antigen have been used to control specific clonal outbreaks in Cuba, Chile, Brazil, New Zealand, France and Norway. Various other subcapsular antigens have been investigated (10-11). A genomic method known as reverse vaccinology led to the development of 4CMenB, which is the only vaccine that has been shown to generate antibody responses against genetically heterologous serogroup B strains in Phase 3 trials in both infants and adolescents and has been submitted for approval to the European Medicines Agency. 4CMenB is a multicomponent vaccine that combines factor H binding protein, Neisserial adhesin A, and *Neisseria* heparin binding antigen with OMV from the New Zealand outbreak strain. The vaccine promises to be an important advance in vaccine practice (11, 63-65). Other serogroup B vaccines are under development.

An optimal strategy for meningococcal disease control would include broad-coverage vaccines in infants where the disease incidence is highest coupled with immunization of adolescents (where peak carriage occurs) to induce herd effects and prevent secondary peak disease. Vaccine availability, implementation issues and cost have driven meningococcal vaccine policies, which tend to be narrow in scope (65).

4. Policy decisions for the prevention of meningitis

Strategies and policies to prevent and control meningitis tend to be pathogen-specific, because differences in epidemiology, available vaccines, cost and the complexity of instituting large scale programs would make general guidelines unhelpful. Nevertheless, the vision of a meningitis free world is most likely to be realized from innovative approaches to integrated meningitis prevention and control.

Implementation of vaccines against meningitis-causing organisms has been a major priority of global health funding organizations such as the Gates Foundation and the Global Alliance for Vaccines and Immunisation (GAVI). The Gates Foundation alone has committed more than 14 billion dollars toward vaccines for developing countries (66). Investments such as these have led to innovative strategies and partnerships toward vaccines against meningitis. Early efforts focused on introducing existing vaccines, such as *Haemophilus influenzae* type b and pneumococcal conjugate vaccines, to developing countries, while more recent efforts include the development of specialized low-cost vaccines targeted to the needs of developing nations.

A notable GAVI initiative was the introduction of *Haemophilus influenzae* type b vaccine to the world's poorest countries, which began in 2005, on the heels of the WHO global *Haemophilus influenzae* type b vaccine recommendation. By 2008, half of eligible countries, representing 42% of eligible infants, had access to free or subsidized vaccine (67). GAVI has also funded 7-valent pneumococcal vaccine, which has been adopted by a number of countries, the first being Rwanda (68). The Meningitis Vaccine Project recently supported the development of a low-cost (40 cents a dose) tetanus toxoid conjugate vaccine against serogroup A meningococcal disease for use in the meningitis belt. This project was an innovative multi-stakeholder partnership including the WHO, UNICEF, the US Centers for Disease Control, the US Center for Biologics Evaluation and Research (CBER), and the Serum Institute of India. This vaccine has dramatically reduced disease and associated morbidity and mortality after immunization of 19 million residents of Burkina Faso, Mali and Niger in the course of a few weeks (8, 68).

4.1 Considerations for the design of preventative interventions

Vaccine policy for meningitis, as for most infectious diseases, is determined by the burden of disease, public awareness of the problem, availability of vaccines and the ability to fund vaccination campaigns. Yet even with compelling disease burden, clear epidemiologic justification and ample funding, difficulties in vaccine formulation or adding vaccines to crowded schedules may present significant barriers to implementing vaccine policies. The prevention of bacterial meningitis requires vaccinating a large proportion of the community and immunization against relatively rare diseases, thus such programs might not meet pharmacoeconomic parameters in all nations as it did recently in the African meningitis belt (69).

Routine immunization implementation may be necessary to assess clinical effectiveness, cost effectiveness and herd effects; therefore, effective vaccine policies must consider multiple variables in the use of health care resources. The perceived and actual burden of disease may vary because public perception can be skewed by reports of epidemics or small numbers of cases of severe disease. Or, the true burden of disease may be masked by

Epidemiology
Populations suffering from disease
Populations carrying or transmitting the causative organism
Genetic, group, and strain diversity of the organism
Genetic, strain, or serogroup shifts over time and space
Escape mutants
Serogroup or serotype replacement over time and as a result of vaccination campaigns
Proximity of populations (potential for herd effects)
Vaccines
Number and type of available vaccines
Ability for vaccines to protect against circulating pathogens in a given region
Effects on immunogenicity and efficacy when given with existing vaccine schedules
Duration of immunity
Effects in target age groups
Policy
Existing vaccine schedules
Timing of doses
Need for booster doses or catch-up campaigns
Funding
Ability to reach key populations to administer vaccines
Possibility for herd effects
Reduction of the risk for developing antibiotic resistance

Table 9. Considerations for developing vaccine policy

under-diagnosis, under-reporting or, if early antibiotic treatment prevents case confirmation by culture (70-71). Thus, public awareness of disease burden should precede explanations of new vaccines. Media reports may occasionally be counter-productive, especially when considering their treatment of vaccine safety (72).

Vaccine availability can be limited by logistical factors like the lack of a universally protective antigen. Thus, not all meningitides are vaccine-preventable in practice (e.g. serogroup B meningococcus, group B streptococcus), nor are many of the encephalitides. Vaccines cannot be considered available unless they have been approved for licensure, yet licensure is necessary but not sufficient for availability to the general public because funding sources have a strong impact on policy decisions. In the public market, pharmacoeconomic considerations may appear calculating or callous to the general public. In a "private" market, the vaccinee must willingly obtain and pay for the vaccine. Although in this context, the decision to receive vaccine is less likely to be driven by a sense of public-mindedness, the near-universal uptake of pneumococcal conjugate vaccine in Portugal indicates that collective responsibility may be powerful in some regions.

4.2 Policy approaches to vaccine against meningitis-causing pathogens

Universal (age-based) routine immunization is a primary model for limiting or eliminating meningitis globally. Prevention in the context of disease outbreaks involves antibiotic chemoprophylaxis as well as targeted vaccine use, generally in the setting of meningococcal disease. Universal vaccination approaches require multiple considerations because successful prevention arises only from a clear understanding of several key factors including the populations at greatest risk of disease, the population where carriage occurs, the features of available vaccines, the feasibility of implementation of immunization policies (Figure 3).

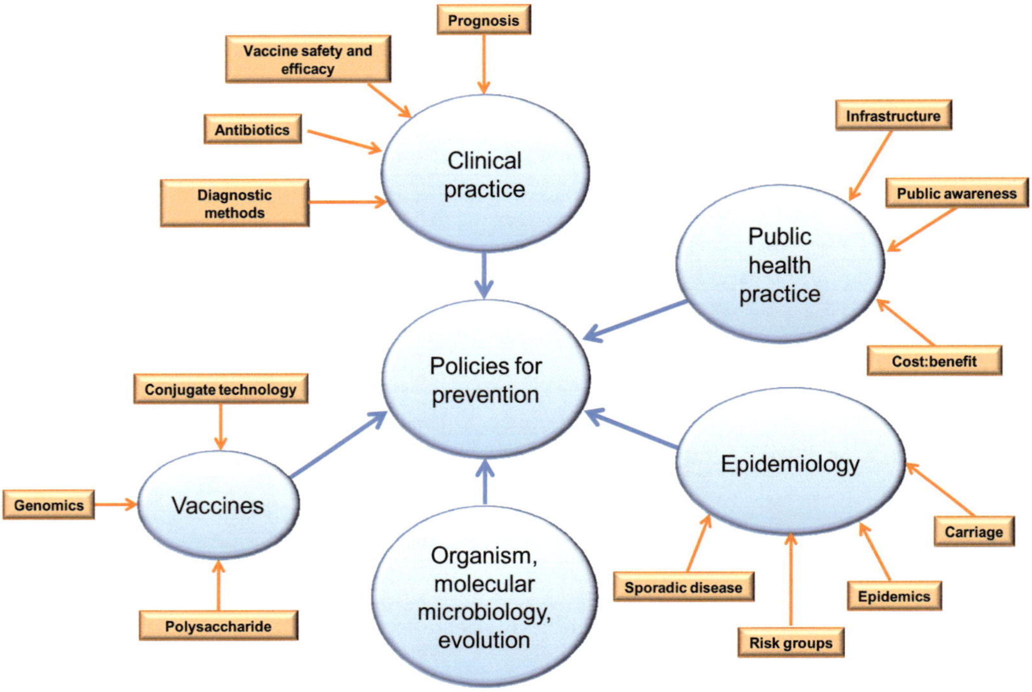

Fig. 3. Considerations that inform policymaking decisions for meningitis prevention

Universal immunization against *Haemophilus influenzae* type b , meningococcal serogroup C and pneumococcal disease stand as exceptionally noteworthy successes in the primary prevention of meningitis. These universal policies are more likely to protect high-risk individuals than selective programs in part because risk factors may be poorly understood. Debates about selective versus universal or voluntary and compulsory vaccination policies remain unresolved.

Primary prevention of other causes of meningitis is somewhat more complex. Control of meningococcal serogroup C resulted through the expansion of the immunization schedule to include older children and adolescents, reducing carriage to provide adequate herd effects and the use of catch-up campaigns to ensure vaccine coverage.

Secondary prevention of meningitis can include interventions, like antibiotic chemoprophylaxis, that can operate at the population level or for an individual. Targeted use of vaccines within communities or geographic areas can also control epidemic as shown

Young children were at the highest risk of disease and also comprised the primary population where carriage occurs
Glycoconjugate vaccines enabled direct protection and reduction in carriage that provided further herd effects in the critical at-risk population simultaneously
Implementation of immunization was straightforward because vaccines fit well into the existing routine infant immunization schedules
Herd effects extended beyond the vaccinated population and into the general population because primary vaccination reduced carriage in the key reservoir for the causative disease pathogens.

Table 10. Considerations that led to the success of universal vaccination policies against *Haemophilus influenzae* type b and pneumococcal diseases

in Cuba, Norway and New Zealand by the use of tailor-made outer membrane vesicle vaccines against meningococcal serogroup B (73). Policy focus in the Middle East has been directed toward the control of meningococcal disease Hajj pilgrims (62, 74). Globally, routine infant immunization schedules commonly include *Haemophilus influenzae* type b and pneumococcal conjugate vaccines within the first six months of life, with a booster in the second year of life, which is important to long-term protection. Meningococcal vaccine schedules are more variable and routine recommendations may target infants, older children, adolescents, or some combination of these.

4.3 Expert commentary and five year view

Where meningitis prevention and control is concerned, optimally, vaccine innovation will involve the development of broadly protective vaccines that are safe and immunogenic across the age spectrum. From a pure feasibility point of view, combining antigens will be critically important given the increasingly crowded immunization schedules. Cost and the crowded immunization schedules are typically cited as the major impediments to making progress in the area of meningitis prevention and control.

The recent advent of vaccines to prevent meningitis and sepsis caused by *Haemophilus influenzae* type b, the pneumococcus and the meningococcus further completes a general picture of universal vaccination to promote public health, beginning with vaccine policies against diseases like measles, mumps, polio, and diphtheria. Yet most of the world's children remain unprotected, which underscores the work of organizations like the WHO, the Gates Foundation and GAVI in limiting infectious disease.

The effects of vaccine programs depend on many factors. Antibody concentration wanes rapidly in infants, and more slowly in toddlers and young children while persons 10 years of age and older can have antibody persistence for five years or more (75). Herd protection may depend on booster dosing in various age groups or catch-up campaigns. Similarly, continued vaccination of infants may be necessary to protect the vulnerable elderly population from pneumococcal disease. Yet, with the dramatic reduction of cases, the political will to support booster vaccinations may be lacking.

Compliance, and therefore vaccine coverage, may be an issue for adolescents, who traditionally visit medical practitioners infrequently, and who often refuse vaccines but represent an important population for meningococcal carriage and also have an increased risk for case fatality. Combined vaccination with other routine vaccinations for this age group, such as Tdap and HPV, may help overcome this difficulty, and are supported by clinical studies (22-23, 76-78). Booster immunizations with DT/IPV/aP combinations, catch-up for MMR/V and depending on the country, catch-up vaccination for hepatitis A or for hepatitis B may provide additional opportunities for vaccination of adolescents. Suboptimal coverage rates, especially for newer vaccines, place substantial numbers of adolescents at risk. One approach to increase adolescent vaccination is to establish routine school-based adolescent immunization programs by primary care trusts, school nursing teams and similar facilities.

In a recent survey analyzed by the Federal Center for Health Education (Bundeszentrale für gesundheitliche Aufklärung) in Germany, 64% of parents had a positive opinion on vaccination, 35% declined individual vaccines due to various reservations and only 1% generally dismissed vaccines. About 50% of the parents with reservations reported that the reason for their reservation was that they assessed the vaccine to be unnecessary, vaccination was discouraged by the physician (41%) or they were afraid of side reactions (40%). The survey data reveal the central role of the medical profession (79).

Education of adolescents, their parents and/or guardians, health care providers, policy makers and physicians is vital to successful implementation of adolescent immunizations and it has to be considered that the role of pediatricians gradually decreases for adolescents older than 14 years, while the role of the family practitioner, internist, and gynecologist increases. Of note, 35% of the preventive care visits made by late adolescent females (18-21 years old) are to obstetricians and gynecologists, which provides an opportunity for concomitant HPV and quadrivalent meningococcal vaccines. Obstetricians may be particularly well positioned to intervene in meningitis affecting the very young infant in the future by administering vaccines to pregnant women to limit infections such as Group B streptococcus, a leading cause of neonatal meningitis. For various reasons, family practitioners are often slower than pediatricians to accept new universal vaccine recommendations (80-81), which might require adjustments in communication about new products.

Achieving reductions in meningitis has to remain a top priority for the modern world. Within this context, a vaccine with the following properties might be considered a magic bullet were it to be developed:

- Multicomponent vaccine with coverage against *Haemophilus influenzae* type b, and PCV (23 - valent), and meningococcus (5 valent: A, B, C, W-135, and Y)
- Safe, immunogenic, and effective in young infants, children, adolescents and adults
- Ability to reduce or eliminate carriage

Such a vaccine, if used appropriately, could help bring us closer to a "meningitis free world". Although a singular such vaccine is not likely to be developed within the next five years, incremental progress is inching us closer toward such broad vaccines. Admittedly, Group B streptococcus remains a critical target, and the new paradigm of maternal immunization will be required for successful control of that disease. Moreover, listerial, viral, fungal, mycobacterial and other rare forms of meningitis will remain with us for some time to come albeit at low rates. The world is now positioned with an ever growing armamentarium of preventative tools the likes of which physicians and public health officials of past generations could only have dreamed.

5. Acknowledgements

All authors are full time employees of Novartis Vaccines and Diagnostics (a manufacturer of meningococcal vaccines) or were full time employees of Novartis Vaccines and Diagnostics at the time this chapter was written. The authors are grateful to Johanna Pattenier MD, Karen Slobod MD, James Wassil MS, and Mahlet Woldemariam MS, all of Novartis Vaccines and Diagnostics, for scientific and editorial review. We thank Giorgio Corsi for supporting us with the art work in figure 3.

6. References

[1] Tan LK, Carlone GM, Borrow R. Advances in the development of vaccines against Neisseria meningitidis. N Engl J Med. 2010 Apr 22;362(16):1511-20.

[2] Tyler KL. Chapter 28: a history of bacterial meningitis. Handb Clin Neurol. 2010;95:417-33.

[3] Meningitis Research Foundation. Awareness and Education. Accessed 5 August 2011. http://www.meningitis.org/awareness-education.

[4] Schuchat A, Robinson K, Wenger JD, Harrison LH, Farley M, Reingold AL, Lefkowitz L, Perkins BA. Bacterial meningitis in the United States in 1995. Active Surveillance Team. N Engl J Med. 1997 Oct 2;337(14):970-6

[5] Thigpen MC, Whitney CG, Messonnier NE, Zell ER, Lynfield R, Hadler JL, Harrison LH, Farley MM, Reingold A, Bennett NM, Craig AS, Schaffner W, Thomas A, Lewis MM, Scallan E, Schuchat A; Emerging Infections Programs Network. Bacterial meningitis in the United States, 1998-2007. N Engl J Med. 2011 May 26;364(21):2016-25.

[6] Kutty PK, Kyaw MH, Dayan GH, Brady MT, Bocchini JA, Reef SE, Bellini WJ, Seward JF. Guidance for isolation precautions for mumps in the United States: a review of the scientific basis for policy change. Clin Infect Dis. 2010 Jun 15;50(12):1619-28.

[7] Gold R. Epidemiology of bacterial meningitis. Infect Dis Clin North Am. 1999 Sep;13(3):515-25, v.

[8] Sow SO, Okoko BJ, Diallo A, Viviani S, Borrow R, Carlone G, Tapia M, Akinsola AK, Arduin P, Findlow H, Elie C, Haidara FC, Adegbola RA, Diop D, Parulekar V, Chaumont J, Martellet L, Diallo F, Idoko OT, Tang Y, Plikaytis BD, Kulkarni PS, Marchetti E, LaForce FM, Preziosi MP. Immunogenicity and safety of a meningococcal A conjugate vaccine in Africans. N Engl J Med. 2011 Jun 16;364(24):2293-304.

[9] Harrison LH, Trotter CL, Ramsay ME. Global epidemiology of meningococcal disease. Vaccine. 2009 Jun 24;27 Suppl 2:B51-63.

[10] Zollinger WD, Poolman JT, Maiden MC. Meningococcal serogroup B vaccines: will they live up to expectations? Expert Rev Vaccines. 2011 May;10(5):559-61.

[11] Sadarangani M, Pollard AJ. Serogroup B meningococcal vaccines-an unfinished story. Lancet Infect Dis. 2010 Feb;10(2):112-24.

[12] Melin P. Neonatal group B streptococcal disease: from pathogenesis to preventive strategies. Clin Microbiol Infect. 2011 May 7, 17:1294-1303.

[13] English, M et al. Causes and outcome of young infant admissions to a Kenyan district hospital. Arch Dis Child 2003 88 438.

[14] Berkley, JA et al. Bacteremia among Children admitted to a rural hospital in Kenya. N Engl J Med 2005 352 39.

[15] Centers for Disease Control and Prevention Public Health Image Library. Accessed 5 August 2011. http://phil.cdc.gov/phil/home.asp

[16] Arkwright PD, Abinun M. Recently identified factors predisposing children to infectious diseases. Curr Opin Infect Dis. 2008 Jun;21(3):217-22.

[17] Hosseininasab A, Alborzi A, Ziyaeyan M, Jamalidoust M, Moeini M, Pouladfar G, Abbasian A, Kadivar MR. Viral etiology of aseptic meningitis among children in southern Iran. J Med Virol. 2011 May;83(5):884-8.

[18] Goldberg M, Fremeaux-Bacchi V, Koch P, Fishelson Z, Katz Y. A novel mutation in the C3 gene and recurrent invasive pneumococcal infection: A clue for vaccine development. Mol Immunol. 2011 Jun 13, 48:1926-1931.

[19] Ku CL, Picard C, Erdös M, Jeurissen A, Bustamante J, Puel A, von Bernuth H, Filipe-Santos O, Chang HH, Lawrence T, Raes M, Maródi L, Bossuyt X, Casanova JL.IRAK4 and NEMO mutations in otherwise healthy children with recurrent invasive pneumococcal disease. J Med Genet. 2007 Jan;44(1):16-23.

[20] Brouwer MC, de Gans J, Heckenberg SG, Zwinderman AH, van der Poll T, van de Beek D. Host genetic susceptibility to pneumococcal and meningococcal disease: a systematic review and meta-analysis. Lancet Infect Dis. 2009 Jan;9(1):31-44.

[21] Tully J, Viner RM, Coen PG, Stuart JM, Zambon M, Peckham C, Booth C, Klein N, Kaczmarski E, Booy R. Risk and protective factors for meningococcal disease in adolescents: matched cohort study. BMJ. 2006 Feb 25;332(7539):445-50.

[22] Cooper B, DeTora L, Stoddard J. Menveo®: a novel quadrivalent meningococcal CRM197 conjugate vaccine against serogroups A, C, W-135 and Y. Expert Rev Vaccines. 2011 Jan;10(1):21-33.

[23] Bröker M, Cooper B, DeTora LM, Stoddard JJ. Critical appraisal of a quadrivalent CRM197 conjugate vaccine against meningococcal serogroups A, C W-135 and Y (Menveo®) in the context of treatment and prevention of invasive disease. Infect Drug Resist 2011, 4:137-147

[24] Gardner P. Clinical practice. Prevention of meningococcal disease. N Engl J Med. 2006 Oct 5;355(14):1466-73.

[25] Zuckerman JN, Bröker M, Worth C. 2010 FIFA world cup South Africa: travel health issues and new options for protection against meningococcal disease. Travel Med Infect Dis. 2010 Mar;8(2):68-73.

[26] Kyaw MH, Lynfield R, Schaffner W, Craig AS, Hadler J, Reingold A, Thomas AR, Harrison LH, Bennett NM, Farley MM, Facklam RR, Jorgensen JH, Besser J, Zell ER, Schuchat A, Whitney CG; Active Bacterial Core Surveillance of the Emerging Infections Program Network. Effect of introduction of the pneumococcal conjugate vaccine on drug-resistant Streptococcus pneumoniae. N Engl J Med. 2006 Apr 6;354(14):1455-63.

[27] Centers for Disease Control and Prevention. Prevention of Perinatal Group B Streptococcal Disease. Revised Guidelines from CDC, 2010. MMWR 2010;59(No. RR-10):1-32.

[28] Furyk JS, Swann O, Molyneux E. Systematic review: neonatal meningitis in the developing world. Trop Med Int Health. 2011 Jun;16(6):672-9. doi: 10.1111/j.1365-3156.2011.02750.x.

[29] Sanders MS, van Well GT, Ouburg S, Morré SA, van Furth AM. Genetic variation of innate immune response genes in invasive pneumococcal and meningococcal disease applied to the pathogenesis of meningitis. Genes Immun. 2011 Jul;12(5):321-34. doi: 10.1038/gene.2011.20.

[30] Gaschignard J, Levy C, Romain O, Cohen R, Bingen E, Aujard Y, Boileau P. Neonatal Bacterial Meningitis: 444 Cases in 7 Years. Pediatr Infect Dis J. 2011 Mar;30(3):212-7

[31] Caugant DA, Maiden MC. Meningococcal carriage and disease-population biology and evolution. Vaccine. 2009 Jun 24;27 Suppl 2:B64-70.

[32] Kristiansen PA, Diomandé F, Wei SC, Ouédraogo R, Sangaré L, Sanou I, Kandolo D, Kaboré P, Clark TA, Ouédraogo AS, Absatou KB, Ouédraogo CD, Hassan-King M, Thomas JD, Hatcher C, Djingarey M, Messonnier N, Préziosi MP, LaForce M, Caugant DA. Baseline meningococcal carriage in Burkina Faso before the introduction of a meningococcal serogroup A conjugate vaccine. Clin Vaccine Immunol. 2011 Mar;18(3):435-43.

[33] Close RM, Ejidokun OO, Verlander NQ, Fraser G, Meltzer M, Rehman Y, Muir P, Ninis N, Stuart JM. Early diagnosis model for meningitis supports public health decision making. J Infect. 2011 Jul;63(1):32-8.

[34] Alkholi UM, Abd Al-Monem N, Abd El-Azim AA, Sultan MH. Serum procalcitonin in viral and bacterial meningitis. J Glob Infect Dis. 2011 Jan;3(1):14-8.

[35] Dubos F, Korczowski B, Aygun DA, Martinot A, Prat C, Galetto-Lacour A, Casado-Flores J, Taskin E, Leclerc F, Rodrigo C, Gervaix A, Leroy S, Gendrel D, Bréart G, Chalumeau M. Serum procalcitonin level and other biological markers to distinguish between bacterial and aseptic meningitis in children: a European multicenter case cohort study. Arch Pediatr Adolesc Med. 2008 Dec;162(12):1157-63

[36] DE Gaudio M, Chiappini E, Galli L, DE Martino M. Therapeutic management of bacterial meningitis in children: a systematic review and comparison of published guidelines from a European perspective. J Chemother. 2010 Aug;22(4):226-37.

[37] Visintin C, Mugglestone MA, Fields EJ, Jacklin P, Murphy MS, Pollard AJ; Guideline Development Group; National Institute for Health and Clinical Excellence. Management of bacterial meningitis and meningococcal septicaemia in children and young people: summary of NICE guidance. BMJ. 2010 Jun 28;340:c3209.

[38] Saha SK, Darmstadt GL, Baqui AH, Hossain B, Islam M, Foster D, Al-Emran H, Naheed A, Arifeen SE, Luby SP, Santosham M, Crook D. Identification of serotype in culture negative pneumococcal meningitis using sequential multiplex PCR: implication for surveillance and vaccine design. PLoS One. 2008;3(10):e3576.

[39] Chalupa P, Beran O, Herwald H, Kaspříková N, Holub M. Evaluation of potential biomarkers for the discrimination of bacterial and viral infections. Infection. 2011 Jul 1, 39:411-417.

[40] Plotkin SA, Orenstein WA, Offit PA. Vaccines. Fifth ed. New York: Elsevier, 2007.

[41] Stoddard J, Dougherty N. Universal immunization of infants against Neisseria meningitidis: Addressing the remaining unmet medical need in the prevention of meningitis and septicemia. Hum Vaccin. 2011 ;6(2).

[42] Fitzwater SP, Watt JP, Levine OS, Santosham M. *Haemophilus influenzae* type b conjugate vaccines: considerations for vaccination schedules and implications for developing countries. Hum Vaccin. 2010 Oct;6(10):810-8

[43] Ojo LR, O'Loughlin RE, Cohen AL, Loo JD, Edmond KM, Shetty SS, Bear AP, Privor-Dumm L, Griffiths UK, Hajjeh R. Global use of *Haemophilus influenzae* type b conjugate vaccine. Vaccine. 2010 Oct 8;28(43):7117-22.

[44] Zwahlen A, Kroll JS, Rubin LG, Moxon ER. The molecular basis of pathogenicity in *Haemophilus influenzae*: comparative virulence of genetically-related capsular transformants and correlation with changes at the capsulation locus cap. Microb Pathog. 1989 Sep;7(3):225-35.

[45] Swift AJ, Moxon ER, Zwahlen A, Winkelstein JA. Complement-mediated serum activities against genetically defined capsular transformants of *Haemophilus influenzae*. Microb Pathog. 1991 Apr;10(4):261-9.

[46] Fitzwater SP, Watt JP, Levine OS, Santosham M. *Haemophilus influenzae* type b conjugate vaccines: considerations for vaccination schedules and implications for developing countries. Hum Vaccin. 2010 Oct;6(10):810-8.

[47] Dhillon S. Spotlight on DTPa-HBV-IPV/Vaccine (Infanrix hexa). BioDrugs. 2010 Oct 1;24(5):299-302.

[48] O'Loughlin RE, Edmond K, Mangtani P, Cohen AL, Shetty S, Hajjeh R, Mulholland K. Methodology and measurement of the effectiveness of *Haemophilus influenzae* type b vaccine: systematic review.Vaccine. 2010 Aug 31;28(38):6128-36.

[49] Shetty S, Cohen AL, Edmond K, Ojo L, Loo J, O'Loughlin R, Hajjeh R. A systematic review and critical evaluation of invasive *Haemophilus influenzae* type b disease burden studies in Asia from the last decade: lessons learned for invasive bacterial disease surveillance. Pediatr Infect Dis J. 2010 Jul;29(7):653-61.

[50] Johns TL, Hutter GE. New combination vaccines: DTaP-IPV (Kinrix) and DTaP-IPV/(Pentacel). Ann Pharmacother. 2010 Mar;44(3):515-23.

[51] Dhillon S. DTPa-HBV-IPV/Vaccine (Infanrix hexa): A Review of its Use as Primary and Booster Vaccination. Drugs. 2010 May 28;70(8):1021-58.

[52] Gómez de León Cruces P, Díaz García J, Santos JI. Effect of the DTwP *Haemophilus influenzae* b conjugate vaccination in Mexico (1999-2007). Arch Med Res. 2010 May;41(4):281-7.

[53] McIntosh ED, Reinert RR. Global prevailing and emerging pediatric pneumococcal serotypes. Expert Rev Vaccines. 2011 Jan;10(1):109-29.

[54] Rendi-Wagner P, Paulke-Korinek M, Kundi M, *et al*. National pediatric immunization program of high risk groups: no effect on the incidence of invasive pneumococcal disease. Vaccine 2009; 27: 3963-3968.

[55] Whitney C, Farley M, Hadler J *et al.* Decline in invasive pneumococcal disease after the introduction of protein–polysaccharide conjugate vaccine. N Engl J Med 2003; *348*; 1737–1746.

[56] Madhi SA, Klugman KP; Vaccine Trialist Group. A role for *Streptococcus pneumoniae* in virus-associated pneumonia. Nat Med 2004; 10: 811-3.

[57] Silfverdal SA, Berg S, Hemlin C, Jokinen I. The cost-burden of paediatric pneumococcal disease in Sweden and the potential cost-effectiveness of prevention using 7-valent pneumococcal vaccine. Vaccine 2009; 27: 1601-1608.

[58] Hsu HE, Shutt KA, Moore MR, *et al.* Effect of pneumococcal conjugate vaccine on pneumococcal meningits. New Engl J Med 2009; 360: 244-256.

[59] Heijstek MW, Ott de Bruin LM, Bijl M, Borrow R, van der Klis F, Koné-Paut I, Fasth A, Minden K, Ravelli A, Abinun M, Pileggi GS, Borte M, Wulffraat NM. EULAR recommendations for vaccination in paediatric patients with rheumatic diseases. Ann Rheum Dis. 2011 Aug 3.

[60] Levy C, Varon E, Bingen E, *et al.* Pneumococcal meningitis in French children before and after the introduction of pneumococcal conjugate vaccine. Pediatr Infect Dis J 2011; 30: 168-170.

[61] Gessner BD, Mueller JE, Yaro S. African meningitis belt pneumococcal disease epidemiology indicates a need for an effective serotype 1 containing vaccine, including for older children and adults. BMC Infectious Diseases 2010; 10: 22.

[62] Memish ZA, Goubeaud A, Bröker M, Malerczyk C, Shibl AM. Invasive meningococcal disease and travel. J Infect Public Health. 2010 Dec;3(4):143-51.

[63] Su EL, Snape MD. A combination recombinant protein and outer membrane vesicle vaccine against serogroup B meningococcal disease. Expert Rev Vaccines. 2011 May;10(5):575-88.

[64] Bai X, Findlow J, Borrow R. Recombinant protein meningococcal serogroup B vaccine combined with outer membrane vesicles. Expert Opin Biol Ther. 2011 Jul;11(7):969-85.

[65] McIntosh D, Safadi M. Policies for Meningococcal Vaccination (accepted)

[66] Bill and Melinda Gates Foundation. Global Health program Overview. Accessed 5 August 2011. http://www.gatesfoundation.org/global-health/Documents/global-health-program-overview.pdf.

[67] Johns Hopkins. Bloomberg School of Public Health. Pneumo Action. Accessed 5 August 2011. http://www.preventpneumo.org/

[68] Laforce FM. Technology transfer to developing country vaccine manufacturers to improve global influenza vaccine production: A success story and a window into the future. Vaccine. 2011 Jul 1;29 Suppl 1:A1.

[69] The Hib initiative. Frequently asked questions. Accessed 5 August 2011. http://www.hibaction.org/hibactivities/HibFAQ.pdf

[70] Bröker M. Burden of invasive disease caused by Haemophilus influenzae type b in Asia. Jpn J Infect Dis. 2009 Mar;62(2):87-92. Review.

[71] Bröker M. Burden of invasive disease caused by Haemophilus influenzae type b in Africa. Minerva Pediatr. 2008 Jun;60(3):337-42. Review.

[72] Nigrovic LE, Thompson KM. The Lyme vaccine: a cautionary tale. Epidemiol Infect. 2007 Jan;135(1):1-8.

[73] Holst J, Martin D, Arnold R, Huergo CC, Oster P, O'Hallahan J, Rosenqvist E. Properties and clinical performance of vaccines containing outer membrane vesicles from Neisseria meningitidis. Vaccine. 2009 Jun 24;27 Suppl 2:B3-12.

[74] Memish ZA. The Hajj: communicable and non-communicable health hazards and current guidance for pilgrims. Euro Surveill. 2010 Sep 30;15(39):19671.

[75] de Whalley PC, Snape MD, Kelly DF, Banner C, Lewis S, Diggle L, John TM, Yu LM, Omar O, Borkowski A, Pollard AJ. Persistence of Serum Bactericidal Antibody One Year After a Booster Dose of Either a Glycoconjugate or a Plain Polysaccharide Vaccine Against Serogroup C Neisseria meningitidis Given to Adolescents Previously Immunized With a Glycoconjugate Vaccine. Pediatr Infect Dis J. 2011 Jun 13.

[76] Pace D. MenACWY-CRM, a novel quadrivalent glycoconjugate vaccine against Neisseria meningitidis for the prevention of meningococcal infection. Curr Opin Mol Ther. 2009 Dec;11(6):692-706.

[77] Pace D, Pollard AJ, Messonier NE. Quadrivalent meningococcal conjugate vaccines. Vaccine. 2009 Jun 24;27 Suppl 2:B30-41.

[78] Pace D. Quadrivalent meningococcal ACYW-135 glycoconjugate vaccine for broader protection from infancy. Expert Rev Vaccines. 2009 May;8(5):529-42.

[79] Bundeszentrale für gesundheitliche Aufklärung. Elternbefragung zum Thema "Impfen im Kindesalter". Ergebnisbericht. May 2011. Accessed 4 August 2011. http://www.bzga.de/forschung/studien-untersuchungen/studien/?sid=10&sub=64

[80] Clevenger LM, Pyrzanowski J, Curtis CR, Bull S, Crane LA, Barrow JC, Kempe A, Daley MF. Parents' acceptance of adolescent immunizations outside of the traditional medical home. J Adolesc Health. 2011 Aug;49(2):133-40.

[81] Vitek WS, Akers A, Meyn LA, Switzer GE, Lee BY, Beigi RH. Vaccine eligibility and acceptance among ambulatory obstetric and gynecologic patients. Vaccine. 2011 Mar 3;29(11):2024-8.

14

Laboratory Diagnosis of Meningitis

S. Nagarathna, H. B. Veenakumari and A. Chandramuki
Department of Neuromicrobiology,
National Institute of Mental Health and Neurosciences (NIMHANS),
Bengaluru Karnataka,
India

1. Introduction

Meningitis is an infection of the membranes (meninges) surrounding the brain and spinal cord. Meningitis is usually of multiple etiology-bacterial, fungal or viral yet bacteria remain the common etiological agent (Reid & Fallon, 1992). Meningitis can be acute, with a quick onset of symptoms, or chronic, lasting a month or more, or can be mild or aseptic, but the emphasis should be on identification of cause so that appropriate interventions can be applied.

Bacterial meningitis continues to be a potentially life threatening emergency with significant morbidity and mortality throughout the world and is an even more significant problem in many other areas of the world, especially in developing countries (Carbonnelle, 2009, Brouwer et al., 2010).

Types of bacteria that cause bacterial meningitis vary by age group. Currently, the average age of contracting meningitis is above 25 years with Streptococcus pneumoniae, Neisseria meningitidis and Haemophilus influenzae being the most common pathogens (Ogunlesi et al., 2005, Brain, 2004 as cited in Maleeha Aslam et al., 2006). Trauma to the skull gives bacteria the potential to enter the meningeal space. Similarly, individuals with a cerebral shunt or related device are at increased risk of infection through those devices. In these cases, infections with Staphylococci, Pseudomonas aeruginosa and other gram-negative bacilli are more likely. Recurrent bacterial meningitis may be caused by persisting anatomical defects, either congenital or acquired, or by disorders of the immune system. (Brouwer et al., 2010)

Tuberculous meningitis (TBM), is common in those from countries where tuberculosis is common, and is also encountered in those with immune problems, such as AIDS.

Despite advancement in vaccine development and chemoprophylaxis bacterial meningitis remains a major cause of death and neurological disabilities which can be prevented by rapid and accurate diagnosis with prompt treatment which is essential for good outcome (Carbonnelle, 2009).

Viral meningitis is generally less severe and clears up without specific treatment. Viral ("aseptic") meningitis is serious but rarely fatal in people with normal immune systems. Usually, the symptoms last from 7 to 10 days and the patient recovers completely. Often, in early phases of viral meningitis and bacterial meningitis, the symptoms are almost similar (Carbonnelle, 2009).

Fungal meningitis is rare, but can be life threatening. Although anyone can get fungal meningitis, people at higher risk are those who have AIDS, leukemia, or other forms of immunodeficiency. The most common cause of fungal meningitis in HIV, is Cryptococcus spp. In the last two decades, more elaborative use of intensive care units for serious medical disorders, advancements in transplant procedures and concomitant use of immunosuppressive therapies as well as the pandemic spread of HIV, etc. have increased the incidence of Central Nervous System (CNS) fungal infections which present with various clinical syndromes: meningitis commonly. The clinical picture may mimic TBM and therefore, needs careful evaluation. The CNS mycoses carry higher risks of morbidity and mortality as compared to other infective processes and therefore promptly require precise diagnosis and appropriate medical and/or surgical management strategies to optimize the outcome (Raman Sharma, 2010).

Chemical meningitis can develop after neurosurgical procedures and can be differentiated from bacterial meningitis by Cerebrospinal fluid (CSF) glucose levels and CSF White Blood Cell (WBC) values.

The causes of non-infectious meningitis include cancers, systemic lupus erythematosus, drug induced, head trauma, brain surgery etc.

2. Collection, transportation, receipt and storage of CSF

Direct testing of CSF is the most accurate way to confirm the diagnosis of bacterial meningitis. CSF should be collected from all the cases with suspected meningitis before commencement of antimicrobial therapy, unless lumbar puncture (LP) is contraindicated.

Petechial fluid can be another specimen in cases with meningococcal meningitis. Petechial lesions, if present, may be gently irrigated by injecting 0.2 ml of sterile saline solution using a small syringe with a fine needle and the fluid collected for smear and culture.

Early diagnosis is essential and is best established by laboratory examination of CSF. However, therapy should not be dependent or delayed pending lumbar puncture or laboratory results (WHO).

To initiate the definitive identification of a bacterium responsible for meningitis, CSF specimens should be obtained from patients with clinical signs and symptoms of meningitis and should be transported to the laboratory without delay. N.meningitidis, S.pneumoniae, and H.influenzae are fastidious organisms that may not survive long transit times.

The processing of a CSF specimen is one of the few clinical microbiology procedures that must be done immediately. Laboratorians should always record the date and time a specimen was received. Usually, three or more tubes of CSF are collected during a LP procedure.

The tubes should be numbered in sequential order with tube number one containing the first sample of CSF obtained. The CSF in tubes 1, 2, and 3 most often are examined for chemistry, microbiology, and cytology, respectively (Gray & Fedorko, 1992). However, the particular tests performed on tubes 2 and 3 are subjective and probably best determined by the laboratarians.

Contamination with skin flora and disinfectant will be ruled out after the first tube of CSF is collected. The probabilities of detecting microorganisms by staining and by culturing are related to the volume of specimen that is concentrated and examined (Tenney et al., 1982 as cited in Gray & Fedorko, 1992)

CSF volumes of 2 to 3 ml are usually sufficient to detect bacteria, but for mycological and mycobacterial investigations a minimum of 5 ml (preferably 10 to 15 ml) of CSF is required. If only a small amount of CSF is received with requests for multiple assays, the order of priority of the tests is determined after discussion with the physician.

The specimen should not be refrigerated before subjecting to microbiological tests as it may prevent the recovery of the organisms; fastidious organisms may not survive variations in temperature (Kasten, 1990 cited in Gray & Fedorko, 1992)

CSF specimens should be stored at room temperature or at 37°C if they cannot be processed immediately or till microscopy and bacterial cultures are performed, after which it can be refrigerated for further use (WHO).

3. Laboratory diagnosis of bacterial meningitis

Bacterial meningitis is a significant cause of mortality and morbidity worldwide. Neurological outcome and survival depend largely on damage to CNS prior to effective antibacterial treatment. Quick diagnosis and effective treatment is the key to success. The diagnostic dilemma in acute pyogenic meningitis is due to large spectrum of signs and symptoms.

3.1 Examination of CSF

The CSF should arrive still warm and either be examined immediately or placed in an incubator for examination within an hour. If delay is anticipated either in transportation to the laboratory or for examination, CSF should be divided into two containers: one in a plain bottle and the other in a bottle having a few drops of glucose broth. In the laboratory, CSF from the plain bottle can be used for making smears for staining whereas cultures are done from containers having CSF in glucose broth. The residual CSF should be preserved frozen in the CSF bank for further assessment and evaluation with evolving /additional contributory findings.

An examination of CSF involves the following:

3.1.1. Macroscopic examination.
3.1.2. Cytological examination.
3.1.3. Examination of Gram stained smear.
3.1.4. Culture and antimicrobial susceptibility testing.
3.1.5. Latex agglutination test for antigen detection.
3.1.6. Other diagnostic methods.

3.1.1 Macroscopic examination

By appearance, the CSF is normally clear like water; cloudy, purulent, bloody or pigmented CSF as per the disease states.

Hazy, cloudy, turbid CSF indicates either metastatic spread of tumors into the CNS or pleocytosis or severe meningeal infection; Opalescent CSF may be suggestive of cryptococcal meningitis. The turbid nature of the CSF is attributable to both the bacteria and leukocytes present.

Hemorrhagic CSF may be indicative of Anthrax meningitis with supportive clinical findings.

Frank clots or pellicles in CSF occur only if protein concentration exceeds 15g/L.

Xanthochromia of CSF is seen within 4 weeks of a cerebral hemorrhage.

In evaluating patients with suspected meningitis or encephalitis, a careful history along with biochemical and cellular analysis of CSF is required.

3.1.1.1 CSF glucose

CSF glucose concentrations <45 mg/dL are indicative of bacterial meningitis. (Bonadio, 1992) CSF glucose concentrations depend on serum concentrations and should always be tested on paired samples. A CSF/serum ratio cut-off of <0.4 is helpful in distinguishing between bacterial and aseptic meningitis with a sensitivity and specificity of 91% and 96%, respectively. (Genton & Berger 1990)

The individual predictors of bacterial meningitis consists of a glucose concentration of less than <40 mg/dl and a ratio of CSF to blood glucose of <23 mg/dl (Brouwer et al., 2010, Gray & Fedorko, 1992).

Chemical meningitis can be differentiated from bacterial meningitis by CSF glucose levels (< 10 mg/dL) and CSF WBC values (>7500 cells/µL) (Forgacs et al., 2001).

3.1.1.2 CSF protein

Despite typical CSF findings, the spectrum of CSF values in bacterial meningitis is so wide that the absence of one of more of the typical findings may not affect the diagnosis. In community-acquired bacterial meningitis, (CABM) only 50 percent may have a CSF glucose above 40 mg/dL (2.2 mmol/L), less than half cases may have a CSF protein below 200 mg/dL, CSF protein measurements of >55 mg/dL are diagnostic of bacterial, fungal and tubercular meningitis (Bonadio, 1992)

3.1.2 Cytological examination

In untreated bacterial meningitis, the WBC count is elevated, usually in the range of 1000–5000 cells/mm3, although this range can be quite broad (<100 to >10, 000 cells/mm3).

Bacterial meningitis usually leads to a neutrophil predominance in CSF, typically between 80% and 95%; 10% of patients with acute bacterial meningitis present with a lymphocyte predominance (defined as >50% lymphocytes or monocytes) in CSF (Tunkel et al., 2004). Preponderance of CSF polymorphonuclear cells may be used to distinguish bacterial meningitis from other causes. It is important to note that a false-positive elevation of the CSF WBC can be found after traumatic lumbar puncture, or in patients with intracerebral or subarachnoid hemorrhage in which both red blood cells and white blood cells are introduced into the subarachnoid space. In these instances, the following formula can be used as a correction factor for the true WBC count in the presence of CSF red blood cells (RBC).

$$\text{True WBC in CSF} = \text{Actual WBC in CSF} - \frac{\text{WBC in blood x RBC in CSF}}{\text{RBC in blood}}$$

Generalized seizures may also induce a transient CSF pleocytosis (primarily neutrophilic), although the CSF WBC count should not exceed 80/microL in this setting. However, CSF pleocytosis should not be ascribed to seizure activity alone unless the fluid is clear and colorless, the opening pressure and CSF glucose are normal, the CSF Gram stain is negative, and the patient has no clinical evidence of bacterial meningitis.

Since the CSF is hypotonic neutrophils may lyse, and counts may decrease by 32% after 1 hour and by 50% after 2 hours in CSF specimens, held at room temperature (Steele et al, 1986, as cited in Gray & Fedorko., 1992), hence a delay may produce a cell count that does not reflect the clinical situation of the patient.

Characteristic CSF findings for bacterial meningitis consist of polymorphonuclear pleocytosis, hypoglycorrhachia, and raised CSF protein levels (Van De Beek et al., 2006, as cited in Brouwer et al., 2010). However, low CSF WBC do occur, especially in patients with septic shock and systemic complications (Heckenberg et al, 2008 and Weisfelt, et al., 2006 as cited in Brouwer et al., 2010). A relationship between a large bacterial CSF load, lack of leukocytes response (Tauber, et al., 1992 as cited in Brouwer et al 2010.,), probably indicating excessive bacterial growth and poor cell response, is well known especially in cases of pneumococcal meningitis. (Brouwer et al., 2010)

In CABM, 10-15 percent have a CSF WBC below 100/microL (Durand et al 1993). In some proportion of the patients of CABM, around 15 percent may not exhibit characteristic CSF findings (Van de Beek et al 2004).

Some patients have milder CSF abnormalities, which cannot usually be identified. Potential causes include early presentation, recent prior antibiotic therapy etc

WBC differential may be misleading early in the course of meningitis, as in small proportion there may be an initial lymphocytic predominance and viral meningitis may initially be dominated by neutrophils. (Arevalo, 1989, as cited in Seehusen, 2003).

In our study, the cell counts of the CSF samples ranged from acellular to sheets of cells, not countable on the hemocytometer. A predominance of polymorphonuclear cells was the common feature in all cases with high cell counts.

In some facilities, clinical and management decisions are made on the cell type and the number. Thus, patients with cerebrospinal fluid pleocytosis, on further assessment, may have a preponderance of polymorphonuclear cells that would prompt a diagnosis of bacterial meningitis. 14 cases in our study had a CSF cell count of < 100 cells/cumm, 2 of which had a cell count of 10 cells/cmm and one had no cells.All these cases yielded S.pneumoniae on culture. Normal or marginally elevated CSF white cell counts are known to occur in 5-10% patients and are associated with an adverse outcome. (Van De Beek et al., 2004, as cited in Mani et al 2007)

3.1.3 Examination of Gram stained smear

It is preferable to make a smear from CSF at the time of collection itself, for direct demonstration of organisms.

The Gram stained smear made either directly from the CSF or from the centrifuged deposit can reveal not only the Gram character of the causative organism, but can also clinch the diagnosis in some cases. Gram stain may not be interpretable in grossly blood-stained samples.

Although Gram staining of CSF sediment is a very useful, cheap and fairly rapid method of identification of organism, the sensitivity in developing countries is only 25-40% (Singh, 1988, as cited in Sanya, 2007) when compared to 80-85% in developed countries (Gray & Fedorko, 1992).

CSF Gram staining may swiftly identify the causative microorganism for patients with suspected bacterial meningitis. The additional value of Gram staining for CSF culture negative patients is elucidative (Brouwer et al 2010). In 1/3rd of the cases with bacterial meningitis defined by CSF parameters may have negative CSF cultures; around 50% of the CSF culture negative patients have a positive Gram stain with equal percent of patients being pretreated with antibiotics (Bryan, 1990, as cited in Brouwer et al., 2010).

The Gram stain is positive in 10 to 15 percent of patients who have bacterial meningitis but with negative CSF cultures (Durand 1993).

In developing countries among suspected meningitis cases, CSF Gram staining can identify the causative organisms in 2/3rd, and CSF culture is positive in 1/10th of the pretreated patients (Shameem et al., 2008 as cited in Brouwer et al, 2010).

Gram staining correctly identifies the pathogen in 69 to 93% of patients with pneumococcal meningitis.

The reported yield for meningococcal meningitis is highly variable and may range from 30-89%, in a spectrum of all-ages, paediatric and untreated adult patients; (Brouwer et al., 2010)

The reported sensitivities of CSF Gram staining vary considerably for different microorganisms. CSF Gram staining correctly identifies the organism in 50 to 65% of children and in 25 to 33% in adults with H. influenzae meningitis (Brouwer et al.,).

The reported sensitivity of Gram stain for bacterial meningitis has varied from 60 to 90 percent; however, the specificity approaches 100 percent (van de Beek et al., 2004, Fitch &Van de Beek 2007). In CABM, CSF Gram stain had a sensitivity of 80 percent and specificity of 97 percent (Van de Beek 2004).The yield of both Gram stain and culture may be reduced by prior antibiotic therapy.

In our study, Gram stain provided an evidence of the causative bacteria in 253 (65.7%) patients. Our relatively high yield of pathogens on Gram stain can be attributed to the routine use of cytospin to concentrate the smear. (Mani et al 2007). The chances of recovery of bacteria in CSF Grams up to 100-fold, can be intensified by replacing conventional centrifugation with cytospin centrifugation. (Shanholtzer, et al 1982., as cited in Gray & Fedorko., 1992,). This increase is comparable to the concentration of 100 ml of CSF to a volume of 1.0 ml by conventional centrifugation. Cytospin-prepared smears not only increased the positivity of the smears, the morphology of the cells were well preserved with uniform distribution of the cells. This is especially helpful in partially treated pyogenic meningitis, which can mimic TBM posing a diagnostic dilemma for clinicians.

It is to be noted that the preliminary report of Gram staining should be conveyed immediately on the basis of initial observations.

3.1.4 Culture and antimicrobial susceptibility testing

Culture is the gold standard for determining the causative organism in meningitis. Culture of CSF is also infrequently performed in many health institutions in developing countries.

After the receipt, specimen should be cultured at the earliest. CSF should also be inoculated into enrichment medium like sodium thioglycollate broth along with solid media like enriched, selective or differential media. Incubate in air plus 5-10% carbon dioxide.

Aerobic CSF culturing techniques are obligatory for CABM. Anaerobic culture may be important for postneurosurgical or posttraumatic meningitis or for the investigation of CSF shunt meningitis.

Sensitivity of CSF culture does not exceed 40% with results available only after 2-3 days (Singh, 1988 and Gray & Fedorko, 1992 as cited in Sanya et al., 2007) While CSF culture are only positive in about 80% of the time(Coyle, 1999, Zunt, & Marra 1999), negative or inconclusive culture results may be seen in patients with partially-treated meningitis and those with atypical bacteria, and Mycobacterium tuberculosis.

In a series of 875 meningitis patients for whom the diagnosis was defined by a CSF WBC count of over 1, 000 cells per mm3 and/or more than 80% polymorphonuclear cells, the CSF culture was positive for 85% of cases in the absence of prior antibiotic treatment. CSF cultures were positive for 96% of patients if meningitis was due to H.influenzae, 87% of patients with pneumococcal meningitis, and 80% of patients with meningococcal meningitis (Bohr, et al., 1983 as cited in Brouwer et al., 2010)

The yield of CSF culture is lower for patients who have been pretreated before lumbar puncture. Pretreatment for more than 24 h is associated with a further decrease of positive CSF cultures.Two large case series reported decreases in yield from 66 to 62% and 88 to 70% if patients were pretreated with antibiotics (Bohr, et al., 1983, Nigrovic, et al.. 2008 as cited in Brouwer et al 2010,.).

A decrease in culture positivity can be expected for pretreated patients with clinically defined meningitis. Meningococcal meningitis diagnosed either by culture or by PCR can show positive CSF cultures though in low percentage of patients receiving pretreatment and 4-5 times more for those who did not receive any treatment (Bronska, 2006 as cited in Brouwer et al., 2010). In our study, 40.8% of culture positivity was noted (Mani et al., 2007) and 10% in a similar study (Shameem et al., 2008 as cited in Brouwer et al., 2010).

For patient management, physicians hardly wait for antimicrobial susceptibility reports, as the treatment is usually initiated with more than one antimicrobial agent. Nevertheless, the laboratory must have its policy regarding testing and reporting for antimicrobial susceptibility. For organisms such as N. meningitidis and beta-haemolytic streptococci with predictable susceptibility patterns, there is no need of performing antimicrobial susceptibility testing. For all other organisms antimicrobial susceptibility tests have to be performed, as per standard methodology or automated systems according to accessibility and affordability to enhance the turnaround time.

In a world of increasing resistance to antibiotics and emerging pathogens, culture combined with susceptibility testing remains the gold standard for diagnosis (Brouwer et al., 2010).

3.1.5 Latex Agglutination Test (LAT) for antigen detection

Tests are available to detect antigen in the CSF which are feasible at peripheral as well as intermediate laboratories where fundamental, preliminary facilities are not available.

Of all these tests latex agglutination is a tool for screening and is rapid, sensitive, and specific less labour-intensive, are highly sensitive and specific much more expensive than routine culture and are not available for routine use in developing countries(Sanya et al., 2007).

Kits are commercially available containing reagents for detecting antigens and the test can be performed under field conditions.

LAT detects the antigens of the common meningeal pathogens in the CSF, although these tests are not routinely recommended.

LAT is a diagnostic test that has been utilized for providing speedy results.These tests utilize serum containing bacterial antibodies or commercially available antisera directed against the capsular polysaccharides of meningeal pathogens (Tunkel et al., 2004). Agglutination with the respective latex reagents indicates presence of corresponding antigen in CSF and is diagnostic.

Antigen testing may result in few indeterminate, false negatives, and false-positives. True-positive results do not appear to modify the decision to administer antimicrobial therapy, therefore reserved for specific clinical circumstances. The suggested indications are-

- Initial negative CSF Gram staining and CSF cultures;
- Partially-treated and pretreated patients with negative CSF culture (Shivaprakash et al., 2004)

The false-negative LAT could be possibly because of low antigen titres in the CSF. It is possible that the antiserum in diagnostic LAT kits does not detect all the capsular serotypes prevalent in the particular geographical area or probably as yet unrecognized serotypes are the causative agents in such cases.

The reported sensitivities of LAT of CSF samples from patients with bacterial meningitis ranged from 78 to 100% for H. influenzae type b meningitis, 59 to 100% for pneumococcal meningitis, and 22 to 93% for meningococcal meningitis (Brouwer et al 2010.,).

In negative CSF cultures with clinical presentation and CSF parameters compatible with bacterial meningitis, CSF latex agglutination has a lower sensitivity for detecting bacteria (Tarafdar et al 2001 as cited in Brouwer et al 2010,.).

In CSF specimens positive for the causative microorganism, the positivity of the LAT can be upto 100% (Perkins, etal., 1995 as cited in Brouwer et al., 2010).

A strong decline in the sensitivity of LAT is expected among patients with antibiotic pretreatment prior to lumbar puncture (Bronska, et al., 2006, as cited in Brouwer et al 2010.,). The additional value of LAT is therefore limited.

In our study, the LAT was positive in 54.6% of cases. In the culture negative cases, LAT was positive in 49.6%, wherein 82% of these positive cases were also positive by Gram's stain, but 18% samples which did not show any evidence of the pathogen on either Gram's stain or culture, were positive by LAT, thus helping clinch the diagnosis.

A negative test does not rule out pyogenic meningitis and should be considered as an adjunct test and needs to be interpreted cautiously, considering the patient clinical condition and several other factors into consideration.

3.1.6 Other laboratory tests

3.1.6.1 Blood cultures

Blood cultures can be useful in a situation where CSF cannot be obtained before the administration of antimicrobials. Blood cultures can enhance the identification of the causative organism which follow haematogenous route to reach the meninges (WHO).

Blood cultures are often positive and valuable to detect the causative organism and establish susceptibility patterns if CSF cultures are negative. Majority of the patients with bacterial meningitis have positive blood cultures.

Blood culture positivity differs for each causative organism:

- 50 to 90% of H. influenzae meningitis
- 75% of pneumococcal meningitis and
- 40% of children and 60% of adult patients with meningococcal meningitis

Extended culture is preferred and the inoculated media should not be discarded before seven days of incubation.

Cultures obtained after antimicrobial therapy are much less likely to be positive, the yield will be decreased by 20% for pretreated (Brouwer et al 2010.,) and could be even higher in developing countries.where the patients are partially treated either by the local practitioners or due to availability of drugs over the counter because of not-so stringent policies, before they approach the referral centres.

The automated blood culture systems for example BACTEC system available in less-developed countries, has time-to-detection advantages with reasonable turnaround time, and has to be compared with standard culture techniques available at most health facilities in such countries. Therefore, culture results might be overly sensitive. Hence excluding cultures of presumed contamination and also to note what proportion of the cultures are contaminated, is of primary importance.

3.1.6.2 Polymerase Chain Reaction (PCR)

Diagnosis of bacterial meningitis has long been based on classical methods of Gram stain, culture of CSF, and serological tests. The performance of these methods, especially culture and direct smear, is thwarted by failure to detect bacteria in pretreated cases and reluctance to perform lumbar punctures at admission. Indeed, patients with meningitis frequently receive antibiotics orally or by injection before the diagnosis is suspected or established. Thus an alternative method has become necessary to help clinicians and epidemiologists for the management and control of bacterial meningitis. Nucleic acid amplification tests such as

PCR assays are highly sensitive and specific and have been evaluated for their effectiveness in detecting the presence of bacterial DNA in CSF from patients with suspected and proven bacterial meningitis.

PCR-based assays are useful adjuncts to conventional bacterial culture and antigen detection methods in establishing the bacterial etiology in meningitis in settings where substantial numbers of specimens are culture negative.

With the advent of quantitative PCR methods, monitoring prognosis of patients on therapy is possible with a greater degree of accuracy. The high sensitivities of PCR protocols ensure detection even with a minimal amount of the DNA or RNA present.

PCR may play a greater role in the diagnosis of bacterial meningitis. It has been suggested that PCR is useful in establishing the diagnosis of viral meningitis in CSF culture negative patients (Kaplan, 1999).

A study including culture-confirmed CABM evaluated the diagnostic accuracy of a broad-range PCR for H. influenzae, S. pneumoniae, and N. meningitidis had an overall specificity of 100 percent The sensitivity for H. influenzae, S. pneumoniae and N.meningitides, was 92%, 100%, and 88%; respectively (Corless et al., 2001 as cited in Brouwer et al 2010.,).

By multiplex assay, it is found that in bacterial meningitis patients defined by positive CSF culture, positive CSF Gram stain, and based on clinical suspicion with negative cultures, PCR has high sensitivities for H. influenzae, S. pneumoniae, and N. meningitidis with a specificity of 100% for all three microorganisms (Tzanakaki et al 2005., as cited in Brouwer et al.,).

In an another, study the sensitivities and specificities of multiplex PCR for CSF diagnosed by CSF culture, latex agglutination test, PCR, or Gram stain may be comparatively lower for H. influenzae, S. pneumoniae, and, N. meningitides.

The incremental value of PCR next to culture, Gram stain, and latex agglutination is high.(Parent du Châtelet et al 2005 as cited in Brouwer et al.,).

Meningococcal DNA detection by PCR has been used widely and is performed routinely for patients with suspected meningococcal meningitis and negative CSF cultures in many parts of the world (Welinder-Ol et al., 2007 as cited in Brouwer et al.,). In the United Kingdom, a large proportion of meningococcal disease cases are now diagnosed by PCR without culture (Gray et al., 2006 as cited in Brouwer et al.,) PCR detection of meningococcal DNA requires special techniques and is expensive.

Pretreatment with antibiotics may decrease the sensitivity of PCR of CSF samples compared to untreated patients (Bronska et al 2006., as cited in Brouwer et al.,). PCR can also be a useful tool for the swift typing of meningococcal strains in an evolving epidemic.

A high bacterial load determined by quantitative PCR has been associated with unfavorable outcomes of both pneumococcal and meningococcal disease (Brouwer et al 2010.).

Data on PCR detection of group B streptococci in CSF are limited, and group B streptococci have been tested only with multiplex PCR detection assays (Chiba et al 2009 as cited in Brouwer et al.,).

An initial study of the PCR detection of L. monocytogenes in patients with bacterial meningitis showed that a high concentration of bacteria in the CSF is needed for PCR detection. Recent studies of multiplex PCRs including L. monocytogenes showed lower detection thresholds. The sensitivity, specificity, and incremental value of PCR in L. monocytogenes meningitis are unclear, as only one patient was included in each of these studies (Brouwer et al., 2010).

Problems with false-positive results have been reported. In our study, PCR assay showed an overall sensitivity of 100% by positively identifying all the culture, smear and antigen positive cases. Additional cases, which could not be diagnosed by the conventional techniques, were also picked by this assay. Out of the 32 controls, the assay showed a positive result in only two cases of autopsy proven TBM cases, suggesting the possibility of a mixed underlying infection in those particular patients (Mani et al., 2007).With high prevalence of tuberculous infection in developing countries and the impaired immune status of patients, co- existent pneumococcal and tubercular meningitis may not be so uncommon (Garg et al., 2008). However, further refinements may make PCR a more useful tool in the diagnosis of bacterial meningitis in a clinical setting especially when results of CSF Gram stain and culture are negative.

3.1.6.3 Flow cytometry

Recently, flow cytometry with a dedicated bacterial channel has (Sysmex UF-1000i) possible application in automated cell counting and this novel approach in the differential diagnosis of meningitis has been explored.(Nanos, and Delanghe 2008.)

3.1.6.4 Inflammatory markers

Diagnosis and management of bacterial meningitis require various biological tests and a multidisciplinary approach.

Occasionally, there is difficulty in distinguishing bacterial meningitis from aseptic meningitis on the basis of commonly used laboratory tests. A number of recent studies strongly suggest that measurements of C- reactive protein (CRP) in CSF could reliably discriminate between them (Singh 1994). Its advantages include its very low serum levels in normal individuals, a rapid rise within 12 to 24 hours of infection and a large incremental increase thereafter. Qualitative assay of CRP is simple to perform at the bedside by medical staff. Sound clinical judgement combined with qualitative CRP assay as an adjunctive test should provide a rational basis for treatment decision in the management of bacterial meningitis. This will significantly reduce unnecessary antimicrobial therapy, ensure adequate dosage of antibiotics and will also prevent emergence of resistant strain of microorganisms (Col PL Prasad et al., 2005) especially in those situations where facilities for performing bacterial cultures of antibiotic susceptibility testing are not available (Singh 1994).

Several other analytes are reported to be of significance in the diagnosis of meningitis including adenosine deaminase, cytokines, and lactate concentrations although their diagnostic significance has yet to be established. CSF β_2-microglobulin and neopterin concentrations are used in the diagnosis of AIDS dementia complex with some success.(McArthur, et al., 1992, Watson & Scott 1995).

The limited diagnostic utility of most CSF biochemical analytes is attributable to several causes including timing of sample acquisition and the need for serial determinations of analytes. Most of these markers lack neurospecificity and in patients with a damaged blood-brain barrier, diagnostic values of intrathecal concentrations are questionable. Organism-specific antibody index evaluation is useful in determining whether the specific viral or bacterial antibody under evaluation is being synthesized intrathecally and is of tremendous diagnostic significance. (Reiber and Lange 1991). Measurements of all biochemical analytes in the CSF should be reviewed in conjunction with the albumin index; an elevated albumin index is evidence of a compromised blood-brain barrier and leakage from the serum into the CSF. Furthermore, contamination by erythrocytes from a traumatic spinal tap or intracerebral hemorrhage will cause variations in measurements; therefore, an isolated determination of CSF analytes can be an adjunctive tool for the differential diagnosis of unknown CNS disease (Thompson 1995).

Patients with listerial meningitis often do not have characteristic CSF findings, with relatively low CSF leukocyte counts and high CSF protein concentrations (Brouwer, et al., 2006 as cited in Brouwer et al., 2010). A mononuclear cell predominance in the CSF is found more frequently than for other types of bacterial meningitis (Clauss, and Lorber 2008 as cited in Brouwer etal., 2010).Listeria demonstrates "tumbling motility" in wet mounts of CSF. The yield of Gram staining for Listeria meningitis is low, ranging from 23 to 36% for both children and adults, CSF Gram stain that show diphtheroids should prompt heightened awareness for the possibility of Listeria infection, particularly in immunocompromised patient. The sensitivity, specificity, and incremental value of PCR in L. monocytogenes meningitis are unclear, as only few cases have been studied (Brouwer et al 2010).

Nocardial meningitis results in findings typical of bacterial meningitis. Since nocardiae grow slower than common bacteria, the microbiology laboratory should always be notified when nocardiosis is clinically suspected.

Meningitis caused by anaerobic bacteria is rare. It is advisable to perform anaerobic culture on cerebrospinal fluid from patients with identifiable risk factors such as when sinus, otitic or mastoid symptoms precede or accompany the onset of meningitis in children or adults. The presence of irregularly stained gram negative rods in the CSF or meningitis unresponsive to empiric antibiotics should also raise the suspicion of anaerobic infection (sree neelima et al., 2004).

CSF analysis has been reported to be normal for 20% of patients with culture-proven nosocomial meningitis (Weisfeltet al., 2007).

In case of anthrax meningitis, the CSF is grossly hemorrhagic with few PMN neutrophils and numerous gram-positive bacilli.

In patients with purulent CSF indices with no evidence of bacteria on Gram smear it is very important to examine a wet mount of CSF for amebic trophozoites. Molecular methods have also been developed for the rapid identification of meningoencephalitis caused by Naegleria.

Adults with S. agalactiae meningitis have typical CSF findings(Domingo, 1997and Dunne and Quagliarello, 1993, as cited in Brouwer et al 2010).CSF WBC counts are inconclusive for many neonates with meningitis due to S. agalactiae with a normal CSF examination in a very small proportion of patients (Ginsberg, 2004, as cited in Brouwer et al, 2010).

Lyme disease is caused by Burkohlderia burgdorferi (B. burgdorferi) and is known to be neurotropic. The results of laboratory testing among patients with neurologic Lyme disease vary depending on the stage of the illness. In very early CNS involvement (meningismus) or late-stage infection (encephalopathy), the CSF may appear normal.When clinical signs of meningitis or encephalitis are present, CSF may reveal a mononuclear pleocytosis, mildly increased protein, and, in some cases, an elevated IgG index or oligoclonal immunoglobulins. Intrathecal anti- B. burgdorferi antibody production is present in 70%-90% of patients with Lyme meningitis (Coyle 1992 as cited in Brian and Jenifer1994). Given the limitations of diagnostic tests, clinicians need to consider clinical factors that would aid in the diagnosis of Lyme disease. These include a history of an erythema migrans rash or Ixodes tick bite, exposure to a Lyme endemic area, and the combination of neuropsychiatric and extraneural symptoms as it is a multisystemic illness. Once in the CNS, B. burgdorferi, like T. pallidum, may remain latent, only to cause illness months to years later. (Logigian 1990 as cited in Brian and Jenifer 1994).

4. Important points in diagnosis

Acute bacterial meningitis is a life threatening condition and specimen deserves immediate processing and diagnosis is best established by laboratory examination of CSF.

If there is an insufficient volume of sample for carrying out all the investigations, prioritize the tests as per the medical advice.

The CSF should be examined fresh at the earliest, as on storage cells disintegrate and produce a cell count that does not reflect the true clinical situation.

Cell count to be performed on the uncentrifuged CSF specimen.

When a clot is present in CSF, it invalidates the CSF cell count.

Results of cell count and type, Gram stain, antigen detection assays etc. and positive cultures must be conveyed to the physician caring for the patient (if possible) as soon as the results are available, and a permanent record of the communication and the name of the person who was notified of the initial results should be made.(WHO)

The management of the patient should be based on immediate cell-count and Gram stain smear results.

Notify to the public health authorities on isolation/detection of any epidemic prone pathogens (e.g. N.meningitidis).

5. Tuberculous meningitis (TBM)

The non-specific clinical and cerebrospinal fluid (CSF) features have made TBM often difficult to diagnose with certainty, especially at early stages and has to be differentiated from a plethora of other infectious and non-infectious meningitis such as viral, bacterial cryptococcal or carcinomatous meningitis, often resulting in diagnostic dilemma.TBM is usually diagnosed when irreversible neurologic damages have already taken place and on firm clinical suspicion, immediate anti-tuberculosis therapy is recommended, regardless of the results of the tests. Early and reliable diagnosis of TBM still poses a great challenge though delay in diagnosis and treatment is regarded as major contributing factor.

In cases of TBM, the CSF pressure is typically higher than normal, appear clear or slightly turbid. If the CSF is left to stand, a fine clot resembling a pellicle or cobweb may form. This faintly visible "spider's web clot" is due to the very high level of protein in the CSF, typical of this condition. In proven cases of TBM, hemorrhagic CSF also has been recorded attributing to fibrinoid degeneration of vessels and hemorrhage.

CSF typically has lymphocytic pleocytosis.In adults, the mean WBC count averages around 223 cells/µL (range, 0-4000 cells/µL), while the proportion with neutrophilic pleocytosis (>50% neutrophils) averages 27% (range, 15-55%) and the proportion with normal cell count averages 6% (range, 5-15%). In children, these numbers are 200 cells/µL (range, 5-950 cells/µL), 21% (range, 15-30%), and 3% (range, 1-5%), respectively. (Gracia - monco 1999)

Usually, there is shift to lymphocytic predominance over the ensuing 24 to 48 hours (Verdon et al., 1996 as cited in Gracia - monco 1999), although occasionally neutrophils persist, resulting in the so called persistent neutrophilic meningitis (Peacock as cited in Gracia - monco 1999). This syndrome can also occur in HIV infected patients, particularly when meningitis is caused by multidrug resistant mycobacteria (Sánchez-Portocarrero et al 1996., as cited in Gracia - monco 1999). In 20-25 % of HIV negative patients neutrophilic predominance is present (Verdon et al 1996., as cited in Gracia - monco 1999). It has also been described in immunocompromised patients who are not infected with HIV with TBM. (Mizullani et al 1993 as cited in Gracia - monco 1999).

For patients with HIV and/or immunosuppression, while the mean WBC count in the CSF is 230 cells/µL, as many as 16% of HIV-infected patients may have acellular CSF, compared with 3-6% of HIV-negative patients. Patients whose CSF samples are acellular may show pleocytosis if a spinal tap is repeated 24-48 hours later. The proportion who have neutrophilic pleocytosis of the CSF (>50% neutrophils) is 42% (range, 30-55%). (Gracia - monco 1999).

Within a few days after commencement of anti-TB therapy, the initial mononuclear pleocytosis may change briefly in some patients to one of polymorphonuclear predominance, which may be associated with clinical deterioration, coma, or even death. This therapeutic paradox has been regarded by some authors as virtually pathognomonic of TBM. (Smith1975 as cited in Gracia - monco 1999). This syndrome is probably the result of an uncommon hypersensitivity reaction to the massive release of tuberculoproteins into the subarachnoid space. (O Toole et al., 1969 and Udani et al., 1971 as cited in Gracia - monco 1999).

CSF cell counts and cell morphology by cytospin studies form an important preliminary step in TBM diagnosis.Identifying the atypical polymorphonuclear predominance and at times acellular forms of TBM is essential. The appearance of reactive monocytes and floating tubercles, which are clumps of reactive monocytes with mononuclear cells such as small lymphocytes and polymorphonuclear cells, are diagnostic of TBM. Giant cells are multinucleated inflammatory cells and are observed in 5 % and floating tubercles in 23 % of cases of TBM by routine CSF cytospin studies, as per the experience of studying a large number of CSF samples of TBM cases.

The proportion with depressed glucose levels (< 45 mg/dL or 40% of serum glucose) averages 72% (range, 50-85%) for adults and 77% (range, 65-85%) for children. (Gracia - monco 1999)

CSF typically has an elevated protein level, and marked hypoglycorrhachia. The mean protein level in adults averages 224 mg/dL (range, 20-1000 mg/dL), and in children it is 219 mg/dL (range, 50-1300 mg/dL). The proportion with a normal protein content averages 6% (range, 0-15%) for adults and 16% (range, 10-30%) for children.

While HIV-infected patients generally have a mean protein level of 125 mg/dL (range, 50-200 mg/dL), as many as 43% of the patients may have a normal CSF protein content. The proportion who have depressed CSF glucose levels (< 45 mg/dL or 40% of serum glucose) averages around 69% (range, 50-85%).

If tuberculosis is suspected, the presence of normal protein and glucose levels, and even the absence of white cells in the CSF, should not be considered a reason for not processing with a search for tubercle bacilli both on stained CSF specimens and in culture. (Gracia - monco 1999)

Direct Ziehl-Neelsen (ZN) staining of the cerebrospinal fluid for acid-fast bacilli remains the cornerstone of rapid diagnosis, but this technique lacks sensitivity, but requires large volumes of CSF, and meticulous microscopy to achieve the best results. One of the underlying difficulties is due to the fact that tubercle bacilli are paucibacillary and are shed intermittently in the CSF.It has been recommended that collection of three to four serial samples and spinning of large volumes of CSF for 30 minutes may enhance the rate of detection of AFB in smear microscopy. However, repeat collection of such large volume of CSF is practically impossible. Though less sensitive, smear microscopy is a simple, rapid, cost effective adjunct for the diagnosis of TBM.

A positive smear result is present in an average of 25% (range, 5-85%) of adults and only 3% (range, 0-6%) of children, whereas the numbers with a positive CSF culture average 61% (range, 40-85%) and 58% (range, 35-85%) for adults and children, respectively. (Gracia - monco 1999).

Cultures of CSF by the conventional method using Lowenstein Jenseen(LJ) medium can take 4 to 8 weeks. Automated AFB culture system provides a highly sensitive and rapid tool for the isolation and drug susceptibility testing of MTB, from CSF of TBM patients. Use of a solid medium in conjunction with the automated systems like BACTEC 12B medium is essential for optimal recovery of MTB from CSF specimens. (Venkataswamy et al., 2007 and Jalesh et al., 2010). Drug-resistant tuberculosis is an increasing problem worldwide. MDR TBM was observed in 2.4% of cases (Nagarathna et al., 2008) Several PCR-based tests are also designed for the rapid detection of MDR TB Strains.

Among HIV, on an average the number of positive CSF culture is 23%.

CSF culture for mycobacteria (Gracia - monco 1999) must be processed in a biological safety cabinet.

Indirect modes of diagnosing TBM are by the use of immunodiagnostic methods. These are alternative and adjunctive tests and not confirmatory for TBM diagnosis. These methods have been evaluated, but there are variable immune responses in TBM patients at different stages of the infection posing a barrier to the detection of mycobacterial antibodies in CSF samples. The patients at the chronic stages of TBM have a myriad of antibody responses to all major antigens of MTB, while patients at the early stages have lower detectable antibody response. In addition, interpretation of mycobacterial antibodies in the CSF must take into account the contribution of antibodies from the plasma for correlative interpretation.

Genomic analysis and antigen mining of MTB have yielded novel, more specific antigens, such as early secretory antigenic target 6 (ESAT-6), 38-kDa antigen, 11kda. One approach to provide direct evidence of existing infection is the detection of the presence of specific antigens in the circulating CSF. The immunological tests especially the ELISA can be used to detect MTB antigens such as Lipoarabinomannan (LAM) 38 kDa antigen, A60 antigen, antigen 5 and 6 by use of epitope specific monoclonal antibodies. Nevertheless, the diagnostic efficiency of the antigen-based approach is still unsatisfactory.

The antibody detection ELISA are the more popular test utilized in immunodiagnosis. These can be utilized to detect either the total antimycobacterial Antibodies using the MTSE (MTB soluble extract) or specific antibody to defined antigens such as LAM, 38 kDa, A 60, 30kDa 1,6kDa. There are several secretory MTB antigens defined to detect humoral immune responses: some of these are early secretory antigenic target 6 (ESAT-6), ag85 complex, MPT63, MPT 64, MPT 70, 14 kDa, 19KDa, 38 kDa, 85B, 45/47, ORF 9, ORf 10 and culture filtrate (CF) antigens. The overall percentage of TBM diagnosis, by immune diagnosis, does not exceed 70 to 87 % (Akepati 1989, Chandramuki 1989, Akepati et al., 2002) Detection of mycobacterial immune complexes (IgG and IgM) also aid in the diagnosis of large proportion of TBM cases (Patil et al., 1996).

A number of strategies have been attempted to improve the laboratory diagnosis of TBM. Nucleic acid amplification tests (NAAT) show potential roles in confirming the diagnosis of TBM.

PCR is the most widely applied alternative rapid diagnostic technique for TBM. A prospective large scale study to evaluate the efficacy of an in-house developed IS6110 uniplex PCR in the diagnosis of clinically suspected of TBM showed all culture-positive samples were positive by the PCR assay. The assay was found to be positive in 70% of the samples with a clinical diagnosis of TBM with an observed sensitivity of 76.37% (negative predictive value 59.90%) and a specificity of 89.18% (positive predictive value 94.69%). A diagnostic accuracy of 80% was seen in patients with a clinical diagnosis of TBM. Patients with a clinical diagnosis of TBM were found to be 9.38 times more likely to be PCR-positive (Rafi et al., 2007).

MTB belongs to the group of intracellular bacteria, which replicate within resting macrophages. During the early stages of the CNS infection, the tubercle bacilli in the CSF are immediately phagocytosed by the macrophages, leading to the scarcity of mycobacterial markers in the circulating CSF. Thus, no such tests have yet become available for early diagnosis of active TBM with the requisite sensitivity and specificity.

Use of neurochemical markers has been investigated in patients with TBM wherein decreased levels of taurine and vitamin B-12 and increased levels of phenylalanine were noted in patients with TBM. Levels of nitrite, its precursor arginine and homocysteine were significantly higher in patients with TBM.

Adenosine deaminase activity measurement could be an inexpensive, valuable tool in the diagnosis of early TBM. (Janvier et al., 2010). Despite its many limitations, tuberculin skin test an indirect test to demonstrate the cell mediated immune response in the body to mycobacterial antigens which by necessity, remains in widespread use. The Centers for Disease Control and Prevention, the American Thoracic Society, and the Infectious Disease Society of America have updated the guidelines, and they are quite useful in practice. Cutoff points for induration (5, 10, or 15 mm) for determining a positive test result vary based on the pretest category into which the patient falls. Negative results from the purified protein derivative test do not rule out tuberculosis, if the 5-tuberculin test skin test result is negative, repeat the test with 250-tuberculin test. Note that this test is often nonreactive in persons with TBM.

A combination of direct microscopy on ZN staining, culture by conventional LJ media and automated culture system in clinically suspected cases, supported by other laboratory parameters increases the sensitivity of diagnosing TBM as compared to any single method.

TBM still remains a diagnostic challenge because of inconsistent clinical presentation and lack of rapid, sensitive and specific tests. The ideal diagnostic test for TBM should combine acceptable sensitivity and specificity with speed, low cost and ease of execution in a clinical laboratory in developing countries where the disease is more prevalent.Finally the success of TBM diagnosis depends on continued dialogue and collaboration between attending physician and/or laboratarian, medical microbiologist, immunologist, chemical analyst, molecular biologist and pathologist.

Failure to respond to treatment should prompt a search for fungal infections or malignancy.

6. Fungal meningitis

Fungal meningitis is rare, but can be life threatening. The most common cause of fungal meningitis among people with immune system deficiencies, like HIV, is Cryptococcus, Candida, which can lead to meningitis in rare cases, especially in pre-mature babies with very low birth weight. People with immunodeficiencies are at a higher risk for histoplasma meningitis. Histoplasma is found primarily in soil or bird/bat droppings in the Midwestern United States, although it can be seen in other places. Soil in Southwestern United States and northern Mexico contain the fungus Coccidioides, which can cause fungal meningitis. People at higher risk include African Americans, Filipinos, pregnant women in the third trimester, and immunocompromised persons.

Lumbar puncture is also part of the routine evaluation. CSF is tested for opening pressure WBC and differential, glucose, protein, culture, antibodies/antigens, India ink stain (Cryptococcus). However, repeated sampling is often required because diagnosis of non-HIV-associated cryptococcal meningitis, coccidioidal meningitis, histoplasmosis, and candidal meningitis can be difficult.

Up to three sets of blood cultures should be taken in all patients; they may be positive when candidal, histoplasmal, or cryptococcal meningitis is associated with disseminated disease.

CSF analysis usually reveals lymphocytic pleocytosis with raised protein and low sugar levels. In our study, 52% of the patients had < 20 cells/cmm while only 20% had > 100 cells/cmm. The diagnosis of cryptococcal meningitis can be established with India ink stain in > 50% of the cases of cryptococcal meningitis in HIV-negative cases and in > 90% of patients with AIDS (Satishchandra et al., 2007).

The India ink or Nigrosin should be shaken well before every wet mount preparation. Too much stain makes the background too dark and the stain should be regularly checked for quality control, contamination by examining just the stain under a microscope. It will be positive when about 10^3 -10^4 colony-forming units (CFU)/ml are present in a CSF sample.

AIDS patients have larger concentrations of yeast ranging between 10^{5}-10^{7} CFU/ml (Satishchandra et al., 2007)

False positive readings may occur with air bubbles, myelin globules or RBC and leukocytes. Air bubbles under high power, will be hollow and will not show the typical cell with characteristic nuclei. Monocytes and neutrophils have a crenated margin (and not the entire margin as is seen in cryptococcal cell) and will not show the characteristic refractive cell inclusions, and the luminous halo around the cell is not well demarcated like in Cryptococcus. Centrifuging the CSF to 500 rpm for about 10 minutes and performing India ink stain on the pellet can improve the sensitivity of this test. (Casadevall and Perfect.1998, as cited in Satishchandra et al., 2007)

The CSF sample should also be evaluated for cryptococcal antigen assay that is positive in almost all cases except very early in the disease or in those with very high titers due to prozone effect and in certain patients with cryptococcomas. (Brew BJ 2001, as cited in Satishchandra et al., 2007)

The methods used for antigen detection are latex agglutination test and enzyme immunoassay and are > 90% sensitive and specific. Cryptococcal antigen titers usually decrease with treatment, but it can remain at low titers for long periods even after effective therapy. (Lu, 2005 as cited in Satishchandra et al., 2007)

Antigen testing should go hand in hand with culture, since low levels of antigen titre persist for a long time even after clearance of the organism from CSF. Occasional false positive reaction is also encountered, particularly in the presence of rheumatoid factor or infection with the yeast Trichosporon spp. Pronase treatment is necessary when serum, instead of CSF, is to be tested.

A positive fungal culture is the gold standard for diagnosis of Cryptococcal infection and CSF samples show fungal growth in almost all the cases. In our series, fungal cultures grew C. neoformans in 100% of the cases. Fungal cultures also help to determine the species of the infecting organism and sensitivities to various antifungal agents. Globally, all cases of Cryptococcosis in AIDS patients are due to var grubii, followed by var neoformans. Our observations highlight the fact that the rate of C.gattii in this part of the country is comparatively low (2.8%) (Nagarathna et al., 2010). Drug susceptibility testing of the fungal isolates is not routinely done except in cases of recurrent disease. (Satishchandra et al., 2007) and has become important due to emerging antifungal resistant fungi causing infections in patients with AIDS. However, in a pilot study conducted by us did not reveal resistance to any of the routine antifungal drugs.

The routine processing of CSF for chronic meningitis and subacute meningitis cases for fungal culture is a good surveillance procedure so as not to miss any Cryptococcal, Candidial and occasionally the Cladosporial CNS infections This is more essential because of the incidence of HIV. In disseminated Cryptococcal infections, additional sampling of sputum, urine and blood is useful. The fungus often isolated is Cryptococcus. The other CNS fungal agents are almost never isolated except rarely the Cladosporium. Cytospin studies can identify the yeasts when India ink preparation is negative.

Pan-fungal PCR has been a promising aid in rapid, early diagnosis of invasive fungal infection (IFI).On the other hand, it has the potential to detect all fungal species.

Epidemiological studies now indicate that the spectrum of fungal pathogens has expanded well beyond Aspergillus fumigatus and Candida species (Pfaller and Diekema. 2004. as cited in Lau et al., 2007). However, current culture-based phenotypic methods are insensitive and slow, may initially be nonspecific, and require considerable expertise for correct morphological identification of less common or unusual fungi (Alexander, and Pfaller. 2006, Chen et al., 2002 as cited in Lau et al., 2007). Additional drawbacks of conventional culture include the failure of zygomycetes to grow

- when hyphal cells have been damaged during processing (Larone, 2002 as cited in Lau et al., 2007)
- or the collection of tissue biopsy specimens directly into formalin fixative for paraffin embedding when IFIs are not suspected clinically (Iwen 2002 as cited in Lau et al., 2007)
- or when limited material is available.

Recent efforts to improve the sensitivity and specificity of diagnostic tests have focused on culture-independent methods, in particular nucleic acid-based methods, such as PCR assays. These can be applied to fresh and formalin-fixed, paraffin-embedded sections. Numerous studies have highlighted the advantages of using PCR technology to detect viable and nonviable fungal pathogens in a variety of clinical specimens. The majority of assays target multicopy genes, in particular the ribosomal DNA (rDNA) genes (18S, 28S, and 5.8 S) and the intervening internal transcribed spacer (ITS) regions (ITS1 and ITS2), in order to maximize sensitivity and specificity.

To date, most assays have been designed to detect Candida or Aspergillus species only. Given that more than 200 fungal species have been reported to cause disease in humans and companion animals, the clinical utility of a species-specific or even a genus-specific assay is limited. Sequence-based identification of PCR products is a sensitive alternative, provided that accurate sequences have been submitted to public databases, e.g., GenBank. A panfungal PCR assay targeting the internal transcribed spacer 1 (ITS1) region of the ribosomal DNA gene cluster successfully detected and identified the fungal pathogen in 93.6% and 64.3% of culture-proven and solely histologically proven cases of IFI, respectively. A diverse range of fungal genera were identified, including species of Candida, Cryptococcus, Trichosporon, Aspergillus, Fusarium, Scedosporium, Exophiala, Exserohilum, Apophysomyces, Actinomucor, and Rhizopus. The results support the use of the panfungal PCR assay in combination with conventional laboratory tests for accurate identification of fungi in tissue specimens. (Lau et al., 2007).

Galactomannan(GM) is a component of the cell wall of the mould Aspergillus and is released during growth. Detection of GM in blood is used to diagnose invasive aspergillosis infections in humans. Eg Platelia galactomannan enzyme immunoassay (Bio-Rad). Although the test is approved by the FDA for use with patients with neutropenia and those undergoing stem cell transplantation, controversy about the test's utilization exists. Although initial results were promising, various sensitivities and specificities (29 to 99%) have been reported recently in prospective studies (Zedek and Miller 2006). The Aspergillus GM test was performed on CSF and serum. Detection of Aspergillus GM in CSF may be diagnostic of cerebral aspergillosis. It is suggested that the Aspergillus CSF GM index might be diagnostic for cerebral aspergillosis in patients at high risk for aspergillosis and with a compatible neurological disease. (Claudio Viscoli et al., 2002).

A positive result supports a diagnosis of invasive aspergillosis (IA) and should be considered in correlation with clinical condition, microbiologic culture, histological examination of biopsy specimens, and radiographic evidence, and other laboratory parameters.

A negative result does not rule out the diagnosis of IA.When there is a strong suspicion of IA, repeat testing is recommended. Patients at risk of IA should have a baseline serum tested and should be monitored twice a week for increasing GM antigen levels. GM antigen levels may be useful in the assessment of therapeutic response. Antigen levels decline in response to antimicrobial therapy. False-positive results are reported to occur at rates of 8% to 14%.

The Glucatell (1r3)-β-D-glucan (BG) detection assay was studied as a diagnostic adjunct for IFIs and a serum BG level of 60 pg/mL was chosen as the cutoff. IFIs included candidiasis, fusariosis, trichosporonosis, and aspergillosis. Absence of a positive BG finding had a 100% negative predictive value, and the specificity of the test was 90% for a single positive test result and 96% for 2 sequential positive results. The Glucatell serum BG detection assay is highly sensitive and specific as a diagnostic adjunct for IFI.

Glucatell assay may be a useful diagnostic adjunct for the diagnosis of invasive fungal infection, particularly in high-risk populations. The positivity of this test, particularly when used in a serial fashion, often precedes the microbiological or clinical diagnosis of invasive fungal infection. This cell wall component has the advantage of being present and detectable in a variety of fungal infections. (Zekaver etal., 2004).

7. Cysticercal meningitis

At NIMHANS, at the department of Neuromicrobiology, the neurocysticercal immunology has revealed anticysticercal antibody in CSF of approximately 5-10 % of cases, involves the use of whole cyst antigen often called porcine cyst sonicated, partially purified antigens such as antigen B, defined antigens such as 8-10 kDa, 23kDa, 64-68 kDa by EITB, antigens secreted while cysts are maintained invitro, namely excretory /secretory (E/S) antigens. Qualitative ELISA kit for the detection of anticysticercal antibodies in CSF, which uses purified E/S antigens of Cysticercus cellulosae maintained *in vitro,* was developed by the department of Neuromicrobiology in collaboration with Astra Research laboratory/organization E/S antigens of Cysticercus cellulosae for use in immunodiagnosis and vaccine preparation (CYSTI-CheX) *European patent WO/90/08958, 1990-dtd 9/7/1991.*The inclusion of anticysticercal antibody especially applied to CSF in endemic countries should form a routine laboratory test, as Neurocysticercosis can have protean clinical manifestations.

8. Carcinomatous meningitis

Leptomeningeal carcinomatosis occurs in approximately 5% of patients with cancer. The shedding of atypical and malignant cells into the subarachnoid space can itself trigger meningitic inflammation which is influenced by the inflammatory cells such as polymorphonuclear cells and mononuclear cells along with atypical CSF cells. The definitive identification of the tumour cells in CSF can provide useful information about the cause of chronic meningitis and nature of the malignant meningitis whether primary or secondary metastasis.

The best mode available is the cytological examination of CSF by cytospin in all cases of chronic meningitis. Atypical or definitive malignant cells in the CSF can arise from primary

CNS tumours such as ependymoma, choroids plexus papilloma, pinealoma, medulloblastoma, glioblastoma multiforme and many other tumors or secondary metastasis in the CNS, originating from bronchopulmonary, breast, or ovarian malignancies.

- Tests to aid in the diagnosis of TBM-
- CSF cell analysis using cell counting chamber and cytospin, acid fast smear examination of cytospin smear, either by Kinyouns or Ziehl Neelsen stain, or auramine O staining, CSF culture by conventional methods on LJ slopes or Middlebrook liquid media, and or by using automated systems. Detection of Mycobacterial DNA by polymerase chain reaction, adjunctive add on tests by immunological modes to detect mycobacterial antigens, antimycobacterial antibodies / mycobacterial immune complexes.Multimodal approach is essential in the diagnosis of TBM.
- Tests to detect anticysterical antibodies in CSF and / serum samples.
- Serum /CSF VDRL and Treponema pallidum particle agglutination test tests to rule out or establish Neurosyphilis.
- CSF cytospin to detect atypical / malignant cells to aid in diagnosis of secondary or primary CNS neoplasia.
- Mycological exercises on CSF 1 by India ink, Cryptococcal antigen tests and culture to establish Cryptococcal aetiology
- CSF C- reactive protein assay to establish chronic microbial aetiology especially partially treated pyogenic meningitis.
- Additional tests to rule out /establish neurobrucellosis, neuroborreliosis, neuroaids.
- Wetmout preparation to detect motile acanthamoeba species in CSF t establish cases of primary amoebic granulomatous meningitis.
- Meningeal biopsy and histology, only in exceptional cases of idiopathic chronic meningitis.Microarrays, or biochips, are a new technology that can allow rapid detection of bacterial genetic materials. The microarray method provides a more accurate and rapid diagnostic tool for bacterial meningitis compared to traditional culture methods. Clinical application of this new technique may reduce the potential risk of delay in treatment. (Ben et al., 2008)

Inadequacy of current diagnostic tools for bacterial meningitis is typical of less-developed countries. Properly interpreted test is a key tool in the diagnosis of a variety of diseases. Proper evaluation of CSF depends on knowing which tests to order, normal ranges for the patient's age, and the test's limitations. Diagnostic uncertainty can be decreased by using accepted corrective formulae. (carbonnelle.E). Although improvement in diagnosis is urgently required, the emphasis should be on identification of causes so that appropriate interventions can be applied. (GE Enwere)

9. Quality assurance (QA)

Follow manufacturer's instructions for media and diagnostic kits.
Follow standard QA procedures for laboratory equipment and test methods.

10. Biosafety

- Perform all work on suspected isolates in a safety cabinet.
- Wash hands particularly after collection and handling of the clinical specimen.
- Use leak proof containers in sealed plastic bags for transportation of the sample.

11. Referral and notification

Isolates associated with clustering, outbreaks, diagnostic dilemma, epidemiological importance, with unusual or unexpected resistance patterns have to be notified/referred, for confirmation, strain characterization antimicrobial susceptibility testing, serotyping etc.

12. Acknowledgement

Dr P Satishchandra Director and Vice-Chancellor, Professor of Neurology NIMHANS Bengaluru Karnataka, India.

13. References

Akepathi. C., Bothamley, GH., Brennan, PJ., Ivanyi.J., 1989 M Levels of antibody to defined antigens of Mycobacterium tuberculosis in tuberculous meningitis. *J Clin Microbiol,.* Vol, 27, 5, May;:821-25.

Akepati, C., Konstantin, L., Haradara Bahubali, V., Khanna, N., Pier, NB., Mandavalli, G., Parthasarathy, S., Sursarla Krishna, S., Vasanthapuram, R., Philip, A., Vishnu, KG., & Gennaro, ML 2002 Detection of Antibody to Mycobacterium tuberculosis Protein Antigens in the Cerebrospinal Fluid of Patients with Tuberculous Meningitis.*J Infect Dis,* 186, vol 5, 678-683.

Ben RJ, Kung S, Chang FY, Lu JJ, Feng NH, Hsieh YD 2008.Rapid diagnosis of bacterial meningitis using a microarray. *J Formos Med Assoc.* 107, 6, Jun, 448-53.

Blood Safety and Clinical Technology Guidelines on Standard Operating Procedures for Microbiology Chapter 13-Pyogenic Meningitis world health organization.

Bonadio WA. 1992 The cerebrospinal fluid: physiologic aspects and alterations associated with bacterial meningitis. *Pediatr Infect Dis J,* 11:423-32.

Brouwer, MC., Tunkel, AR., van de Beek D.and van de Beek D 2010. Epidemiology, Diagnosis, and Antimicrobial Treatment of Acute Bacterial Meningitis. *Clin Microbiol Rev,* Vol. 23, No. 3 July pp. 467-492.

Carbonnelle E. (2009) Laboratory diagnosis of bacterial meningitis: usefulness of various tests for the determination of the etiological agent. *Med Mal Infect.* Vol 39, Issue (7-8), Jul-Aug; PP 581-605.

Chandramuki A., 1989., Rapid diagnosis of tuberculous meningitis by ELISA to detect mycobacterial antigen and antibody in the cerebrospinal fluid *J Infect Dis.* Vol 160, 2, Aug;343-4.

Claudio, V., Marco, Machetti, M., Gazzola., P., Maria, De Andrea.., Paola, D., Maria Van Lint, MT., Gualandi, F., Truini, M., & Bacigalup, 2002 Aspergillus Galactomannan Antigen in the Cerebrospinal Fluid of Bone Marrow Transplant Recipients with Probable Cerebral Aspergillosis *Journal of Clinical Microbiology,* Vol. 40, No. 42., Apr, p. 1496–1499

Col Prasad, PL., Brig Nair, MNG., Lt Col Kalghatgi, AT. 2005, Childhood Bacterial Meningitis and Usefulness of C - reactive protein *MJAFI;* 61, 13-15.

Coyle PK. 1999; Overview of acute and chronic meningitis. *Neurol Clinics,* vol 17, (4), 691-710.

Durand, ML., Calderwood, SB., Weber, DJ., Miller SI, Southwick FS, Caviness VS Jr, Swartz MN.1993; Acute bacterial meningitis in adults. A review of 493 episodes. *N Engl J Med,* 328(1), Jan 7, 21-8.

Enwere GE Obaro SK 2001, Diagnosis of bacterial meningitis.*The Lancet*, Vol 358, Issue 9292, 3 November Pp1549,

Fitch MT, van de Beek D. 2007; Emergency diagnosis and treatment of adult meningitis. *Lancet Infect Dis* 7:191-200.

Forgacs, P., Geyer, CA and Freidberg, SR. 2001; Characterization of chemical meningitis after neurological surgery. *Clin Infect Dis* 32:179-85.

Garcia -Monco Juan C.1999Central nervous system tuberculosis *Neurologic clinics* vol 17 no4 pp737-759.

Garg, N., Rafi, W., Nagarathna, S., Chandramuki, A., Seshagiri, SK., Pal, Pramod K.& Satish, S. 2008 Co-existent pneumococcal and tubercular mixed meningitis in heterozygous sickle cell disease: a case report. *Int J Infect Dis*, Sep;12(5):560-2..

Genton, B.&Berger JP.1990. Cerebrospinal fluid lactate in 78 cases of adult meningitis. *Intensive Care Med*, 16, 196-200.

Gray, LD.& Fedorko, DP.1992, Laboratory Diagnosis of Bacterial Meningitis *Clinical Microbiology Reviews*Vol.5, No.2 p 130-145.

Jalesh NP., Nagaraja, D.,.Subbakrishna, K., Venkataswamy, MM., &Chandramuki, A. 2010 Role of the BACTEC radiometric method in the evaluation of patients with clinically probable tuberculous meningitis *Ann Indian Acad Neurol*, vol13(2): Apr-Jun 128–131

Janvier F, Servonnet A, Delacour H, Fontan E, Ceppa F, &Burnat P. 2010 Value of assaying adenosine deaminase level in patients with neuromeningeal tuberculosis. *Med Trop (Mars)*, ;70, Feb 1, 88-93.

Kaplan SL 1999 Bacterial meningitis -Clinical presentations, diagnosis, and prognostic factors of bacterial meningitis. *Infect Dis Clin North Am*; 13(3):579-94

Lau, A., Chen, S., Sorrell, T., Carter, D., Malik, R., Martin, P, &Halliday, C. 2007 Development and Clinical Application of a Panfungal PCR Assay To Detect and Identify Fungal DNA in Tissue Specimens *Journal of Clinical Microbiology*, Vol. 45,, No. 2,. Feb380-385.

Maleeha, A., Rubeena, H., & Tahir, M.2006 Bacterial meningitis:A diagnostic approach Biomedica Vol.22 Jul. - Dec/Bio-13 (A)

Mani, R., Pradhan, S., Nagarathna, S., Wasiulla, R., Chandramuki, A. 2007. Bacteriological profile of community acquired acute bacterial meningitis.A ten-year retrospective study in a tertiary neurocare centre in South India. *Indian J Med Microbiol* 25:108-14

McArthur JC, Nance-Sproson TE, Griffin DE, Hoover D, Selnes OA, Miller EN, Margolick JB, Cohen BA, Farzadegan H, Saah A. 1992The diagnostic utility of elevation in cerebrospinal fluid beta2- microglobulin in HIV-1 dementia. *Neurology*, 42, 1707-12.

Nagarathna S, Veena Kumari, HB., Arvind, N., Divyalakshmi, A., Chandramuki, A., Satishchandra, P. and Ravi, V.2010Prevalence of Cryptococcus gattii causing meningitis in a tertiary neurocare center from south India, a pilot study. *Indian J Pathol Microbiol*, 53, 4, 855-56

Nagarathna S, Rafi W, Veenakumari HB, Mani R, Satishchandra P, Chandramuki A. 2008 Drug susceptibility profiling of tuberculous meningitis.*Int J Tuberc Lung Dis*, vol12, (1), Jan, 105-7

Nanos NE, Delanghe JR. 2008 Evaluation of Sysmex UF-1000i for use in cerebrospinal fluid analysis *Clin Chim Acta*. Jun;392(1-2):30-3.

Patil SA, Gourie-Devi M, Anand AR, Vijaya AN, Pratima N, Neelam K, Chandramuki A. 1996 Significance of mycobacterial immune complexes (IgG) in the diagnosis of tuberculous meningitis *Tuber Lung Dis*. Apr;77, 2, 164-7.

Rafi W, Venkataswamy MM, Nagarathna S, Satishchandra P, Chandramuki A. 2007

Raman Sharma R, 2010 Fungal infections of the nervous system: current perspective and controversies in management *Int J Surg*, Vol 8(8), 591-601.

Reiber H, Lange P. 1991 Quantification of virus-specific antibodies in cerebrospinal fluid and serum. Sensitive and specific detection antibody synthesis in the brain. *Clin Chem*, 37, 1153-60

Reid, H. and R.J. Fallon. Bacterial infections, 1992, pp: 302-334. In J.H. Adams and L.W. Duchen (ed), Green Field's Neuropathology. Oxford University Press, New York.

Role of IS6110 uniplex PCR in the diagnosis of tuberculous meningitis experience at a tertiary neurocentre. *Int J Tuberc Lung Dis*. 11, 2, Feb, 209-14.

Sanya, EO., S., Taiwo, S.S., Azeez O.I. & Oluyombo R. 2007.Bacteria Meningitis: Problems of Empirical Treatment in a Teaching Hospital in the Tropics. *The Internet Journal of Infectious Diseases*Vol 6 No 1.

Satishchandra, P., Mathew, T., Gadre, G., Nagarathna, S., Chandramukhi, A., Mahadevan, A. & Shankar, SK. 2007 Cryptococcal meningitis: clinical, diagnostic and therapeutic overviews *Neurol India* 55(3):226-32.

Seehusen, DA., Reeves, MM., Fomin, DA2003. Cerebrospinal fluid analysis. *Am Fam Physician*, 15; 68(6): Sep 1103-8.

Shivaprakash MR, Rajagopal V, Nagarathna S. 2004 Latex agglutination test in the diagnosis of pyogenic meningitis.*J Commun Dis*, 36, (2)jun, 127-31.

Singh 1994.Cerebrospinal fluid C reactive protein in the diagnosis of meningitis in children *Indian paediatrics* vol 31august 939 -942.

SreeNeelima, G., Aparna, Inaparthy., & Thomas, H., 2004, Meningitis due to Fusobacterium necrophorum in an adult.*BMC Infect Dis*. 4: 24.

Thomspon EJ. 1995 Cerebrospinal fluid. *J Neurol Neurosurg Psychiatry*, 59, 349-57

Tunkel, AR., Hartman, BJ., Kaplan, SL., Kaufman, AB., Roos, KL., Scheld, WM& Whitley, RJ., 2004. Practice guidelines for the management of bacterial meningitis*clin Infect Dis*, vol 39, 9, 1267–84.

Van de Beek D, de Gans J, Spanjaard L, Weisfelt, M., Reitsma, JB., & Vermeulen, M.et al. 2004.Clinical features and prognostic factors in adults with bacterial meningitis. *N Engl J Med*, oct 351, 1849-1859.

Venkataswamy MM, Rafi W, Nagarathna S, Ravi V, Chandramuki A. 2007; Comparative evaluation of bactec 460tb system and lowenstein-jensen medium for the isolation of M. tuberculosis from cerebrospinal fluid samples of tuberculous meningitis patients. *Indian J Med Microbiol* 25:236-40

Watson MA, Scott MG. 1995 Clinical utility of biochemical analysis of cerebrospinal fluid. *Clin Chem*;41:343-60.

Weisfelt, M., D. van de Beek, L. Spanjaard, and J. de Gans. 2007. Nosocomial bacterial meningitis in adults: a prospective series of 50 cases. *J.Hosp. Infect.* 66, 71–78.

Zedek DC and Miller MB 2006 Use of Galactomannan Enzyme Immunoassay for Diagnosis of Invasive Aspergillosis in a Tertiary-Care Center over a 12-Month Period. *J Clin Microbiol*, April, 44, 4, 1601

Zekaver O., Gloria, M., Elihu, E., Hagop, K., Fumihiro, S., Richard, JR., Paul, AK., Malcolm, AI., John, HR., a, and Luis, OZ.2004 -d-Glucan as a Diagnostic Adjunct for Invasive Fungal Infections: Validation, Cutoff Development, and Performance in Patients with Acute Myelogenous Leukemia and Myelodysplastic Syndrome *Clin Infect Dis*.vol 39 (2): 199-205.

Zunt, JR& Marra CM 1999 Central nervous system infections –Cerebral spinal fluid testing for the diagnosis of central nervous system infection. *Neurol Clin*, 17(4), 675-89.

15

Role of Dexamethasone in Meningitis

Emad uddin Siddiqui
and Ghazala Irfan Qazi
Aga Khan University Hospital
Pakistan

1. Introduction

The inflammatory cascade in acute bacterial meningitis leads to tissue damage and exudates accumulation especially in H. influenza, pneumococcal meningitis and in tuberculous meningitis. The administered antibiotics will also exaggerate the formation of inflammatory exudates from tissue destruction and endotoxins from bacterial lysis, resulting in edema formation. Accumulation of these inflammatory substrates, neutrophils and edema ultimately results in ischemia and pressure effect on neurons and nerve fibers with worsening of neurological signs and symptoms.

Despite the effective antibiotic therapies, bacterial meningitis still has considerable morbidity and mortality in both adult and pediatric population. (Brouwer MC et al., 2010). Other than the definitive treatment with appropriate antibiotics, supportive and adjuvant therapy has its own characteristic role in the improved outcome of disease. Evidence from experimental models also support the role of adjuvant therapy like, early administration of glucocorticoids in selective cases of pyogenic meningitis, however most modalities investigated so far have not been sufficiently supportive for their routine use in the management of all cases of meningitis.

2. Pathophysiology

According to Monro-Kellie doctrine (Morki B, 2008), if there is an increasing size of one constituent or a mass within the cranial vault, the pressure will be shared by either brain, arterial and venous blood flow and/or the CSF. Similarly, if there is trauma or inflammation to brain parenchyma or meninges, exudates will accumulate with oedema, and edematous and inflamed brain causes either partial or complete obstruction of CSF flow which may results in hydrocephalus. Edematous and inflamed brain reduces the venous blood flow from cranial vault, leading to venous congestion and edema, on the other hand, it also hampered arterial blood supply and hence reduce brain perfusion, and oxygenation which may further aggravate hypoxic inflammation and hence worsening of edema, thereby further increasing intra cranial venous congestion and pressure, consequently compromising the brain parenchyma results in different clinical presentation like altered mental status.

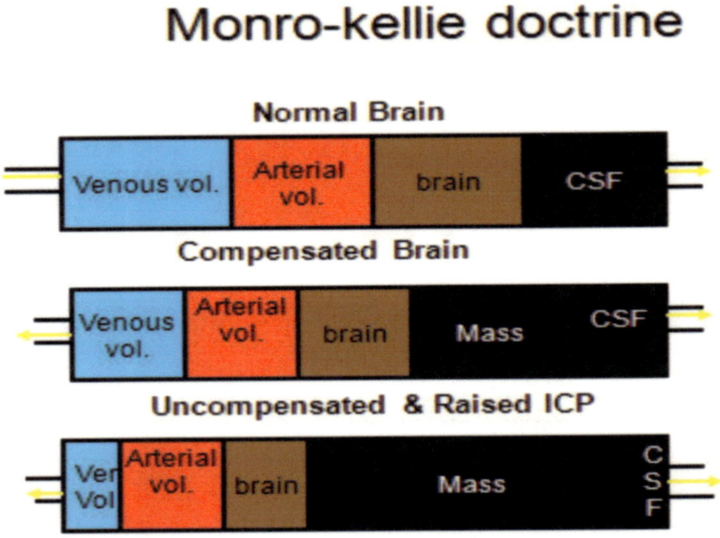

Fig. 1. Monro-Kellie hypothesis: Increase in volume (mass effect) of cranial constituents (blood, CSF, and brain tissue) must be compensated by a decrease in volume of another.

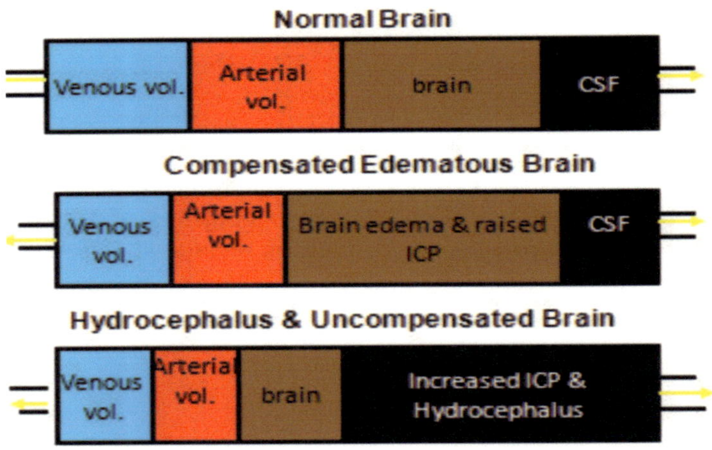

Fig. 2. Monro-Kellie hypothesis in case of increase intracranial pressure and hydrocephalus, compromising arterial and venous blood and compressed brain parenchyma and CSF.

3. Role of anti inflammatory agents

There are wide spectrum of complications associated with meningitis, these may be neurological and non neurological (systemic). Systemic complications relate with bacteremia and related toxins, which ranges from sepsis to septic shock, disseminated intravascular coagulation, respiratory distress syndrome and respiratory arrest, while prolong fever, vasomotor collapse, pericardial effusion, arthritis, hypothalamic and other endocrine dysfunction including hyponatremia and bilateral adrenal hemorrhage are also not uncommon. Anemia may also manifest as a part of meningitis.

Several anti inflammatory agents have been studied in reducing the inflammatory exudates in animal model of pyogenic and other type of meningitis. Indomethacin, platelet factor inhibitors and pentoxifylline, recombinant protein C, intravenous immunoglobulin and monoclonal antibodies, have been evaluated for their isolated and combine anti inflammatory properties in reducing the CSF inflammation and edema, but none of them have evident promising results. (Singhi P et al., 2008)

Though the role of glucocorticoids in systemic complications of meningitis is not discussed in the literature as extensively as it has been described for neurological outcomes, especially in reducing the incidence of hearing loss and other acute or chronic neurological sequel, on the contrary, use of glucocorticoids did not reduce overall mortality in most cases of meningitis. Cochrane review data supports its use in patients with bacterial meningitis in high-income countries, but results were not found to be beneficial from low-income countries. (Daoud AS et al., 1999). Bacterial immunogenicity, host immunity and response, timing and efficacy of antibiotics and steroids used and susceptibility of organism all account for the consequences in low income countries. The adjunctive benefit of corticosteroids during treatment of meningitis caused by other organisms (viral, fungal, and parasitic) is unknown.

4. Role of steroids in meningitis

With its unique anti-inflammatory and immune suppressive properties, efficacy of this drug has been extensively studied in different types of meningitis. Adjuvant therapy of glucocorticoids like dexamethasone is useful in both adult and pediatric meningitis and tuberculous meningitis as evident from experimental studies and vast growing clinical data. (Friedland IR et al., 1994).

Steroid limits the production of inflammatory mediators like IL-1, IL-6 and TNF and exudates and help in reduction of edema, resulting in the decrease cerebral pressure and hence improve CSF flow within the cistern thus helps in stabilizing the blood brain barrier (BBB), this in turn leads to improvement of neurological symptoms. (Karen & Tyler 2008). Dexamethasone also inhibits the production of TNF by macrophages and microglia, but only if it is administered before these cells are activated by endotoxin.

A meta-analysis conducted in 2010 on the role of dexamethasone in pediatric meningitis has shown that dexamethasone did not improve overall mortality; however it can reduces severe hearing loss in children. (Brouwer MC et al., 2010). However, the etiological agents, nutritional status, prior immunity and immunization and demography play an important role in outcome of such meningitis.

Most experts had consensus on the beneficial role of steroid with its maximum benefits when it is used at least one hour prior to recommended antibiotics therapy. (King, 1994: Pickering, 2009). Regarding H. Influenzae meningitis in children older than six week age, the use of steroid prior to antibiotics is recommended by American Academy of Pediatrics and as describe Infectious Diseases Society of America (IDSA) guidelines 2004. (Tunkel AR et al., 2004). In H. Influenzae meningitis steroids significantly reduce the risk of sensorineural hearing loss, while other experts' belief that outcome of meningitis is not dependent on steroids when it was given. Dexamethasone also did not help in ameliorating the other neurologic consequences especially in children. (Brouwer MC et al., 2010).

Beneficial role of dexamethasone in neonatal meningitis has not been evidence from the literature. It is not indicated in bacterial meningitis in children younger than six weeks as it does not shown promising results in different past studies. Steroids are also not advised as adjuvant therapy in patients with congenital or acquired CNS anomalies. (Daoud AS et al., 1999).

The severity of illness at the time of presentation may appear to play a prominent role in outcome than just administration of adjuvant therapy with dexamethasone. (Peltola H et al., 2010). On the other hand dexamethasone may also mask the clinical presentation of meningitis, or any of its associated sequels like abscess, empyema, subdural collection, tuberculous meningitis, resistant meningitis. Routine administration of dexamethasone is also not recommended in developing countries as most patients got their first few doses of antibiotics before the diagnosis of meningitis. Still dexamethasone has a role in reducing the inflammatory exudates if given with or given soon after the initial antibiotics preferably within one hour, but this time interval is not clearly defined in literature. (King SM et al., 1994).

With the advent of effective immunization against H. Influenzae globally, Streptococcal Pneumoniae is becoming the common organism causing meningitis. Resistant of S. pneumonia to cephalosphorins group is also evidently increasing from literature. Widespread use of susceptible vancomycin against these resistant species of S. pneumonae is increasing. At the same time studies had shown an increasing number of therapeutic failures when dexamethasone is combine with vancomycin and various other antibiotics like rifampicin and cephalosporin etc. steroids may reduce the penetration of these antibiotics in CSF or it may lead to decrease level of some antibiotic (eg, vancomycin, ceftriaxone, and rifampin) within the CSF, mechanism is not clear. (Friedland, 1994: Moellering, 1984).

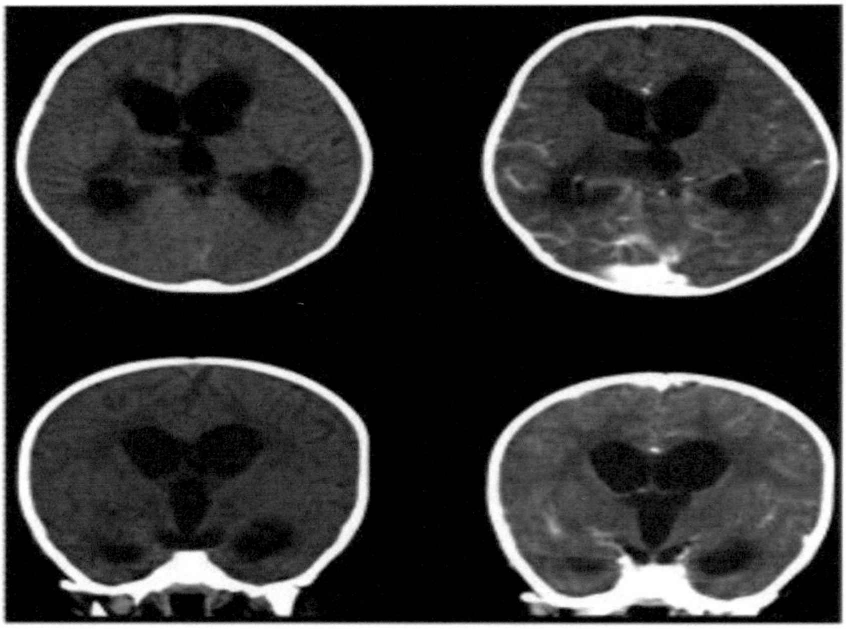

Fig. 3. CT scan brain showing low attenuated areas and increase enhancements with hydrocephalus in patient with pneumococcal meningitis

Dexamethasone in case of pneumococcal meningitis should be use after considering the risks and benefits. In adults with pneumococcal meningitis; dexamethasone has shown to have clinical benefits in term of neurological outcomes, but in children its use is controversial in pneumococcal meningitis. On the other hand few experts recommend that it should be used in all cases of confirm or suspected pneumococcal meningitis even if they are previously vaccinated, while other focused on the risk and benefits. However experts' consensus that steroid is only effective in reducing hearing loss if given before antibiotics. (Pickering 2009).

In patients with hypo spleenism, sickle cell disease and complement and immune deficiency, corticosteroids should be use cautiously. Thus controversies for its use in pneumococcal meningitis still persist. Dexamethasone is also not recommended in patients with aseptic meningitis, nonbacterial, or meningitis with gram-negative enteric bacteria. In such cases dexamethasone if started before should be discontinued as soon as a diagnosis of nonbacterial or gram-negative enteric meningitis is confirmed. (Tunkel AR et al., 2004).

Randomized controlled trials from low income country with steroid therapy in tuberculosis meningitis for initial 6-8 weeks of anti tubercular treatment were found to have significantly reduced mortality in patients who present with stage I disease; there was also reduce mortality noticed in patients who present with stage II disease. (Thwaites, GE. et al., 2008). However there was no significant long term reduction in the residual neurologic deficits and disability among survivors. Prednisone as compare to dexamethasone is associated with a significant reduction in mortality in children with tuberculous meningitis as compare to adults. (Thwaites, GE. et al., 2008).

5. Doses of dexamethasone in meningitis

In case of pyogenic meningitis dexamethasone should be used at 0.15 mg/kg per dose (10 mg intravenously in adults) every six hours for two to four days (Tunkel AR et al., 2004). Two days of dexamethasone appear to be as effective as and less toxic than longer courses. (Syrogiannopolus GA et al., 1994)

Steroids should be started at presentation or before or with the commencement of anti tubercular therapy. Dexamethasone, dose of 8 mg/day for children weighing <25 kg, 12 mg/day for adults and children >25 kg, for 3 weeks, and then tapered off gradually over the following 3 to 4 weeks. Prednisone, dose of 2 to 4 mg/kg/day for children and 60 mg/day for adults, for 3 weeks, then tapered off gradually over the following 3 weeks.

6. Complication of dexamethasone

Problems related with the glucocorticoids use are usually associated with it prolong duration. There may be complexity in clinical assessment and response to therapy, gastrointestinal bleeding, secondary fever, hypertension, hyperglycemia, leukocytosis etc. It may also impair antibiotic penetration into the cerebrospinal fluid (CSF) that can lead to therapeutic failure, particularly in areas with increasing rates of penicillin-resistant S. pneumonia. (Thomas R et al., 1999).

Corticosteroids do not reverse CNS damage that has already resulted from the pathophysiologic consequences of bacterial meningitis (e.g., cerebral edema and increased intracranial pressure). However, even in children with bacterial meningitis in the developing world, use of adjunctive dexamethasone should be considered, because no adverse effects were attributable to its administration in this trial and its use may benefit some of the children with this devastating disorder. (Mongelluzo J et al., 2008)

7. Dexamethasone in adult meningitis

Clinical trials of corticosteroids (dexamethasone) as adjuvant therapy have been conducted in different centers all over the world with inconsistent results. However studies shown that corticosteroids significantly reduced severe hearing loss and other neurologic sequel, while on other hand, it is also helpful in reducing the overall mortality. Meta analysis using dexamethasone in adult meningitis demonstrates favorable outcomes in terms of both morbidity and mortality especially in cases of pneumococcal meningitis. It also reduces mortality in adult onset streptococcal pneumonae meningitis. (Daniel J S et al., 2010). Dexamethasone is also associated with reduce rate of acute neurological and hearing defect, however there was no difference in long term neurological sequelae, (Brouwer MC et al., 2010) although some experts recommend to discontinue dexamethasone if S. pneumonia was not found in the CSF culture, but others still recommend the use of adjunctive dexamethasone regardless of microbial etiology in conjunction with the first dose of antimicrobial therapy. (de Gans & Van de, 2002)

8. Dexamethasone in pediatric meningitis

The role of dexamethasone use in cases of pediatric meningitis is more controversial, it must be individualized according to the organism especially in case of H. influnzae and pneumococcal meningitis. Even though, a better outcome can only be attained if dexamethasone is use before or at the same time of first dose of antibiotics. (Tunkel AR et al., 2004). Routine use of dexamethasone in pediatric population is not recommended, potential risk and benefits must be taken in to account as it may not reverse neuronal damage that has already resulted from the pathophysiologic consequences of bacterial meningitis.

However, even in children with bacterial meningitis in the developing world, use of adjunctive dexamethasone should be considered, because no adverse effects were attributable to its administration in different trials and its use may benefit some of the children with this devastating disorder.

9. Dexamethasone in neonatal meningitis

The administration of dexamethasone did not significantly affect mortality or neurologic outcome in small children up to two years of age, hence it is not currently recommended. (Daoud AS et al., 1999).

10. Acknowledgment

I would like to thanks Ms Uzma Siddiqui who gave me enormous moral assistant in writing this book chapter. I am also be thankful to Saif ul Islam and Zain ul Islam for their kind support.

11. References

Brouwer, MC. Mcintyre, P. de-Gans, J. Prasad, K. Van-de-Beek, D. (2010). Corticosteroids for acute bacterial meningitis. *Cochrane database systemic review* 2010, Sept 08 ;(09). CD004405.

Daniel, J S. Stephen, B C. Anna, R T. (October 4, 2010). Dexamethasone to prevent neurologic complications of bacterial meningitis in adults. *Up to date on line. Version 18.3: September 2010.* Accessed on 12/06/2011. http://www.uptodate.com/contents/dexamethasone-to-prevent-neurologic-complications-of-bacterial-meningitis-in-adults?source=search_result&selectedTitle=1%7E150

Daoud, AS. Batieha, A. Al-Sheyyab, M. (1999). Lack of effectiveness of dexamethasone in neonatal bacterial meningitis. *Eur J Pediatr* 1999; 158:230-33.

De-Gans, J. Van-de-Beek, D. (2002). Dexamethasone in adults with bacterial meningitis. *N Engl J Med* 2002; 347:1549-1556.

Friedland, IR. Paris, M. Shelton, S. McCracken, GH. (1994). Time-kill studies of antibiotic combinations against penicillin-resistant and susceptible Streptococcus pneumoniae. *J Antimicrob Chemother* 1994; 34:231.

King, SM. Law, B. Langley, JM. (1994). Dexamethasone therapy for bacterial meningitis: Better never than late? *Can J Infect Dis* 1994; 5:210

Mace, SE. (2008). Acute Bacterial Meningitis. *Emerg Med Clin N Am*; 26(2) :2008 281–317

Moellering, RC. (1984). Pharmacokinetics of vancomycin. J Antimicrob Chemother 1984; 14 Suppl D: 43.

Mokri, B. The Monro–Kellie hypothesis. Applications in CSF volume depletion. *Neurology* 2001;56:1746–1748

Mongelluzo, J. Mohamad, Z. Ten-Have, TR. Shah, SS. (2008). Corticosteroids and mortality in children with bacterial meningitis. *JAMA* 2008; 299:2048-2055.

Odio, CM. Faingezicht, I. Paris, M. Nassar, M. Baltodano, A. Rogers, J. Saez-Liorens, X. Olsen, KD. Mccracken, GH. (1991). The beneficial effects of early dexamethasone administration in infants and children with bacterial meningitis. *N Engl J Med* 1991; 30: 324 (22):1525-31

Peltola, H. Roine, I. Fernández, J. Gonzalez Mata, A. Zavala, I. Gonzalez, Ayala, S. Arbo, A. Bolonga, R. Govo, J. Lopez, E. Mino, G. Dourando de Andrade, S. Sarna, S. Jauhianinen, T. (2010). Hearing impairment in childhood bacterial meningitis is little relieved by dexamethasone or glycerol. *Pediatrics* 2010; 125(1): e1-8.

Peltola, H. Roine, I. Fernández, J. Zavala, I. Avala, SG. Mata, AG. Arbo, A. Bolonga, R. Mino, G. Goyo, J. Lopez, E. deAndrade, SD. Sarna, S. (2007). Adjuvant glycerol and/or dexamethasone to improve the outcomes of childhood bacterial meningitis: a prospective, randomized, double-blind, placebo-controlled trial. *Clin Infect Dis* 2007, 15; 45(10):1277-86.

Pelton, SI. Yogev, R. (2005). Improving the outcome of pneumococcal meningitis. *Arch Dis Child* 2005; 90(4):333–4.

Pickering, LK. (2009). Summaries of infectious disease. Haemophilus influenzae infections: Page 314-321. *Red Book: Report of the Committee on Infectious Diseases, 28th ed, American Academy of Pediatrics, Elk Grove Village, IL.*

Pickering, LK. (2009). Summaries of infectious disease. Pneumococcal infections: Page 524-535. *Red Book: Report of the Committee on Infectious Diseases, 28th edi, American Academy of Pediatrics. Elk Grove Village, IL*

Roine, I. Peltola, H. Fernández, J. Zavala, I. González Mata, A. González Ayala, S. Arbo, A. Bologna, R. Miño, G. Goyo, J. López, E. Dourado de Andrade, S. Sarna, S. (2008). Influence of admission findings on death and neurological outcome from childhood bacterial meningitis. *Clin Infect Dis* 2008; 46(8):1248-52.

Roos, Kl. Tyler, TL. (2008). *Harrison's Principles of Internal Medicine.* "Chapter 376. Meningitis, Encephalitis, Brain Abscess, and Empyema" {EDITOR NAME} Fauci AS, Braunwald E, Kasper DL, Hauser SL, Longo DL, Jameson JL, Loscalzo J: Harrison's Principles of Internal Medicine 17e: www.accessmedicine.com/content.aspx?aID=2906668. ISBN 978-0-07-147691-1

Singhi, PD. Singhi, SC. Newton, CRJ. Simon, J. (2008). *Text book of pediatric intensive care, CNS infection, 2008.,* Lippincot Williams and Wilkins. 530 Walnut street Philadelphia, PA 19106 ISBN 970-7817-8275-3.

Syrogiannopoulos, GA. Lourida, AN. Theodoridou, MC. Pappas, IG. Babilis, GC. Economidis, JJ. Zoumboulakis, DJ. Beratis, NG. Matsaniotis, NS. (1994). Dexamethasone therapy for bacterial meningitis in children: 2- versus 4-day regimen. *J Infect Dis* 1994; 169(4):853-8.

Thomas, R. Le Tulzo, Y. Bouget, J. Camus, C. Michelet,. C. Le Corre, P. Bellissant, E. (1999). Trial of dexamethasone treatment for severe bacterial meningitis in adults. *Intensive Care Med* (1999) 25(5): 475-480

Thwaites, GE. Duc Bang, N. Huy Dung, N. Quy, HT. Oanh Do, TT. Cam Thoa, NT. Hien, NQ. Thuc, NT. Hai, NN. Ngoc Lan, NT. Lan, NN. Duc, NH. Tuan, VN. Hiep, CH. Hong Chau, TT. Mai, PP. Dung, NT. Stepniewska, K. White, NJ. Hien, TT. Farrar, JJ. (2008). Dexamethasone for the treatment of tuberculous meningitis in adolescents and adults. *N Engl J Med* 2004; 351:1741-51.

Tunkel, AR. Hartman, BJ. Kaplan, SL. (2004). Practice guidelines for the management of bacterial meningitis. *Clin Infect Dis* 2004; 39:1267. Uploaded from http://www.thecochranelibrary.com/ dated 20/07/2011

Van de Beek, D. Weisfelt, M. De Gans, J. Tunkel, AR. Wijdicks, EFM. (2006). Drug insight: adjunctive therapies in adults with bacterial meningitis. *Nat Clin Pract Neurol* 2006; 2:504–16.

Van-de-Beek, D. Farrar, JJ. De Gans, J. Mai, NT. Molyneux, EM. Peltola, H. Peto,TE. Roine, I. Scarborough, M. Schultsz, C. Thwaites, GE. Taun, PQ. Zwinderman, AH. (2010). Adjunctive dexamethasone in bacterial meningitis: a meta-analysis of individual patient data. *Lancet Neurol* 2010; 9(3): 254–63

16

Treatment of Adult Meningitis and Complications

Sónia Costa and Ana Valverde
Neurology Department, Hospital Professor Dr. Fernando Fonseca EPE, Amadora, Portugal

1. Introduction

The term meningitis implies inflammation of the leptomeninges and cerebrospinal fluid (CSF) in the subarachnoid space. Typically manifests as headache, neck stiffness, light sensitivity, and varying degrees of neurological symptoms and signs.

The most common and often most severe forms of meningitis are due to infections, including bacteria, viruses, fungi, and parasites. Noninfectious causes of meningitis include primary inflammatory syndromes such as vasculitis and connective tissue disease, neoplasms of solid tumor and hematologic forms, and chemical irritants including certain medications, subarachnoid blood, and biologic matter spilling into CSF from tumors.

Although a patient may present with symptoms of meningitis within days of onset, distinguishing acute from subacute or chronic meningitis may not always be possible early in the course. Nevertheless, the distinction is important because of the varying urgency, causes, and treatment strategy involved in each syndrome.

In this review we summarize the current concepts of the approach to the treatment of adult meningitis and management of neurologic complications.

2. Bacterial meningitis

Bacterial meningitis is a medical, neurologic and sometimes neurosurgical emergency that requires a multidisciplinary approach. Bacterial meningitis has an annual incidence of 4 to 6 cases per 100,000 adults, and *Streptococcus pneumoniae* and *Neisseria meningitidis* are responsible for 80 percent of all cases. Recommendations for antimicrobial therapy are changing as a result of the emergence of antimicrobial resistance. (Van de Beek et al., 2004; Schuchat et al., 2005; Van de Beek et al., 2006)

In adults presenting with community-acquired acute bacterial meningitis, the sensitivity of the classic triad of fever, neck stiffness, and altered mental status is low (44%), but almost all such patients present with at least two of four symptoms — headache, fever, neck stiffness, and altered mental status (as defined by a score below 14 on the Glasgow Coma Scale).

2.1 Antimicrobial treatment

The choice of antibiotic for empirical therapy is based on the possibility that a penicillin- and cephalosporin-resistant strain of *S. pneumonia* is the causative organism, and on the patient's age and any associated conditions that may have predisposed to meningitis (table 1).

Predisposing factor	Common bacterial pathogens	Initial intravenous antibiotic therapy
Age: 2-50 years	*N meningitidis* *S pneumoniae*	Vancomycin plus ceftriaxone or cefotaxime*
Age: >50 years	*N meningitidis* *S pneumoniae* *L monocytogenes*, aerobic gram-negative bacilli	**Vancomycin plus ceftriaxone or cefotaxime plus ampicillin
With risk factor present (alcoholism or altered immune status)	*S pneumoniae* *L monocytogenes* *H influenzae*	**Vancomycin plus ceftriaxone or cefotaxime plus ampicillin
*In areas with very low penicillin-resistance rates monotherapy penicillin may be considered **In areas with very low penicillin-resistance and cephalosporin-resistance rates combination therapy of amoxiciclin and a third-generation cephalosporin may be considered		

Table 1. Recommendations for empirical antimicrobial therapy in suspected community-acquired bacterial meningitis (adapted from Van de Beek et al., 2006)

For adults up to 50 years old from countries with high rates of pneumococcal penicillin- or cephalosporin-resistance, this should be a combination of either a third- or fourth-generation cephalosporin plus vancomycin. In countries with very low rates of pneumococcal penicillin-resistance (such as The Netherlands) (Van de Beek et al., 2002), penicillin can still be used safely as a first-line agent. In the UK, the addition of vancomycin is also not considered necessary and is not recommended unless the patient presents from one of the geographic regions associated with high-level ceftriaxone resistance, such as Spain, Southern Africa, and certain parts of the USA. In adults older than 50 years, and in the immunocompromised patient, ampicillin should be added to this combination because of possible *Listeria meningitis*. (Nudelman & Tunkel, 2009; Schut et al., 2008; Van de Beek et al., 2006; Williams & Nadel, 2001)

Once the bacterial pathogen is isolated and the sensitivity of the organism to the antibiotic is confirmed by in vitro testing, antimicrobial therapy should be modified accordingly. Recommendations for antibiotic therapy in bacterial meningitis are summarized in table 2-4 and some important tips are:

a. Bacterial meningitis due to *S. pneumoniae, H. influenzae* and group *B streptococci* is usually treated with intravenous antibiotics for 10–14 days.

b. Meningitis due to *N. meningitidis* is treated for 5–7 days.
c. Patients with clinically suspected meningococcal meningitis who are treated with penicillin must be isolated for the first 24 h after initiation of antibiotic therapy and also treated with Rifampin 600 mg orally every 12 h for 2 days to eradicate nasopharyngeal colonization (penicillin does not eradicate the organisms in the nasopharynx).
d. Meningitis due to *L. monocytogenes* and *Enterobacteriaceae* is treated for 3–4 weeks.
e. Gentamicin is added to ampicillin in critically ill patients with *L. monocytogenes* meningitis.

Pathogen	Recommended therapy	Adult dosage (intravenous)	Days of therapy	Alternative therapy
Streptococcus pneumoniae			10 to 14	Meropenem, moxifloxacib or cloranfenicol
Penicillin MIC: < 0,1 mcg per mL	Penicillin	4 million units every four hours		
Penicillin MIC: 0,1 to 1 mcg per mL	Ceftriaxone	2g every 12 hours		
Penicillin MIC: ≥ 1 mcg per mL	Vancomycin *plus* Ceftriaxone	15 to 22,5 mg per kg every 12 hours 2 g every 12 hours		
Neisseria meningitidis	Ceftriaxone	2 g every 12 hours	5 to 7	Chloranfenicol, meropenem or moxifloxacin
Haemophilus influenza	Ceftriaxone	2 g every 12 hours	7 to 10	Chloranfenicol or moxifloxacin
Streptococcus agalactiae (group B streptococcus)	Ampicillin *plus* Gentamicin	Usually in children	14 to 21	Vancomycin or cefotaxime
Listeria monocitogenes	Ampicillin *with or without* Gentamicin	2 g every four hours 1 to 2 mg per Kg every eight hours	21 First 7 to 10 days	Trimethroprim/sulfamethoxazole
Enterobacteriaceae	Ceftriaxone, ceftazidime or cefepime	varies	21 to 28	Ciprofloxacin, meropenem or Trimethroprim/sulfamethoxazole
Staphylococci			7 to 10 days after shunt removal or cerebrospinal fluid sterilization	Daptomycin or lnezolid. Consider adding rifampicin
Methicillin susceptible	Nafcillin	2 g every four hours		
Methicillin resistant	Vancomycin	15 to 22,5 mg per Kg every 12 hours		

Table 2. Pathogen-specific therapy for common causes of bacterial meningitis

Treatment	Dose
Penicilin	2 million units every 4 h
Amoxiclin or ampicillin	2 g every 4h
Vancomycin	15 mg/Kg every 8h
Third generation cephalosporins	
Ceftriaxone	2 g every 12h
Cefotaxime	2 g every 4-6h
Cefepime	2 g every 8h
Ceftazidime	2 g every 8h
Meropenem	2 g every 8h
Chloramphenicol	1-1, 5g every 6h
Fluroquinolones	
Gatifloxacin	400 mg every 24h
Moxifloxacin	400 mg every 24h
Trimethoprim-sulfamethoxazole	5 mg/kg every 6-12h
Aztreonam	2 g every 6-8 h
Ciprofloxacin	400 mg every 8-12h
Rifampicin	600 mg every 12-24h
Aminoglycoside (gentamicine)	1,7 mg/Kg every 8h

Table 3. General recommendations for intravenous empirical antibiotic treatment

Treatment	Dose
Rifampicin	600 mg twice daily for two days
Ceftriaxone	One dose 250 mg intramuscularly
Ciprofloxacine	One dose, 500 mg orally
Azithromycin	One dose, 500 mg orally

Table 4. General recommendations for chemoprophylaxis

2.2 Adjunctive dexamethasone

A large randomized trial showed that dexamethasone (10 mg IV 15–20 min before or with the first dose of antibiotic and given every 6 h for 4 days) is beneficial in adults with acute bacterial meningitis. It reduced unfavorable outcome from 25% to 15% and mortality from 15% to 7%. The benefits were most striking in patients with pneumococcal meningitis. Furthermore, patients on dexamethasone were less likely to have impaired consciousness, seizures and cardiorespiratory failure. Starting corticosteroids before or with the first dose of parenteral antimicrobial therapy appears to be more effective than starting corticosteroids after the first dose of antimicrobial therapy. For some adults with suspected meningitis, the beneficial effect of adjunctive dexamethasone is less certain, or may even be harmful. Therefore these patients should be carefully monitored throughout treatment. Steroids are not recommended in patients with postneurosurgical meningitis, those with a severe immunocompromised state, or in those who are hypersensitive to steroids. Patients with septic shock and adrenal insufficiency benefit from steroid therapy in physiological doses and longer duration. (Van de Beek et al., 2004; Van de Beek & de Gans, 2006; Fitch & Van de Beek, 2007; Nudelman & Tunkel, 2009; Schut et al., 2008; Van de Beek et al., 2006; Williams & Nadel, 2001; Weisfelt et al., 2006)

2.3 Monitoring of the patient and systemic complications

Patients who are diagnosed with acute bacterial meningitis are at risk of various neurological and systemic complications and to detect them, patients should be admitted to intensive care unit where the following should be monitored: vital signs (blood pressure, heart rate, respiratory rate, temperature), oxygen saturation, level of consciousness, presence or absence of focal neurological signs or symptoms, papillary diameter and certain laboratory parameters, like CRP, leukocyte count, electrolytes, urea and creatinine. Analysis of arterial blood gases and measurement of serum lactate are important in patients in whom septic shock is suspected and the platelet count and coagulation tests are important in those in whom disseminated intravascular coagulation is suspected. (Van de Beek et al., 2006)

Table 5 resumes the management of bacterial meningitis in Adults in the Intensive Care Unit.

Bacterial meningitis is often associated with septic shock, which is an important predictor of outcome. It may manifest in several ways: hypotension (systolic pressure < 90 mm Hg or a reduction of >40 mm Hg from baseline) despite adequate fluid resuscitation, tachycardia (>100/min), tachypnea (>20/min), core body temperature >38°C or <36°C, drowsiness and oliguria (Pfister et al., 1993).

Adrenocorticoid insufficiency in patients with septic shock must be treated with low doses of corticosteroids. Care should be taken to estimate and replace imperceptible fluid loss through the skin and lungs in patients who are febrile.

Dyspnea, labored breathing, agitation, followed by progressive drowsiness, tachycardia, scattered crackles on pulmonary auscultation and hypoxemia point to the diagnosis of adult respiratory distress syndrome (ARDS). The chest x ray usually reveals characteristic diffuse alveolar interstitial infiltrates in all lung fields.

Patients with bacterial meningitis are at risk of acute hyponatremia, although most cases are mild. Hyponatremia (serum sodium <135 mmol/l) on admission to hospital is found in 30% of patients (Brouwer et al,. 2007). Most episodes resolve within a few days without specific treatment and does not influence outcome. Severe hyponatremia (<130 mmol/l) is present in 6% of patients.

An exceptionally high frequency of hyponatremia is seen in meningitis due to *L. monocytogenes* (73%) and *S. pyogenes* (58%). This complication may be a result of cerebral salt wasting, the syndrome of inappropriate antidiuretic hormone secretion or exacerbation by aggressive fluid resuscitation. This lack of clarity about the mechanism has resulted in the clinical dilemma about the management of intravenous fluids in bacterial meningitis (restricted or not). The goal should be to maintain a normovolemic state, and in patients with severe hyponatremia to use fluid maintenance therapy then fluid restriction, although there is no clear evidence supporting this approach.

Hypernatremia (serum sodium >143 mmol/l) is less frequent and found on admission in only 7% of patients with culture-proven bacterial meningitis (Van de Beek et al., 2007). Patients with sodium levels >146 mmol/l (2% of patients) are more likely to have seizures before admission compared to those with lower levels. Sodium levels of >143 mmol/l are

Neurocritical care In patients with a high risk of brain herniation, consider monitoring intracranial pressure and intermittent administration of osmotic diuretics (mannitol [25%] or hypertonic [3%] saline) to maintain an intracranial pressure of <15 mm Hg and a cerebral perfusion pressure of ≥60 mm Hg Initiate repeated lumbar puncture, lumbar drain, or ventriculostomy in patients with acute hydrocephalus Electroencephalographic monitoring in patients with a history of seizures and fluctuating scores on the Glasgow Coma Scale
Airway and respiratory care Intubate or provide noninvasive ventilation in patients with worsening consciousness (clinical and laboratory indicators for intubation include poor cough and pooling secretions, a respiratory rate of >35 per minute, arterial oxygen saturation of <90% or arterial partial pressure of oxygen of <60 mm Hg, and arterial partial pressure of carbon dioxide of >60 mm Hg) Maintain ventilatory support with intermittent mandatory ventilation, pressure-support ventilation, or continuous positive airway pressure
Circulatory care In patients with septic shock, administer low doses of corticosteroids (if there is a poor response on corticotropin testing, indicating adrenocorticoid insufficiency, corticosteroids should be continued) Initiate inotropic agents (dopamine or milrinone) to maintain blood pressure (mean arterial pressure, 70–100 mm Hg) Initiate crystalloids or albumin (5%) to maintain adequate fluid balance Consider the use of a Swan–Ganz catheter to monitor hemodynamic measurements
Gastrointestinal care Initiate nasogastric tube feeding of a standard nutrition formula Initiate prophylaxis with proton-pump inhibitors
Other supportive care Administer subcutaneous heparin as prophylaxis against deep venous thrombosis Maintain normoglycemic state (serum glucose level, <150 mg per deciliter), with the use of sliding-scale regimens of insulin or continuous intravenous administration of insulin In patients with a body temperature of >40°C, use cooling by conduction or antipyretic agents

Table 5. Management of Bacterial Meningitis in Adults in the Intensive Care Unit.

associated with a higher heart rate, lower CSF protein and lower CSF glucose levels. Hypernatremia is independently predictive of unfavorable outcome and mortality, however it is unclear if it reflects severe disease or directly contributes to the poor outcome. Physicians should be aware of the potential importance of hypernatraemia in patients presenting with bacterial meningitis and care should be taken in the fluid management.

The coexistence of bacterial meningitis and arthritis has been described in several studies. It occurs in 7% of patients overall, more in meningococcal meningitis (12%) (Likitnukul et al., 1986; Weisfeit et al., 2006). It is caused either by haematogenous bacterial seeding of joints (septic arthritis) or by immune-complex deposition in joints (immunomediated arthritis). A patient with immunomediated arthritis during meningococcal infection typically develops symptoms from day 5 of the illness or during recovery from the infection, generally involving the large joints. A definitive diagnosis of septic arthritis requires identification of bacteria in the synovial fluid by Gram stain or culture. The treatment of acute bacterial arthritis requires antibiotics and joint drainage. Although with some limitation in the range of movement functional outcome is good in most of the patients.

2.4 Deterioration of consciousness

A common cause of a decline in consciousness in bacterial meningitis is clinical evidence of cerebral edema. The release of proinflammatory mediators in the subarachnoid space leads to an inflammatory response in the central nervous system that contributes to an increased permeability of the blood–brain barrier, cerebral edema and increased intracranial pressure. Several supportive therapies have been described, although no therapy has been proved to have clinical efficacy. Nevertheless, in patients with impending cerebral herniation, monitoring of intracranial pressure may be considered, but the outcome is expected to be poor. The use of osmotic diuretics to control intracranial pressure may be an option, although there are no definitive data on the efficacy of this approach. (Figure 1)

Seizures are other frequent cause of deteriorating consciousness with a higher mortality rate. They occur in about 20% of patients, that are older and more likely to have focal abnormalities on brain CT. *S pneumoniae* is the most usual causative micro organism. Patients with seizures or a clinical suspicion of prior seizure should receive anticonvulsant therapy, but the low incidence of this complication does not justify prophylaxis. A rare cause of the deterioration of consciousness in meningitis is nonconvulsive status epilepticus.

Acute hydrocephalus can also complicate meningitis, because the purulent exudate interferes with CSF absorption by the arachnoid villi, resulting in communicating hydrocephalus. When the inflammatory exudate involves the basal cisterns and surrounds the cranial nerves at the base of the brain (basilar meningitis), it may block CSF flow at the foramina of Luschka and Magendie, resulting in obstructive hydrocephalus.

Repeated lumbar puncture or the placement of a temporary lumbar drain may effectively reduce intracranial pressure. In patients with mild enlargement of the ventricular system with no clinical deterioration, a spontaneous resolution may occur, and invasive procedures are therefore withheld.

Cerebral infarction due to arterial occlusion complicates bacterial meningitis in 10–15% of patients. Venous infarction due to septic venous thrombosis occurs in 3–5%. Cerebral infarcts may involve large vascular territories and may cause brain swelling and a mass effect, which may result in a decline in consciousness Arteritis of small and medium-sized arteries and inflammatory involvement of veins is probably caused by tissue destructive agents, such as oxidants and proteolytic enzymes, released by activated leukocytes. Treatment is mainly supportive and these patients have a poor outcome.

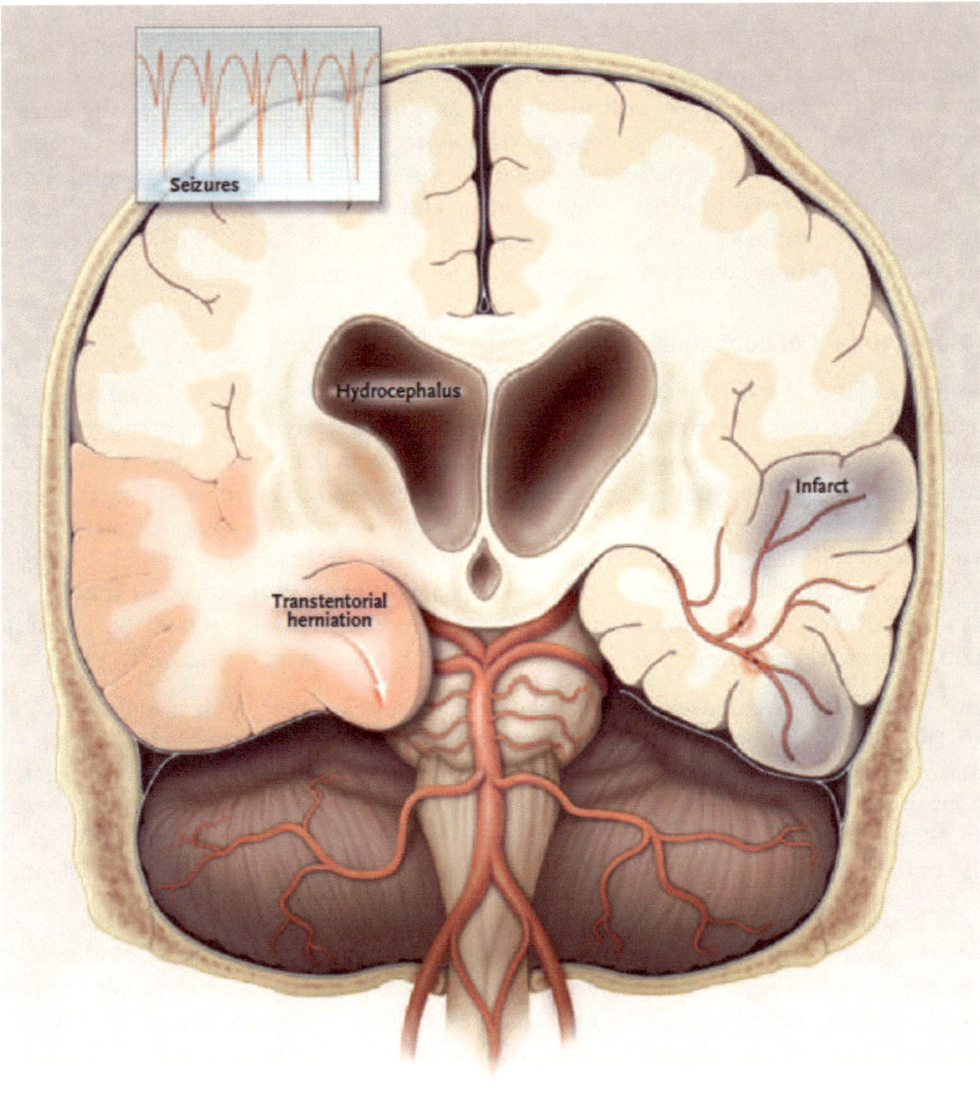

Fig. 1. Major Intracranial Complications in Bacterial Meningitis in Adults.

2.5 Focal neurological complications

In patients who develop focal neurological signs (hemiparesis, monoparesis, aphasia) some entities must be excluded: cerebral infarction (due to inflammatory occlusion of cerebral arteries, septic venous thrombosis), seizures, subdural empyema or a combination of these causes. A brain CT scan is needed to rule out many of these causes.

The possibility of septic intracranial venous thrombosis should be considered in patients with an impaired level of consciousness, seizures, fluctuating focal signs and stroke in non-arterial distributions. MRI with venous-phase studies confirms the diagnosis. Treatment of cerebral thrombophlebitis in bacterial meningitis is directed toward the infection.

Subdural empyema should be suspected in patients who have concomitant sinusitis or mastoiditis or who have recently undergone surgery for either of these disorders. In most cases contrast-enhanced brain CT will reveal the hypodense subdural collections (Figure 2). Brain MRI is more sensitive than CT in detecting subdural empyema along the convexity, and especially for infratentorial subdural empyema. Currently, MRI with diffusion-weighted images (DWI) and apparent diffusion coefficient mapping (ADC) remains the preferred imaging modality for detecting subdural empyema. Subdural empyema should be surgically drained by craniotomy but the outcome is poor if the patient is unconscious.

Abnormalities of the cranial nerves are caused by the meningeal inflammatory process or by an increase in cerebrospinal fluid pressure. The most frequent cranial-nerve abnormality is the involvement of the eighth cranial nerve, which is reflected in a hearing loss in 14 percent of patients. A cochlear implant may eventually be needed by some severely affected patients.

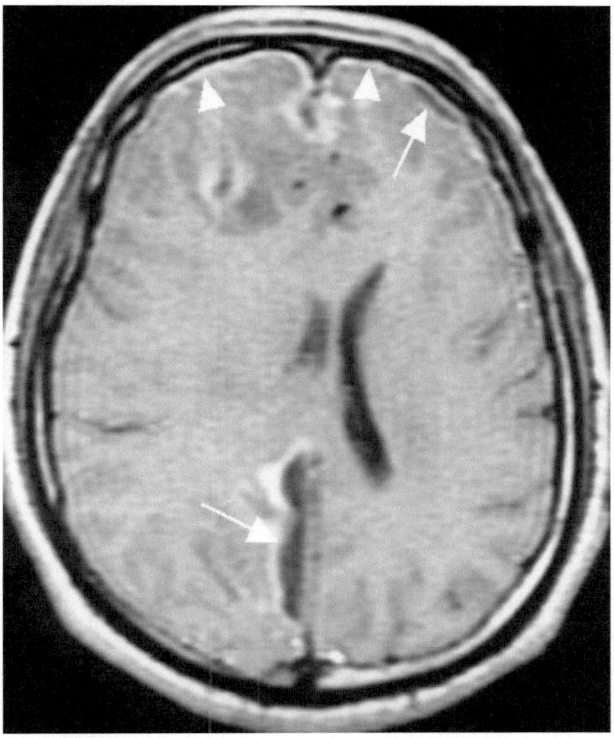

Fig. 2. Frontal sinusitis, empyema, and abscess formation in a patient with bacterial meningitis. This contrast-enhanced, axial T1-weighted magnetic resonance image shows a right frontal parenchymal low intensity (edema), leptomeningitis *(arrowheads)*, and a lentiform-shaped subdural empyema *(arrows)*.

3. Aseptic meningitis

Enteroviruses are the most common etiologic pathogens in persons with aseptic meningitis and do not require specific antimicrobial therapy. They can be diagnosed by CSF polymerase chain reaction testing (Kupila et al., 2006), which is not always needed, but a positive test may be useful in discontinuing antimicrobials initiated presumptively for bacterial meningitis.

Herpes Simplex Virus (HSV) aseptic meningitis is usually a self-limited infection that must be distinguished from HSV encephalitis based on clinical and radiographic features. Therapy with acyclovir can be lifesaving in patients with HSV encephalitis. (Bamberg, 2010)

In contrast with HSV encephalitis, most patients with HSV aseptic meningitis have normal mental status and neurologic function and do not have the temporal lobe enhancement observed on magnetic resonance imaging. Both forms of HSV central nervous system disease are diagnosed by CSF HSV polymerase chain reaction testing. Infection with HSV may cause recurrent disease (e.g., Mollaret meningitis).

Varicella zoster virus infection may cause aseptic meningitis in the absence of cutaneous manifestations. Although it has not been studied in clinical trials, therapy with acyclovir at 10 mg per kg every eight hours is suggested, based on expert opinion.

Lyme disease, a systemic disease with dermatological, rheumatological, neurological, and cardiac manifestations, is caused by *Borrelia burgdorferi* and transmitted by the hard-shelled deer ticks: *Ixodes dammini* in the eastern United States, *Ixodes pacificus* in the western United States, and *Ixodes ricinus* in Europe. The existence of both early and late neurological manifestations, diagnostic uncertainty, and potential for relapse despite therapy have fueled continuing debate over the spectrum of Lyme-related neurological disease. Best agreement exists for the early neurological syndromes, which include lymphocytic meningitis, cranial neuropathy (commonly unilateral or bilateral Bell's palsy), and painful radiculoneuritis, which can occur alone or in combination. Optic neuritis, mononeuritis multiplex, and Guillain-Barré syndrome are other infrequent manifestations of early neurological involvement. Neurological complications of more advanced Lyme disease include encephalomyelitis, with predominant white matter involvement and peripheral neuropathy. Lymphocytic meningitis is usually acute, but may cause chronic or relapsing meningitis and communicating hydrocephalus. Radiculoneuritis, beginning as a painful limb disorder, may continue with exacerbations and remissions for up to 6 months. Encephalopathy with memory or cognitive abnormalities, confusional states, accelerated dementia, and normal CSF study results may occur. Other psychiatric or fatigue syndromes appear less likely to be causally related to Lyme disease.

Borreliosis is treated with parenteral antibiotics if there is evidence that infection has crossed the blood-brain barrier. Ceftriaxone (2 g once daily intravenously) or penicillin (3 to 4 million units intravenously every 3 to 4 hours) for 2 to 4 weeks are first-line drugs. Tetracycline and chloramphenicol are alternatives in penicillin- or cephalosporin-allergic patients. Routine use of corticosteroids is not indicated. Recommendations for the use of corticosteroids in neuroborreliosis generally have been limited to patients treated aggressively with intravenous antibiotics with evidence of severe inflammation that fails to improve. CSF examination should be performed toward the end of the 2- to 4-week treatment course to assess the need for continuing treatment and again 6 months after the conclusion of therapy. Intrathecal antibody production may persist for years following successful treatment and in isolation does not indicate active disease. Patients in whom CSF pleocytosis fails to resolve within 6 months, should be retreated. Peripheral or cranial nerve involvement without CSF abnormalities may be treated with oral agents, either doxycycline, 100 mg twice daily for 14 to 21 days, or amoxicillin, 500 mg every 8 hours for 10 to 21 days.

Up to one third of untreated patients with syphilis develop late syphilis (tertiary syphilis), a slowly progressive inflammatory disease that includes gummatous (granulomatous), cardiovascular, and neurological forms. Early neurological manifestations of tertiary neurosyphilis include pure meningeal or meningovascular disease, with a 3- to 10-year latency period from primary infection, and parenchymal forms, which occur 10 to 30 years after initial infection. General paresis refers to parenchymal cerebral involvement and tabes dorsalis to syphilitic myeloneuropathy. Syphilitic gummas, granulomas that present as space-occupying lesions in brain or cord, may occur at any stage of disseminated disease.

Neurosyphilis spans all stages of disseminated disease. Meningeal, meningovascular, and parenchymal syndromes are perhaps best viewed as a continuum of disease, rather than as discrete disorders. Syphilitic meningitis, meningovascular syphilis, general paresis, and tabes are different clinical expressions of the same fundamental pathological events, specifically meningeal invasion, obliterative endarteritis, and parenchymal invasion. Especially in the antibiotic era, symptomatic neurosyphilis may present, not as one classic syndrome, but as mixed, subtle, or incomplete disease. All of the neurological complications of syphilis have been reported in HIV disease, which may accelerate the onset and progression of neurosyphilis.

Syphilitic meningitis typically occurs earlier than other forms of neurosyphilis and is often asymptomatic. Rare complications of acute syphilitic meningitis include cranial neuropathy, hydrocephalus, myelitis, or lumbosacral radiculitis. Meningovascular syphilis usually occurs 4 to 7 years after primary infection (range, 6 months to 12 years). In addition to stroke, involvement of large and small cerebral vessels also causes headache, vertigo, insomnia, and psychiatric or personality disorders.

Adequate treatment of neurosyphilis is based largely on achieving treponemicidal levels of penicillin in the CSF. *Treponema pallidum* is highly susceptible to penicillin, which is the drug of choice for all stages of syphilis. Serum levels of penicillin should be maintained for many days because treponemes divide slowly in early syphilis (30-33 per hour in experimental settings) and penicillin acts only on dividing cells.

Therapy that is considered standard for non immunocompromised individuals with syphilis meningitis should remain the standard for immunocompromised individuals even with asymptomatic neurosyphilis. Either of the following is acceptable treatment

a. Aqueous (crystalline) penicillin-G at 2-4 million U intravenously every 4 hours; alternatively, continuously for 10-14 days, or
b. Procaine penicillin-G at 2.4 million U/d intramuscularly plus probenecid at 500 mg orally 4 times per day for 10-14 days (probenecid increases brain concentrations of penicillin less than it increases CSF concentrations, but avoid using it if the patient has a history of serious allergy to sulfonamides)

Contraindications include documented hypersensitivity, use of penicillin in pregnant patients (usually safe but benefits must outweigh the risks), and impaired renal function (use caution).

Other antibiotics, as alternative regimens, have not been studied sufficiently, and their routine use is not recommended. If patients are allergic to penicillin, either tetracycline or doxycycline probably is effective. Pregnant women should not receive doxycycline. Typically, tetracycline hydrochloride at 500 mg orally 4 times per day or doxycycline at 100 mg orally twice daily for 4 weeks is prescribed. Defining the efficacy of azithromycin for early syphilis may simplify therapy. Incidentally, the emergence of azithromycin-resistant *T pallidum* has been reported.

4. Tuberculous and cryptococcal meningitis

A high index of suspicion is needed to diagnose tuberculous meningitis because culture results are often delayed and stains are often negative. Empiric therapy may be lifesaving. Polymerase chain reaction testing may be useful. Death may occur as a result of missed diagnoses and delayed treatment.

Most of the guidelines follow the model of short-course chemotherapy of pulmonary tuberculosis: an "intensive phase" of treatment with four drugs, followed by treatment with two drugs during a prolonged "continuation phase". Initial treatment is a combination of isoniazid (5 mg per kg per day); rifampin (10 mg per kg per day, up to 600 mg); pyrazinamide (15 to 30 mg per kg per day, up to 2 g); and ethambutol (15 to 25 mg per kg per day). Streptomycin (20 to 40 mg per kg per day, up to 1 g) should be used instead of ethambutol in young children.

Evidence concerning the duration of treatment is conflicting. The duration of conventional therapy is 6-9 months, although some investigators still recommend as many as 24 months of therapy. No guidelines exist as to the components and duration of treatment in the case of multidrug-resistant TBM.

The use of corticosteroids in adults is controversial; they may be indicated in the presence of increased intracranial pressure, altered consciousness, focal neurological findings, spinal block, and tuberculous encephalopathy. Adding dexamethasone to the treatment regimen seems to improve mortality rate in patients older than 14 years with tuberculous meningitis. Cochrane systematic review concluded that overall adjunctive therapy with corticosteroids reduces the risk of death (relative risk (RR), 0.78).

The potential complications include associated elevated intracranial pressure, hydrocephalus, vasculitis, acute seizures, and hyponatremia. Aggressive and appropriate treatment of these complications can minimize the secondary brain injury and improve the chance of a good outcome. Disturbances of sodium, intravascular volume and water are common in tuberculous meningitis. Hyponatremia occurs in 35% to 65% of patients. Acute seizures occur in about 50% of children and in 5% of adults.

In these patients, associated space-occupying tuberculoma(s) may be the substrate for increased intracranial pressure (Figure 3). Growing evidence suggests that most tuberculomas resolve with antituberculous treatment. However, surgical excision is indicated in: tuberculoma causing obstructive hydrocephalus and significant increased intracranial pressure; tuberculoma causing obstructive hydrocephalus and not resolving on medical treatment; large space-occupying tuberculomas with increased intracranial pressure; and tuberculomas with associated compartmental shifts and not resolving with medical treatment. (Marais, 2010; Murthy, 2010)

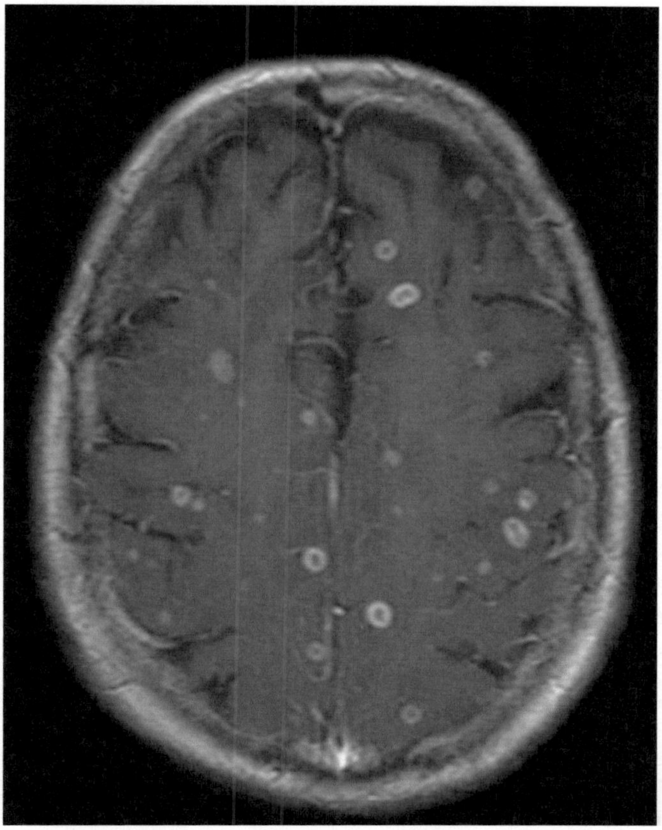

Fig. 3. MRI with contrast showing classical ring enhancing lesions of tuberculomas

Cryptococcal meningitis is the most common fungal meningitis, and usually occurs in patients with altered cellular immunity. It is estimated that the global burden of HIV-associated cryptococcosis approximates 1 million cases annually worldwide. It is relevant that, despite access to advanced medical care and the availability of highly active antiretroviral therapy, the 3-month mortality rate during management of acute cryptococcal meningoencephalitis approximates 20%. Furthermore, without specific antifungal treatment for cryptococcal meningoencephalitis in certain HIV-infected populations, mortality rates of 100% have been reported within 2 weeks after clinical presentation to health care facilities. (Perfect et al., 2010; Saag et al., 2000)

Usually presents with headache, fever, stiff neck and photophobia. However, meningeal symptoms and signs may be minimal or absent in over one half of the cases, and the rather broad clinical spectrum includes personality change, cognitive impairment, cranial neuropathy, altered consciousness and coma.

The CSF profile ranges from striking protein elevation, mononuclear pleocytosis, and hypoglycorrhachia to minimal abnormalities that overlap with those attributable to HIV infection alone. Fungal CSF culture is the gold standard, but the time wasted before a positive result is obtained, limits its clinical utility. India ink smear is helpful when positive, but is too insensitive to exclude the diagnosis if negative. Fortunately, CSF cryptococcal antigen (CrAg) testing is a rapid, specific test with a sensitivity exceeding 90%. The diverse clinical presentations of cryptococcal meningitis enforce CrAg to be performed routinely in CSF of patients with AIDS.

It is apparent that insightful management of cryptococcal disease is critical to a successful outcome. We should divide the treatment in three situations, as follows:

a. **In HIV infected individuals**, the initial treatment (induction regiment) includes amphotericin B (0.7 to 1.0 mg/kg per day IV) with or without flucytosine (25 mg/kg every six hours orally) for 2 to 3 weeks. Renal insufficiency, hypokalemia, and hypomagnesemia may complicate amphotericin B therapy, and the hematological toxicity of flucytosine sometimes precludes its use in patients with AIDS, in whom pancytopenia is common. Patients who are doing well can be switched to fluconazole, 200 mg twice a day for 8 to 10 weeks (maintenance therapy), and then placed on prophylactic therapy of 200 mg daily to prevent relapse. Alternatively Itraconazole can be used (200 mg twice per day orally; drug-level monitoring strongly advised). Active antiretroviral therapy should be initiated 2–10 weeks after the beginning of initial antifungal treatment. Consider discontinuing suppressive therapy during active antiretroviral therapy in patients with a CD4 cell count >100 cells/mL and an undetectable or very low HIV RNA level sustained for >3 months (minimum of 12 months of antifungal therapy); but consider reinstitution of maintenance therapy if the CD4 cell count decreases to <100 cells/mL (B-III).
b. **In organ transplant recipients**, the treatment includes liposomal amphotericin B (3–4 mg/kg per day IV) or amphotericin B lipid complex (5 mg/kg per day IV) plus flucytosine (100 mg/kg per day in 4 divided doses) for at least 2 weeks for the induction regimen, followed by fluconazole (400–800 mg [6–12 mg/kg] per day orally) for 8 weeks initially, and (200–400 mg per day orally) for 6–12 months afterwards.
c. **Non-HIV Infected, Non transplant Hosts,** the treatment includes amphotericin B (0.7–1.0 mg/kg per day IV) plus flucytosine (100 mg/kg per day orally in 4 divided doses) for at least 4 weeks for induction therapy. The 4-week induction therapy is reserved for persons with meningoencephalitis without neurological complications and negative cerebrospinal fluid (CSF) yeast culture results after 2 weeks of treatment. For amphotericin B toxicity issues, lipid formulations of amphotericin B may be substituted in the second 2 weeks. In patients with neurological complications, consider extending induction therapy for a total of 6 weeks, and lipid formulations of amphotericin for the last 4 weeks of the prolonged induction period. Then, start consolidation with fluconazole (400 mg per day) for 8 weeks.

Regarding neurological complications, some of them had already been described in complications of bacterial meningitis, as cerebral edema, increased intracranial pressure, acute hydrocephalus and abnormalities of the cranial nerves. Their management was described above. Poor prognostic features at presentation include impaired level of consciousness, CSF cell count less than 20 cells/µL, and CSF CrAg greater than 1:1024.

Another possible complication is the presence of cerebral cryptococcomas. The treatment consists of induction with amphotericin B (0.7–1 mg/kg per day IV), liposomal amphotericin B (3–4 mg/kg per day IV), or amphotericin B lipid complex (5 mg/kg per day IV) plus flucytosine (100 mg/kg per day orally in 4 divided doses) for at least 6 weeks. Then consolidation and maintenance therapy with fluconazole (400–800 mg per day orally) for 6–18 months. Adjunctive therapies include corticosteroids for mass effect and surrounding edema and/or surgery for large masses (>3 cm lesion).

5. Conclusions

The management approach to patients with suspected or proven bacterial meningitis includes emergent CSF analysis, and initiation of appropriate antimicrobial and adjunctive therapies. The choice of empirical antimicrobial therapy is based on the patient's age and underlying disease status; once the infecting pathogen is isolated, antimicrobial therapy can be modified for optimal treatment.

The most important priority to reduce the burden of bacterial meningitis throughout the world must include the introduction and availability of effective vaccines against the common meningeal pathogens.

Finally a higher index of suspicion is needed to diagnose tuberculous meningitis because culture results are often delayed, stains are often negative and empiric therapy may be lifesaving. A prompt diagnosis of meningitis is specially important in immunosuppressive patients, with high rates of mortality.

6. References

Bamberg DM. Diagnosis, initial management and prevention of meningitis. Americal Family Physician, 2010;82:1491-98

Brouwer MC, van de Beek D, Heckenberg SGB, et al. Hyponatremia in adults with community-acquired bacterial meningitis. Q J Med 2007;100:37–40

Fitch MT, Van de Beek D. Emergency diagnosis and treatment of adult meningitis. Lancet Infectious Dis 2007;7:191-200

Kupila L, Vuorinen T, Vainionpää R, Hukkanen V, Marttila RJ, Kotilainen P. Etiology of aseptic meningitis and encephalitis in an adult population. Neurology. 2006;66(1):75-80

Likitnukul S, McCracken GH Jr, Nelson JD. Arthritis in children with bacterial meningitis. Am J Dis Child 1986;140:424–7

Marais S, Thwaites G, Schoeman JF et al. Tuberculous meningitis: a uniform case definitions for use in clinical research. Lancet Infect Dis 2010:803-12

Murthy JM. Tuberculous meningitis: the challenges. Neurol India. 2010;58(5):716-22

Nudelman Y, Tunkel AR. Bacterial meningitis - Epidemiology, pathogenesis and management update. Drugs 2009; 69(18):2577-96

Perfect JR, Dismukes WE, Dromer F, et al. Clinical Practice Guidelines for the Management of Cryptococcal Disease: 2010 Update by the Infectious Diseases Society of America. Clinical Infectious Diseases 2010; 50:291–322

Pfister HW, Feiden W, Einhaupl KM. Spectrum of complications during bacterial meningitis in adults: results of a prospective clinical study. Arch Neurol 1993;50:575–81

Saag MS, Graybill RJ, Larsen RA, et al. Practice guidelines for the management of cryptococcal disease. Infectious Diseases Society of America. Clin Infect Dis. 2000;30(4):710-8.

Schuchat A, Robinson K, Wenger JD, et al. Bacterial meningitis in the United States in 1995. N Engl J Med 1997;337:970–6

Schut ES, Gans J, Van de Beek D. Community-acquired bacterial meningitis in adults. Practical Neurology 2008;8:8-23

Van de Beek D, de Gans J, Spanjaard L, et al. Antibiotic guidelines and antbiotic use in adult bacterial meningitis in The Netherlands. J Antimicrob Chemother 2002;49:661–6

Van de Beek D, de Gans J, Spanjaard L, et al. Clinical features and prognostic factors in adults with bacterial meningitis. N Engl J Med 2004;351:1849–59 [Erratum, N Engl J Med 2005;352:950]

Van de Beek D, de Gans J, McIntyre P, Prasad K. Steroids in adults with acute bacterial meningitis: a systematic review. Lancet Infect Dis 2004;4:139–43

Van de Beek D, de Gans J. Dexamethasone in adults with community-acquired bacterial meninigitis. Drugs 2006;66:415–27

Van de Beek D, Gans J, Tunkel AR et al. Community-acquired bacterial meningitis in adults. N Engl J Med 2006;354:44-53

Van de Beek D, Weisfelt M, de Gans J, Tunkel AR, Wijdicks EF. Drug insight: adjunctive therapies in adults with bacterial meningitis. Nat Clin Pract Neurol 2006;2:504–16

Van de Beek D, Brouwer MC, de Gans J. Hypernatremia in bacterial meningitis. J Infect 2007;55:381–2.

Weisfelt M, Gans J, Van der Poll T et al. Pneumococcal meningitis in adults: new approach to management and prevention. Lancet Neurology 2006;5:332-42

Weisfelt M, van de Beek D, Spanjaard L, et al. Arthritis in adults with community-acquired bacterial meningitis: a prospective cohort study. BMC Infectious Diseases 2006;6:64

Williams AJ, Nadel S. Bacterial meningitis – Current controversies in approaches to treatment. CNS Drugs 2001:15(12):909-919